SICKLY VAPORS

SICKLY VAPORS

Disease *and* Doctoring
in the Old South

THOMAS HELLING, MD

UNIVERSITY PRESS OF MISSISSIPPI / JACKSON

The University Press of Mississippi is the scholarly publishing agency of
the Mississippi Institutions of Higher Learning: Alcorn State University,
Delta State University, Jackson State University, Mississippi State University,
Mississippi University for Women, Mississippi Valley State University,
University of Mississippi, and University of Southern Mississippi.

www.upress.state.ms.us

The University Press of Mississippi is a member
of the Association of University Presses.

Any discriminatory or derogatory language or hate speech regarding race, ethnicity,
religion, sex, gender, class, national origin, age, or disability that has been retained or
appears in elided form is in no way an endorsement of the use of such language outside
a scholarly context.

Copyright © 2024 by University Press of Mississippi
All rights reserved
Manufactured in the United States of America

∞

Names: Helling, Thomas, 1947– author
http://id.loc.gov/vocabulary/relators/aut
http://id.loc.gov/authorities/names/n2016044078
http://id.loc.gov/rwo/agents/n2016044078
Title: Sickly vapors : disease and doctoring in the Old South / Thomas Helling, MD.
Description: Jackson : University Press of Mississippi, 2024. |
Includes bibliographical references and index
Identifiers: LCCN 2024033904 (print) | LCCN 2024033905 (ebook) |
ISBN 9781496854360 hardback | ISBN 9781496854377 trade paperback |
ISBN 9781496854384 epub | ISBN 9781496854391 epub | ISBN 9781496854407 pdf |
ISBN 9781496854414 pdf
Subjects: LCSH: Diseases—Southern States—History—19th century |
Public health—Southern States—History—19th century |
Medical geography—Southern States—History—19th century
Classification: LCC RA650.5 H45 2024 (print) | LCC RA650.5 (ebook) |
DDC 362.10975—dc23/eng/20240827
LC record available at https://lccn.loc.gov/2024033904
LC ebook record available at https://lccn.loc.gov/2024033905

British Library Cataloging-in-Publication Data available

To TOM HOLDER, southerner, fellow Mississippian, and compassionate practitioner of the healing arts

> There exists among us by ordinary—both North and South—a profound conviction that the South is another land, sharply differentiated from the rest of the American nation, and exhibiting within itself a remarkable homogeneity.
>
> —W. J. CASH, *THE MIND OF THE SOUTH*

CONTENTS

Preface ix

Chapter One: The Congo Is Not More Different 3

Chapter Two: Colonies of Plenty 11

Chapter Three: A Paradise of Ills 19

Chapter Four: Corrupted Air, Putrefied Earth 25

Chapter Five: Doctoring in the Colonial South 41

Chapter Six: Revolution: The Glorious Ally of Disease 51

Chapter Seven: The Ills of Slavery 73

Chapter Eight: Native Healing in Colonial Times 92

Chapter Nine: Southern Medicine for Southern Sickness 104

Chapter Ten: Secession's Vulgar Scourges 136

Chapter Eleven: An Abomination of Health:
Reconstruction of the South 163

Chapter Twelve: Surgery as Southern Medical Redemption 177

Chapter Thirteen: A New South or Still the Old South? 192

Acknowledgments 201

Notes 203

Bibliography 229

Index 253

PREFACE

In January 1866, South Carolinian James Dunwoody Brownson (J. D. B.) De Bow, through his influential southern periodical, *De Bow's Review*, addressed his fellow southerners, now in the wake of the South's ignominious annihilation in their armed rebellion. "The staples of the South are of such inestimable value to the commerce of the world, that they have, in the past, and promise beyond all contingency in the future, to come into triumphant competition with those of every other country upon the face of the earth."[1] Passed were the days of slavery. Whether Blacks would of their own volition provide free labor was an uncertainty. This alone would not restore economic independence. De Bow understood that the commercial recovery of the South, now devoid of slave labor, rested with an influx of immigrants as free labor that might stimulate diversity of market and, at the same time, parcel land to induce yeoman farming and investment of capital, both foreign and domestic, akin to the successes of northern industry and agriculture. In short, he urged a true economic reunification with the North. Only then could there be eventual political and economic reunification.

His aspirations would be a tall order. People of the South had forged a seemingly indelible identity. Interplay of weather, land, and morality had made it so. Rebuked by their northern neighbors but prey to Yankee greed for their produce, the South had rankled at their censure. It was not by design, then, that the southeastern American colonies and, later, states in the Union desired separatism. The same soil, sun, and virtue—however misaligned—added a complexity to health, though, that buttressed their southern uniqueness. Those initial settlers migrating south quickly became aware of a difference. Yes, the earth yielded much—an astounding wealth—but also harbored peculiarities so injurious to planters as to strike down—as if a punishment from God Himself—their unabashed greed. Sicknesses abounded—not those predictable ones of the North, but vicious illnesses much more resistant and resplendent in their malignancy. Health issues now added to a distinctiveness that permeated all aspects of southern society.

Indeed, there had been clear climatic differences that contrasted with the seasonal variations of their northern colleagues, but culturally, at first, both North and South had common origins, populated by Europeans intent on independence from antiquated and oppressive regimes. Yet that same hotter sun, humid air, and fertile soil, so capable of producing crops in lavishness, broke the backs of those industrious European immigrants ill-inclined to toil under that heat. Then did a distinctiveness begin to incubate. Global demands for precious southern harvests of tobacco, rice, indigo, and cotton were too lucrative and irresistible to dismiss. On came white indentured servants, sponsored on their journeys across the Atlantic by rich planters in search of cheap labor. Yet even those workers soon enough were gone, debt paid, drifting southward to lucrative property of their own. Africans, so easily corralled by rival tribes in West Africa, sold to Europeans, and shipped to the New World, provided a sturdy and docile reservoir of labor—not paid for their work or promised freedom but bonded for life. They would tend the soil, endure the heat, and pick the products of this unbelievably rich earth.

The estates of their owners stretched immense across the low country of Virginia, the Carolinas, Georgia, and Louisiana Territory. Awash in wealth, their agricultural windfalls soon became the economic engine of the South—indeed, the entire country. With it developed a peculiar feudal aristocracy. Property, family, and slaves lay at the core of a wayward morality, which emphasized a Christian benevolence that belied its true nature in the subjugation of the Black race; a Christian benevolence whose aim was not the spiritual but the carnal amassing of stupendous affluence. As the North looked to the vast southern prosperity as a revenue source, assessing tariffs and garnishing profits, southerners recoiled, refusing to comply with a North intent on assaulting the very soul of their livelihood. Slavery became the flash point. Above all, abolitionists of the North insisted on its extinction. In it, and in their unique agrarian system, a southern "otherness" grew. They were different. In all their perceived immorality, though, the world needed products from the South, and southern products needed slavery. Historian John Duffy wrote, "As the Western World repudiated slavery, leaving the South isolated and in an almost indefensible moral position, Southerners closed ranks and attempted desperately to rationalize their peculiar institution."[2]

Matters of health then contributed. Fevers and epidemics also prospered in the South. Invisible miasmas liberated by climate itself seemed to circulate, infect, and bring down even the sturdiest of inhabitants. Of their enslaved labor, peculiarities of illness arose, challenges also to traditional medicine. The South had become a repository for sickness, too, and physicians claimed a distinctiveness of their own, a southern brand of medicine diverse from the North. Historian Todd L. Savitt contended that "[t]he South's unique health history undoubtedly contributed to making the region a distinctive national subculture in two principal ways." He asserted first that poor health (by reputation) "perpetuated a negative image of the South that retarded regional development by discouraging immigration and investment" and, second, that prevalence of diseases promoted the idea of the South as a place of "poverty, ignorance, backwardness, and insularity."[3] It also resided in the cabins and lodgings of their shackled servants, who, while tolerant of some New World illnesses, fell victim to numbers more. Here, too, physicians insisted on southern distinctiveness.

Of course, in those early colonial days and first years of the Republic, it all made sense. Illnesses were likely due to bad air, bad earth, or bad behavior—which the South cultivated in great quantity. The humors of Hippocrates and Galen still reigned supreme and ebbed and flowed with miasmas of indescribable origin. The more intense the heat, the more affected was the atmosphere and the more putrefied the soil. Vapors fomented by it all thus polluted the air and disturbed that fragile equilibrium of living things. Such was the consequence of southern living, scientists surmised. Distempers, fluxes, and plagues abounded and assaulted men, women, and children alike. Doctors were fascinated, diseases and epidemics enough to satisfy any professional curiosity. Indeed, they considered the South a magnet for scientific investigation.

That swirl of fertility, feudalism, and pestilence fermented to besmear the South with an uneasy uniqueness. Then, in the minds of southerners, sectionalism, and eventually separatism, became all encompassing, incorporating hearth, bonded "heathens," and home with health matters that affected all. So adamant were they that an emotional yearning for independence grew, anxious to rid themselves of the irritating moral reminders of an intrusive North. And such sentiments would die hard, especially in the brutality of their War of Rebellion and subsequent occupation by detested Yankees. Their nostalgic autobiography, as historian David Anderson would call it after war's end, "coalesced around an imagined plantation community, a lost feudal kingdom, replete with images, heroic hotspurs, beautiful belles, and steadfast slaves."[4]

White southerners from all walks of life mourned the loss of the Old South and the Confederacy. Lives and properties had been shattered and leveled. Economic ruin was now the rule, and memory was the only tangible comfort. While calming the frustrations, disappointments, and anger of unrepentant southern ladies and gentlemen, such an attitude cultivated looming racism, white supremacy, and social injustice. In contrast, in the eyes of the Union, the Old South was gone. Its anachronistic aristocracy and labor force had been dismantled by a righteous adversary intent on denying secession, erasing southern genteelism, and wiping out the curse of slavery. In the eyes of southerners, though, a history, a heritage, and a culture had been forcefully rejected. There would be no easy reconciliation.

While science soon dispelled notions of humors and miasmas, and the medical distinctiveness of the South vanished with time, there still remained a sentiment that somehow the South was special. Southern medicine remained unique in the hearts of physicians looking to redeem a time of splendor long past but still of grand recollections.

SICKLY VAPORS

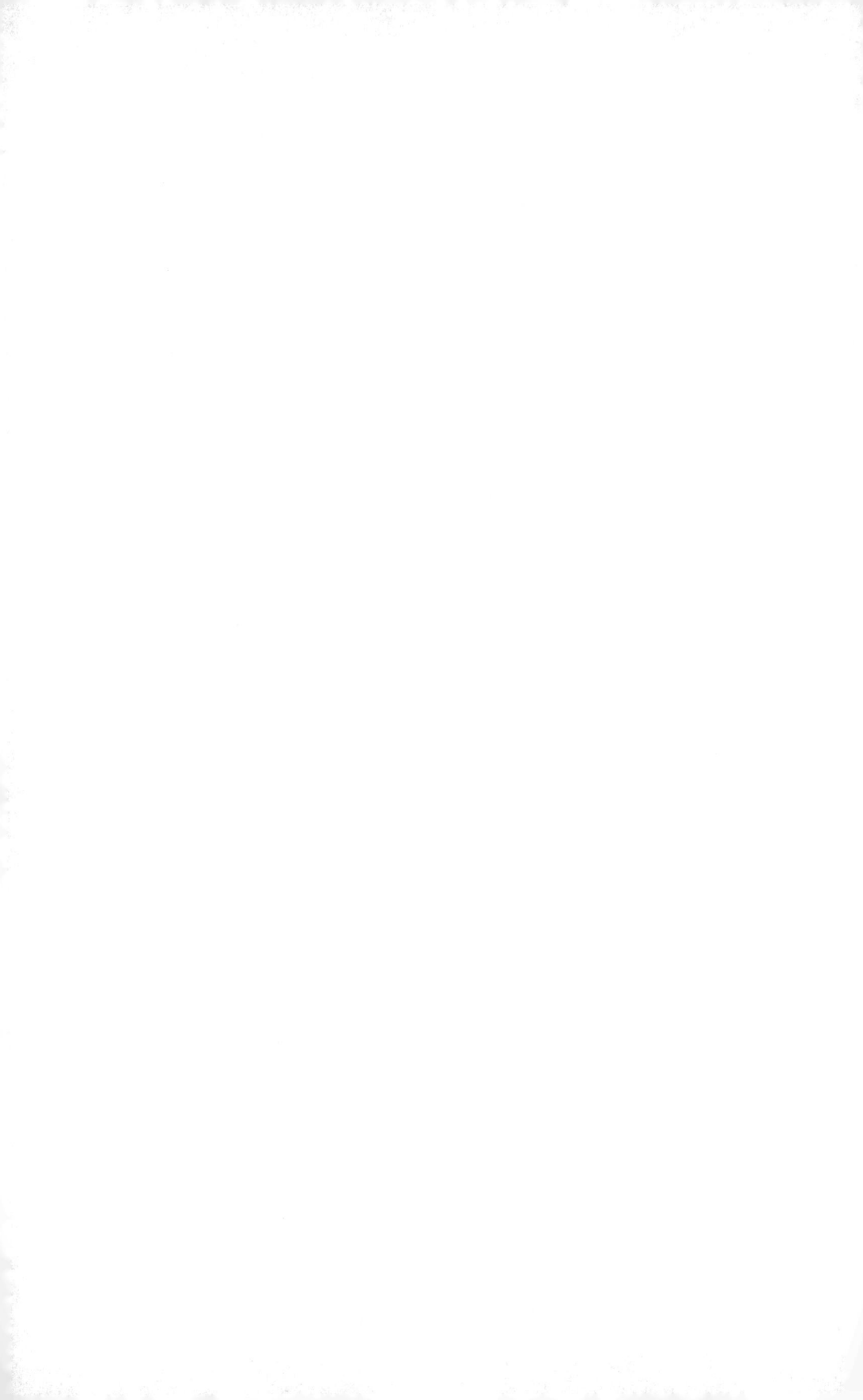

CHAPTER ONE

THE CONGO IS NOT MORE DIFFERENT

> Two distinct peoples, two distinct civilizations.
> —RICHARD N. CURRENT, QUOTED IN WALLERSTEIN,
> "WHAT CAN ONE MEAN BY SOUTHERN CULTURE?"

Almost a century ago, Cornell economist Jesse T. Carpenter wrote of the South: "The roots of Southern unity are grounded in the laws of nature; for soil, climate, and topography had created a South of agriculture as opposed to a North of manufacturing and commerce even before the formation of the present Union."[1] That its peculiar earth, weather, and topography had far-reaching health implications was familiar to southern ancestry. It was stated no better than by the Carolinian physician David Ramsay when he wrote of his home state at the turn of the eighteenth century:

> An opinion prevails that South Carolina is unhealthy. This is neither correctly true or wholly false. A great proportion of the State, especially of the low country, is for the most part inundated. In its sluggish rivers, stagnant swamps, ponds, and marshes are common; and in or near them putrefaction is generated. In all these places, and for two or three miles adjacent to them, the seeds of febrile disease are plentifully sown and from them are disseminated.[2]

Indeed, the Old South[3] was a charmed but capricious land. In its sweltering fecundity—its grasslands and wetlands and timbered forests—the South was the new frontier, a range of opportunity and, soon, a territory of immense wealth and, for some, lavish culture. Those who sought it, the hordes of transatlantic Europeans migrating inland, became part of its fabric, as much of the soil as the trees they toppled, the acres they plowed, and the seeds they planted. Yet their labors in those antebellum times were at the mercy of a myriad of fevers, dysenteries, and epidemics that added to the complexity of their lifestyle and aided in defining a sectionalism founded on human bondage.

As rich as its acreage proved to be, the South was at first backwater country. Economically, before the Revolutionary War, southern British colonies, new on the world stage, were predominately agricultural export zones but still peripheral on the global market. In contrast, after the Revolution and with the new unity of states, the southern territories generated a distinctiveness that would set them apart from their northern neighbors. More and more, a southern nationalism developed, perhaps agriculturally based, which led slowly to the belief that there were, in the words of historian Richard Current, "two distinct peoples, two distinct civilizations." It was the North, he thought, that intended to remake and assimilate the South in its own image, and southerners, provoked by the idea, who fought fiercely to maintain their own uniqueness.[4] It was their prodigious cultivation of staple crops, vital to foreign economic interests, that forced a truth that the South, in all its distinctiveness, was an indispensable component of the new United States, driving a worldwide commercial engine.

That vast New World encountered by homesteaders in the seventeenth and eighteenth centuries was a stark contrast to the worn and predictable landscapes of England, France, the Netherlands, and Spain from which they sailed. In the southern regions of North America, beyond those earliest primitive hamlets along the James River in Virginia, measureless tracts of land, awash in vegetation and fertility, begged cultivation and drew settlers inexorably southward. But it was not the same air or the same sun in the Southland. Heat and humidity cloaked everything, the climate more reminiscent of the Mediterranean than New England. And it was there that the impact of adventure, opportunity, and fortitude clashed with those invisible vapors seemingly provoked by work of sun and soil that set upon man as awful sicknesses. Corrupted air it must be, so the learned thought. Air so foul, went the reasoning, stirred by the consequence of temperature, humidity, swamps, and vegetation, that it hovered over all and descended, inhaled as breaths of life, into quagmires of suffering. Just like the Italian *mal aria*, it was the Mediterranean climate—hot summers and cool, mild winters—brought home to North America. Long before, the sixteenth-century New World voyager and chronicler George Best argued for caution in facing the dangers of discovery and expressed the climatic fears of the time:

> It is to be confessed, that some particular living creature cannot live in every particular place or region, especially with the same love and felicitie, as it did where it was first bredde, for certain agreement of nature

that is between the place, and the thing bredde in that place ... which being translated and brought out of the second or third climate, though they may live, yet will they never ingender or bring forth young.[5]

Indeed, as explained by historian Karen Kupperman, according to English lore, good health was produced by a balance of the Hippocratic humors—phlegm, blood, black bile, and yellow bile—and any disturbance of this balance by outside malice, such as change of climate (temperature and moisture, chiefly), led to ill health and fostered many sicknesses. Thus, southern latitudes portended trouble. Heat, humidity, and dankness spoke of unfathomable dangers.[6] It was that climate, those invisible, breathable fumes, that plagued settlers far more there than the usual ailments of the North. As early nineteenth-century surveyor Samuel Forry expressed:

> Among the various circumstances connected with the production and diffusion of noxious exhalations from the soil, it is generally believed that the presence of dead animal matter, when mingled with vegetable remains in a state of decay, gives rise, in warm countries or in the hot seasons of temperate climates, to miasmas, especially during humid states of the atmosphere, of a more deleterious character than those resulting from vegetable remains alone.

Forry believed, as did others of the time, that sicknesses were highly dependent on interactions of temperature, prevailing winds, elevation, proximity of large bodies of water, geological formations, soil, and vegetation. This was not, of course, to discount the important influence "exerted on the human frame by occupations, modes of life, and moral agencies, the diversity and importance of the resulting effects can no longer excite surprise."[7]

It was an atmospheric phenomenon, so contemporaries believed. Eighteenth-century Scottish physician John Arbuthnot blamed atmospheric differences on the "oscillatory Motion" of fibers of the human body. "The whole nervous system, and the animal Spirits, are in some measure affected." Woe to him who resides in warm climates, Arbuthnot cautioned. Excessive heat brought forth a laziness and indolence. "From Inactivity and Indolence there will follow naturally a flavish [vile] Disposition."[8] Before the microscope, before discovery of teeming microorganisms, and certainly before the age of antibiotics, doctors could only attribute the sweeping sicknesses to a moody and unfamiliar ambience.

Ill health seeped into everyday life. As planters and yeoman farmers moved into the fertile lands below Virginia, they found in abundance raging fevers, the lassitude of typhus, the dysentery of cholera, the speckled menace of smallpox, and the inexorable wasting of consumption. Importation of enslaved Africans imparted another distinctiveness with their peculiar afflictions heretofore unknown to the European. Here disease played as pivotal a role as armed aggression, and belligerents were careful to select time and place for conflict. It was never so obvious than during the American Revolution when British troops retreated from the Carolinas in 1781, hurrying northward to more favorable climates—and freedom from fevers—only to be trapped and destroyed at Yorktown. Health matters were a developing distinctiveness, most agreed. If disease was different here, then so must be treatments. Southern medicine for southern people became the opinion of practitioners of the art. In the post-Revolutionary United States, separatism in health—as in other matters—gained popularity.

Yet as years passed and crops flourished—the economic windfalls of tobacco, indigo, sugar, rice, and cotton—the South became the commercial engine of the country. Settlers of Scottish, Irish, and English heritage scraped out a comfortable existence of affluence, courtly manners, and aristocratic behavior. In that, an agrarian dynasty far different from the industrialized North, the Old South proudly courted distinctiveness—shaped by myriad socioeconomic factors and, in part, by climate. According to historian Bertram Wyatt-Brown, "early Southern society was crude, hierarchic, racialist, and communally mistrustful," largely due, in his opinion, to "the unpredictability of life and fortune in the malarial subtropical climate." A Protestant, conservative faith was the anchor for all ills, even, as Wyatt-Brown contended, spilling over into the realm of "white magic" spells and charms. It was the centerpiece of family and institutional life for white southerners and defined their sense of honor and respectability.[9]

But such virtuous aspirations were contaminated with the cancer of slavery. Before mechanized planting and harvesting, southern wealth hinged on a stout labor force able to endure those curious vicissitudes of weather and soil. No white man could long suffer the relentless heat and sweltering moisture. Acres and acres of farmland demanded attention and toil, planting and picking: labor so tedious and backbreaking few whites had the stomach for it. As their adaptable solution, southern planters partook of that most odious of business, the international African slave trade—forcibly importing those corralled Black souls thought far more amenable to manual labor than white folk. After all, was the common misconception not as economist Lewis Cecil Gray later said? "The great body of Negroes came to America ignorant savages." And thus, so compliant, it seemed.[10]

Africans spilled from slave ships to be shackled for auction and hustled onto plantations. Pearled cotton fields were peppered with black bodies hunched over and whipped to produce. Slavery changed everything. It fueled a complete restructuring of southern society. Different from the North indeed, it centered on a feudal culture, with the plantation a new manor, planters the new aristocracy, and peasants a large subservient class, the lowest of which were slaves.[11] No longer interested in progressive reforms of the North, southerners were intent on maintaining a status quo of indentured and bonded people whose sole function was to generate windfall profits for landowners. Before long, any aspect of culture aligned with the justification for slavery. Safeguards of family and fortunes required persistence of a rigid hierarchy and specified roles for husband, wife, children, and slave servants. In fact, even non-slave holders could be pacified knowing that, despite their humble status, there were always those lower on the rungs of social inequities—and, by God, it would be kept that way. Revivalist religion played a vital role in shoring up this delicate framework by emphasizing a biblical obligation to do so. In fact, manhood was defined by these terms, so that disruption of the social order would, in essence, emasculate male members and disrupt the family unit itself. Honor, southerners felt, was the demonstrated authority of a man over women, children, and enslaved Africans—whether he owned any or not. Behavior became ritualized by rules and customs. And at the very least, they came to believe, slavery required subjugation simply because, in such a biracial society where Africans often outnumbered whites, the fear of rebellion and retribution loomed large and necessitated sometimes brutal oversight.[12] Here, then, became the core of southern society, so embedded as to be indispensable, but so fragile as to be fiercely protected. There could be no compromise. There could be no thoughts of emancipation. Southern economy, southern religion, and southern family could not allow it.

A figurative and literal pox on the South, slavery ushered in more misery. Africans brought their own brand of sickness and bestowed it on an unsuspecting genteel society or, in turn, were afflicted with white man's troubles. Epidemics swept through communities like crashing surf, leaving white and Black bodies in their wakes. Enticed by the challenges of such flagrant maladies, doctors drifted southward. Armed with the flimsy logic of the day, they tackled the desperately ill, questioning and probing. Their particular brand of treatment seemed distinctly illogical—even brutal—by today's standards but was dispensed liberally to the suffering: bleeding, blistering, purging, sweating. Few so-called pharmaceuticals worked. Most medications simply forestalled—or accelerated—the inevitable. In fact, indigenous methods, those practiced by Native American tribes, often seemed equally efficacious. It was a time of perilous medical training anyway. American methods held no candle to practices of traditional European medical masters. Even so, there developed a feeling that southern illness was peculiar, that teachings of their northern professors simply did not work here. Disease was bitter, stubborn, and unforgiving in the South. And of course, Africans befuddled them. Enslaved people became curiosities, like primal relics, with their own unique behaviors, ailments, and forbearances. Doctoring in the South took on its own personality, soon fueling needs for special southern medical education. No need anymore to go beyond the Mason-Dixon Line for training. Best to stay close to home, where special practicalities mattered.[13]

In contrast, the traveled world was still Euro-centric, and Europe was still a medical mecca. European cities were replete with storied seats of learning and magnanimous charity infirmaries. For example, in 1830 Paris boasted some thirty hospitals housing over twenty thousand patients. Such institutions could provide not only coordinated and even specialized care but immeasurable opportunities for education. During that same year, Paris counted five thousand students of medicine. The flamboyance of surgeons like the great Larrey or Dupuytren or Lisfranc, who carried on with the aplomb of medical royalty itself, held sway in lecture halls and surgical exhibitions.[14] Paris possessed opportunities for learning broadcast far and wide, even reaching across the Atlantic.

Yet although wealthy American physicians traveled to Europe to enhance their training, this was by no means a common practice. In the eighteenth and even early nineteenth centuries, transatlantic voyages were hazardous, time-consuming, and expensive. Only the idle rich seemed to prosper by it, and for them it was a luxury indeed, bathing in the glamor of London or Paris and the parade of patients—and cadavers—on whom the English and French quizzed, probed, cut, and dissected in front of galleries of eager young men. For most, it would be the best of times. As author David McCullough described, "A greater journey had begun . . . and from it they were to learn more, and bring back more, of infinite value to themselves and to their country than they yet knew."[15] On their return, they filtered into the cities and towns of the North and the South and attempted to re-create that wonderful atmosphere of scholarship witnessed abroad. Their newfound talents of bleeding and blistering and butchering fell on populations of settlers and immigrants plagued by mysterious new diseases. In the South, the maladies seemed to propagate and exacerbate as if the heat and swamp and lush vegetation conspired together to hasten the demise of covetous planters and their lucrative farmlands.

For many doctors, though, European schooling in the natural sciences was a distant dream. As educational pioneer John Morgan wrote in his appeal for an American medical school in 1765, "A medical education is at least become much more expensive, and a man has little chance, if he keeps free from empiricism, to get a tolerable living by physic now, unless he has spent some years in an expensive education in Europe."[16]

The less affluent sharpened what skills they could on the coattails of local mentors: watching, listening, mimicking, and reading until they were turned loose with a shadow of confidence on an unsuspecting clientele. And in the southern agrarian culture, so removed from the urban elegance of the North, an intellectual isolation caused physicians to pine for their own fellowship and networks of information, as feelings gathered that, perhaps, southern medicine was not only insular but unique and exceptional.

As a consequence, southern medical practices became a quagmire of talent and ability. Rural in nature, the territory hosted practitioners of all calibers, from uneducated folk doctors to native shamans, wandering quacks, and a sprinkling of educated physicians—and not many at that. According to historian Rosemary Stevens, at the time of the American Revolution there were an estimated 3,500 medical practitioners in the colonies. Not more than 400 had received any formal training, and of these, only about half held a recognized medical degree.[17] For the truly learned, such diversity was a shame on their reputations and a dishonor to their noble profession. The disdain felt by their northern colleagues was palpable—the fate, Yankee doctors said, of a culture mired in slavery and beset by all the encumbrances of an agrarian society and southern humidity. It was almost already a foreign country. Of Alabama, author Carl Carmer had said, "The Congo is not more different from Massachusetts or Kansas or California."[18]

Medical sectionalism became the rhetoric of gentrified southerners. Southern environment spawned peculiarities in health that could only be addressed by southern doctors. It was an attitude that Harvard professor John Harley Warner called "the theoretical foundation for a distinctive Southern medicine." At the core of such pursuits was the personal experience with southern practice.[19] In fact, so southern were the sentiments of local physicians that editorials in the few southern medical journals bemoaned the waste of a northern medical education. "Young and inexperienced physicians," Erasmus Fenner of the journal *Southern Medical Reports* wrote in 1849, "fresh from the [northern] Medical Colleges where they had been taught everything better than the nature and treatment of the very diseases they were to encounter."[20]

But was such sectionalism a practical matter or more of a philosophical scapegoat to permeate the justification of slavery and economic prosperity? And as a corollary, was there any rationale for medical sectionalism? Were physicians arguably righteous in maintaining that their unique region demanded an expertise found only in southern training? In brief, was their "peculiar" institution of slavery so fundamental as to lead to medical practices largely unknown in northern cities? Indeed, in southern minds, the "Negro" was not a "white man ... painted black" as some Northerners claimed. No, the Black man was different, inferior, as demonstrated by southern declaration at the dissecting table.[21] So, in that misdirected thinking, was it all a delusional attempt to isolate from abolitionist feelings and direct a politico-economic course so different from the North as to justify secession and total independence? Or perhaps, was it, as Warner contends, the anxious desires of a remote southern medical community to attain respectability among more scholarly northern colleagues?[22]

And so, an obsession with southern medicine developed, as pronounced as southern culture itself, perhaps part and parcel of it. Into the nineteenth century, little did the medically privileged of the South find value in northern interpretation of diseases, feeling that their peculiar climates and peculiar institutions altered southern sicknesses and compromised traditional treatments. Medical sectionalism became as popular as regional segregation. Southern medicine for southern doctors was the byword. There arose an entire network of specific botanical pharmaceutics, medical exchanges, and, eventually, formal southern medical education. Even the scathing catastrophes of the Civil War, so destructive to the South, failed to completely extirpate a southern medical distinctiveness (or, for that matter, southern culture).

Yet in the destructiveness of war, reality had set in, at least for the medical profession. Following the Civil War, sickly Dixie began the agonizing process of resurrection, paying heed to amendable social factors such as poverty, sanitation, and bigotry—a process not entirely completed even to the present day. Doctors, educated by the filth, mutilation, and carnage of four years of warfare, now turned to each other and their Yankee colleagues to unify—as their southern home must—in hopes of applying the miraculous discoveries of the experimental age to their sick and wounded patients. Southern physicians, particularly that group of more regimented surgical specialists, yearned for parity with their northern brethren. And if there is still any remnant of southern medical exceptionality it would be in the deplorable condition of impoverishment and neglect, fates still shared by the supposed beneficiaries of that bloody war not yet erased from American memory.

CHAPTER TWO

COLONIES OF PLENTY

A "SPACIOUS AND FRUITFUL COUNTRY"

Of the New World of the Chesapeake Bay, first settlers found a profusion of resources. "This spacious and fruitful Country of Virginia, is . . . naturally rich, and exceedingly well watered, very temperate, and healthful to all inhabitants, abounding with as many natural blessings . . . From whence ariseth an affluence." It was said by travelers that furs, commodities, timber, cotton, corn, and cattle flourished in abundance. It was a country that "nothing but ignorance can think ill of."[1]

Beware, though, there was ill to be had. Strange fluxes and agues[2] afflicted the intrepid people of Virginia, wrote the governor of the Jamestown colony to the London Company in England in the 1600s, portending a recurring problem in the southern colonies: that of malicious sicknesses. Early planters, so intrigued by the fecundity of the land, made the best of it, though, minimizing the pesky sicknesses as such minor irritation that not even doctors were needed. Jamestown official Robert Beverley in 1705 wrote of the medical profession in the first published history of a British colony, *The History and Present State of Virginia*: "Their Intermitting Fevers, as well as their Agues, are very troublesome . . . [However,] They have Happiness afford great Plenty. And indeed, their Distempers are not many, and their Cures are so generally known, that there is not Mystery enough, to make a Trade of Physick there, as the Learned do in other Countries, to the great oppression of Mankind."[3] Farmers scurried to accommodate. Local remedies prevailed instead. The ubiquitous tobacco was touted as a cure-all, purging gross humors, opening pores and passages, healing gout and ague, curing hangovers, and reducing fatigue. Ordinary medicine as peddled by physicians held little interest for settlers and planters. In fact, doctors as a whole were held in low regard, so unpredictable was their training and expertise. Better to rely on tried-and-true folk tonics instead.

As the Virginia colony filled with eager planters and yeoman farmers, ambitious eyes turned southward toward the expanse of seemingly limitless land for the taking. This was a country of "large navigable rivers and fertile lands" and held high hopes for development.[4] So persuasive were some of the wealthiest speculators that King Charles II of England had granted a charter in 1663 for territories encompassing the lands of "Carolana" (Carolina) from (north) Currituck Inlet to (south) the present Georgia-Florida border, and (west) to the south seas—the current territories of Georgia, Alabama, Mississippi, and Tennessee—to designated proprietors Sir Anthony Ashley Cooper; Edward Hyde, the Earl of Clarendon; George Monck, Earl of Albemarle; John Lord Berkeley (William's brother); Sir George Carteret; and William Craven, Earl of Craven.

Pioneers had already migrated there, at the mouth of the Roanoke River on the border of Virginia, as early as 1657. Now, more steady migration occurred, and soon Albemarle, named after the British proprietor George Monck, hosted numbers of yeomen planters. To reach there they had traversed an immense freshwater morass known as the "Great Dismal Swamp." This primordial swampland—more of a forested lake of Pleistocene origin—was a huge area forty miles by twenty miles in dimension. Native American tribes once inhabited the periphery, but no one could live within. The early eighteenth-century explorer William Byrd characterized it as "very pleasant to the Eye" but treacherous because of the "Noxious Vapours [that] rise perpetually from that vast Extent of Mire & Nastiness." In his opinion, "Agues and other distempers" were the penalties of transgression.[5] William Drummond, a former indentured servant from Scotland, stumbled onto the place in 1665 and called it that forlorn name, "The Great Dismal Swamp." The going was so trying that even the hardy gave up, declaring it impenetrable on foot or horseback.

Yet penetrate it they did. By 1663, when proprietary rule began, Albemarle was a sizeable community, and explorers ventured even farther south. Coastal regions held the most interest. However, the shores of northern Carolina were treacherous to shipping, and the severe weather and rocky soil were hardly conducive to permanent settlements. Before long, pioneers roamed onward, to the pleasing regions of the Ashley River. Of this territory past the Albemarle settlement little was known prior to 1665. In 1663, the Crown's hired surveyor William Hilton had explored the coast as far south as the Combahee River to Port Royal in his ship *Adventure* just five months after Charles II granted his charter to the lords proprietors. It was bountiful land, he crowed in his report, even more fertile than the headlands of Cape Fear to the north:

The Land generally . . . is good Soil . . . The Indians plant in the worst Land, because they cannot cut down the Timber . . . and yet have plenty of Corn, Pumpkins, Water-Mellons . . . [and] have two or three crops of Corn a year . . . The Country abounds with Grapes, large Figs, and Peaches; the Woods with Deer, Conies, Turkeys, Quails . . . The Land we suppose is healthy.[6]

Soon, a colony developed on land between the Ashley and Wando Rivers, at a place called Oyster Point. Settlers felt the new site would be "free from any noisome vapors and all the Summer long refreshed with continued cool breathings from the sea."[7] In 1679, they named their tiny community Charles Towne, present-day Charleston.[8] By 1700, the town counted almost five thousand people, many scattered on large tracts of land on the banks of the Ashley and Cooper Rivers. It was hardly work for gentlemen, however. Countless enslaved Black people—sold, bonded, and manacled—soon arrived into the colony and filled the fields with their forced endurance, durability, and compulsory docility. At Ashley River the colonists prospered and "arrived to a very great Degree of Plenty of all sorts of Provisions." The soil was fertile, Samuel Wilson, proprietor to William Craven, wrote, trees of all sizes abounded, fauna were numberless and varied, rivers ample, cattle and hogs flourished. "Negroes by Reason of the mildness of the Winter thrive and stand much better than in any of the more Northern Colonies and require less clothes, which is a great charge saved." Wine, olive oil, silk, tobacco, cotton, flax and hemp, and sumac, among other plants, grew exceedingly well. Come hither, was his unmistakable message.[9] By 1708, almost ten thousand people (including those who were enslaved) lived in southern Carolina, mostly around Charleston—in fact, enslaved Africans may have outnumbered their white enslavers (and may not have been counted). It was a sequestered community, though, hemmed in by Spaniards to the south, French and natives to the west, and administered by increasingly distant lords proprietors in London. In 1765 businessman Pelatiah Webster of Philadelphia traveled to Charles Towne and was taken by the bourgeoning commerce and emerging sophistication despite the disagreeableness (he claimed) of the climate: "Now I have left Charlestown an agreeable & polite place in which I was used very genteelly . . . The heats are much too severe, the water bad, the soil sandy, the timber too much evergreen; but with all these disadvantages, 'tis a flourishing place, capable of vast improvement."[10]

The march southward continued. Englishman James Oglethorpe, a prison reformer and advocate of British influence in the New World, was granted permission in 1732 by King George II to found a colony south of Charleston for the benefit of the impoverished and unemployed of England. His initial complement of bricklayers, farmers, and other laborers—thirty-two families in all—landed on territory aptly named the Province of Georgia. The area first settled was known as Yamacraw Bluff, territory inhabited by the Creek Nation a few years earlier. The settlers disembarked there on February 1. Oglethorpe wasted no time. "I marked out the Town . . . the first House was begun yesterday in the afternoon." Already, though, disease had crept in. "Our people are all alive but ten are ill with the bloody Flux which I take to proceed from the cold and their not being accustomed to lie in Tents."[11] Oglethorpe named the settlement "Savannah," a name of curious origin. He may have chosen it because of proximity to the Savannah River, a waterway familiar to the Shawnee tribe, whose name (Ša·wano·ki) was translated variously, including "Savana" or "Savannah."[12]

Cultivation of the fertile land was laborious, ill-suited for white settlers in the hot, sticky climate of their new Georgia. Oglethorpe wrote, "[T]here is a vast Quantity of extraordinary fine Land . . . it will be very difficult for White people to hoe and tend their corn in the Hot weather." Africans, the feelings ran, were accustomed to hot weather and physical labor, ideal for labors such as these. By May the lone physician, William Cox, had died, cause undetermined—probably a local ailment, maybe dysentery. Through the first summer a number of settlers died, either of burning fevers, bloody flux, or the effects of alcohol (apparently some form of rum punch was popular—likely bought from Indigenous people). "We had neither Doctor, Surgeon nor Nurse." By mid-July, Oglethorpe counted sixty people sick or dying.[13] Yet by summer 1734, the tiny settlement seemed secure. Farmers carved out several plantations, and workers built docks for the unloading of water-borne supplies and constructed batteries to command approaches to Savannah upstream and downstream.

The southern coastal lands had become the commercial engine of North America. Locally, a thriving planter culture took root and defined society itself in the Old South. Agrarian and parochial though it proved to be, southern plantations were the focal point of life, the driver behind a burgeoning capitalist marketplace. In the eyes of historian Elizabeth Fox-Genovese, they became the central link to the outside world, providing for most, if not all, foodstuffs, clothing (including that for enslaved persons), dwellings, and, importantly, health matters: "[T]he planter would look on every natural and human-made feature of his property as a part of himself."[14]

To the west was the great waterway that cut North American in half. The tribe of northern Illinois natives had bestowed the name *Mississippi* on the wide river, but along its two-thousand-mile course it was called various names by neighboring tribes. The Natchez tribe south of present-day Arkansas called it *Barbanca*, those at the mouth of the river, *Malbanchia*. But for France, it was the Mississippi and, by their claim, the belt line across North America. And France had also laid claim to that huge swath of middle America from Quebec to the Gulf of Mexico that they called Louisiana. In 1699 Louis Phélypeaux, comte de Pontchartrain, dispatched the French adventurer Pierre Le Moyne, Sieur d'Iberville, accompanied by his younger brother Jean-Baptiste Le Moyne, Sieur de Bienville, on a military mission to reconnoiter the entrance of the great river and build forts as a defense against westward expansion by Englishmen and Spaniards. Yet the mouth of the river and distal egress into the Gulf of Mexico were dozens of miles of tortuous, often flooded, waters filled with "alligators, serpents, and other venomous beasts."[15] It would be much preferable for an overland route from the gulf inlet lakes to the Mississippi River far enough upstream as to avoid this tangled, torturous journey. And a center of commerce near the Mississippi mouth was desirable as the next upstream location was the Natchez district, roughly 180 miles away. Furthermore, the Compagnie d'Occident (Company of the West), responsible for the commercial management of the Louisiana territory, felt that the existing outposts, at Biloxi and Mobile, were simply too far from the Mississippi for transport of cargo into the interior of North America. D'Iberville, while persuaded by such arguments, would never realize that mission. He died, presumably of yellow fever, in 1706. It then fell to d'Iberville's young brother, Jean-Baptiste, to establish a permanent settlement along the lower Mississippi River in 1718. He chose the site visited by the two in 1699, on one of the "most beautiful crescents of the river," which seemed the best location for a new settlement.[16]

Jean-Baptiste would anoint it Nouvelle-Orléans, New Orleans. There began a steady in-migration, settlers from Mobile and Biloxi on the Gulf Coast, emigrants from Europe, and Acadians driven from their homes in Nova Scotia by the British occupation.[17] The census of 1726 detailed that already there were recorded 1,952 "masters," 276 hired men and servants, 1,540 "negro" slaves, and 229 native slaves. By 1729 the town was bordered by levees that offered some protection from disastrous flooding of the Mississippi, woods and brush had been cleared to improve air flow, and the colony was prospering with crops of rice, tobacco, and indigo. Even a shipload of young girls had been brought in to court the colonists.[18]

Yet Louisiana air and Louisiana waters harbored dangerous infestations. Despite the glowing report by the historian Antoine-Simon Le Page du Pratz (1695–1775) of the "perfectly good air" that promoted "few illnesses in the prime of life and no lapse in old age," the swampy, lower Mississippi regions were not always so pleasant.[19] The stagnant bayous gave rise to swarms of hungry mosquitoes whose bite foreshadowed the mysterious distempers of eighteenth-century life: malaria and yellow fever. Epidemics had already appeared, in the settlement of Fort Maurepas, near present-day Biloxi, in 1702 and at the settlement La Mobile, on the Mobile River, in 1704. The Mobile epidemic alone killed thirty-five people.[20]

Urban life accentuated other common ailments. Newly arrived settlers were stricken during their transatlantic voyage with conditions such as scurvy and dysentery, caused by lack of fresh food or rotting meat. Manure of cattle and pigs mixed with human excrement thrown carelessly from chamber pots blended with puddles and, as a consequence, disease ran rampant. Other contagions like smallpox were a constant worry. Venereal disease was unbridled. Arrival of women promoted a rash of not only romance but all sorts of sores, rashes, and discharges emanating from men and women. Syphilis and gonorrhea were accompaniments of a mixed-gender population.

Louisiana's enlarging enslaved population presented additional health concerns. There was no place to examine, quarantine, or care for those already ill from their Atlantic passage. In 1728 the Compagnie d'Occident built a slave hospital on its plantation opposite the city of New Orleans as a way to quarantine newcomers.[21] Compounding the problem was a growing number of impoverished subjects. Often homeless, stricken by all the maladies of eighteenth-century New Orleans, with no provisions for health care, they wandered the streets, lay in gutters, or literally died at the feet of passersby. They had nowhere to go. The Hôpital du Roi, founded by the French Crown for military personnel, could be used only if space was available, but its population soon swelled to over nine hundred patients, filling beds, corridors, and walkways and tended to by the hurried transport of Ursuline nuns from Rouen, France, in 1727. The Hôpital des Pauvres de la Charité (Charity Hospital for the Poor) finally opened in 1737, built by a bequeath from shipbuilder Jean Louis and maintained by private donations.[22] In lusty New Orleans, any variety of self-styled healers filtered in, a few formally trained but most not. Even nearby indigenous tribes offered shamans with remedies and rituals of their own. Even though France's King Louis XV tried to restrict practice of medicine in 1723 to only those officially appointed by Louisiana's *chirurgien major* or who submitted to an examination of competence, his edict was almost impossible to enforce outside urban areas, and itinerant healers flocked in and out of the area.

New Orleans would be the sole prize for French adventurism in their failing expanse of Louisiana Territory. Cultivation of lands along the lower Mississippi would be fraught with inaction and indecisiveness and plagued by internecine struggles with Native American tribes. Yet the French were not ignorant of the region's potential. The two brothers Pierre Le Moyne and Jean-Baptiste Le Moyne had traveled along the Mississippi in their quest for trading sanctuaries. They had been captivated by one potential trading outpost high on the river bluffs among the indigenous tribe of the Natchez. In 1700 they posted a garrison there and erected a town they named La Ville de Rosalie aux Natchez (Village of Rosalie among the Natchez). The alluvial soil seemed unbelievably fertile and, before long, intrepid planters followed.

The village and protective fort of Rosalie became permanent fixtures on the Mississippi and maintained a quarrelsome but tolerable relationship with the neighboring Natchez tribes. That is, until November 28, 1729, when growing hatred of the French and their brutality for minor infractions spilled into a blood-thirsty massacre of more than 250 occupants of the French village. Retaliation by the French was swift, brutal, and relentless, and the Natchez were essentially driven from their homeland. Bienville's troops chased any remaining Natchez and their Chickasaw allies across Mississippi Territory to the Tombigbee woodlands in a frenzy of back-and-forth barbarianism.

Yet in all the cruelty of war, sickness was an equal player, felling French troops in astonishing numbers. Despite their zest for battle, the French had been poor colonizers frittering their effort in meaningless squabbles with the natives and harboring disquieting jealousy for the English. Administrative mismanagement reigned. Even standing on the most fertile of ground, settlers were often at the point of starvation, unable to generate the lucrative commerce of planters to the east and poorly supplied with provisions. The acclaimed historian of New France Pierre François Xavier de Charlevoix (1682–1761) said of France's failure to cultivate their lower Louisiana territory, "I know that commerce is the soul of colonies, and that these are of no use to a country like France but for this end, and to hinder our neighbors from growing too powerful. But if they do not begin by cultivating the lands, commerce, after having enriched some few persons, will soon droop and the colony will fail."[23]

Depleted by the Seven Years' War and petrified of English imperialism, King Louis XV ceded to Spain full ownership all Louisiana territory—and New Orleans—to the west of the Mississippi River and all territory to the east to Great Britain in 1762. Ceded back to France in 1800, Napoleon quickly lost interest in his North American conquest and, belabored by a costly war with England and rebellions in its Caribbean holdings, he sold his territory to the young United States in 1801.

The newly acquired Mississippi Territory in its entirety was on the edge of America's frontier. That soil, awash in the nutrients of the Mississippi River, was untamed and fraught with hazards in its unpredictability and susceptibility to flooding. Within hours spring inundations might wipe out acres of crops. Only the hardy could weather the harsh conditions of farming there. James Ruffin was one such adventurer who held the land valueless. Writing to Thomas Ruffin from Tuscaloosa in April 1833, he expressed his distaste:

> Well authenticated accounts from the Yazoo [district] concur in representing that whole section of country as very sickly, though it is very productive . . . I would go to no sickly country. It is calculated that in the county of Yazoo lying between the Yazoo and Big Black river, the negroes die off every few years . . . the whole extent of country lying between these two rivers.

Ruffin went on to assert that land outside of this river basin was worthless. "[Y]ou are in as poor a region as in No. Ca. [North Carolina] and in that part you are liable at any moment to be taken off by diseases of every kind."[24] Only the stout could endure its climate and geography and the whirlwind of illnesses produced.

Physicians in the area were well aware of the health dangers. One was Daniel Drake, who had a similar experience when traveling to the area. According to Drake, both Natchez and the neighboring town of Washington were subject to "autumnal fever," often so troublesome as to be epidemic in proportions. Drake assumed the mixture of organic matter—vegetable and animal—was a key element in fostering these fevers. Autumnal fevers seemed to arise where collections of this putrefying material were most abundant. Drake gave two opinions as to the mechanism of action: either it supplied the material out of which a poison gas was formed; or it may be the nidus or "hot-bed" of animalcule or vegetable "germs."[25] In terms of that most fruitful but fickle land between the Mississippi and Yazoo Rivers, Drake wrote, "The physicians of Vicksburg informed me, that those who travel or work in this [Yazoo] bottom in autumn, are subject to very malignant attacks, which they are accustomed to call the 'Yazoo swamp fever.'"[26] Pioneers were undeterred, however, even with the unhealthiness of the climate: the mosquitoes, the heat, and the humidity.

According to one medical tourist in the early 1800s, the town of Natchez—that former French settlement of Rosalie—and the broad expanse of the Mississippi Territory afforded ample opportunities for putrefaction and emissions of a dangerous and sickly nature. Its hills and gullies contained amounts of decaying vegetable and animal matter that, with exposure to the unfavorable elements—that Mississippi heat and moisture—gave rise to a noxious discharge as a cause of distempers of a most violent kind. Expect extreme epidemics, such as yellow fever and furious diarrheas, he cautioned. No class of persons were exempt: "whites, mulattoes, negroes, Indians, indigenes, old residents, and strangers" were all afflicted. The habits of residents did not help, the same author reported. There was a "general neglect of cleanliness among the inhabitants in their cellars, yards, out-houses."[27] It was as if the Mississippi Territory remained a curse for foreigners: first the French, then Spanish, and then newly minted "Americans." And into this unfriendly cauldron would be ushered the bondage of Black slavery that conferred a special obscenity, bringing down the wrath of nature and health, and, for a time, masked in the delusion of prosperity. It would not easily relent.

CHAPTER THREE

A PARADISE OF ILLS

[T]he very breaking of the soils seemed to loose disease.
—MARTHA CAROLYN MITCHELL

"We of the South vomit just like the sick of Paris and Boston. We urinate from our bladders and so do they . . . But here, we have Bilious Fever and other diseases incident to our climate, which they have not; and it is these diseases which the Southern student is oftenest called to see and treat when properly in practice, and which he never witnesses in the hospitals of London or the North," so argued the influential Atlanta periodical *Georgia Blister and Critic*.[1] It was promotion of a distinct southern type of medicine, as distinct as the climate, the topography, and the peculiar institution of slavery embraced by southern affluence. On the eve of secession and looming civil strife, it had woven into the fabric of Dixie society. That stamp of southern medicine was now part and parcel of the bid of southern states for their own brand of nationalism.

In the eighteenth and early nineteenth centuries many held as a fundamental principle that geography and climate were instrumental in producing manifestations of diseases with regional distinctiveness. The prolific American physician-writer Daniel Drake began his expansive treatise on the internal medical geography of the Mississippi Valley thusly: "[T]here are diseases which scarcely ever occur but in certain climates, localities, or states of society . . . Here then is the foundation of local medical history and practice; a basis which does not support the whole nosology, and yet is broad enough for a large superstructure, whenever an extended region constitutes the field of inquiry."[2]

One noteworthy physician (and avowed racist), Virginian Samuel Cartwright, invoked Hippocrates as the architect of southern diseases, that they were the direct descendants and beneficiaries of those ailments suffered by ancient Mediterranean Greeks. He contended that the southern districts of Virginia, the Carolinas, Georgia, and Louisiana were the only regions that "afforded a home to the civilized white man proper, and opened the doors to the science of medicine in the South." His conviction was that, because southern states had climates similar to Greece, their ailments were similar and should be treated according to Hippocratic dictates long ignored by erudite northern physicians intent on propagating *northern* European doctrines. As a result, Cartwright was convinced that, regarding medicine, the South remained under the "colonial vassalage" of the North. The fact was, he claimed, the climates of Greece bred a purity in the white human race as they now could do for the southern states. It was incumbent on southern physicians, he maintained, that they learn northern medicine for the valued diploma and then study southern diseases to be successful practitioners. Unsaid but stirring in the back of his mind was the burden of that most exceptional of southern creatures, the enslaved African. On this ethnic group, Cartwright would later insist, heaped a unique set of health dilemmas, perplexing and annoying to his white brethren.[3]

Many agreed with Cartwright. After practicing in the so-called backwaters of the new deeper South (Mississippi), physician Erasmus Darwin Fenner (1807–1866) spoke more effusively in 1849:

> It surely will not be denied that the immense region of country which we have marked out as the scope of our observations, differs sufficiently in its prominent features of soil and climate, from the region lying north of it to be justly entitled the Southern States . . . In like manner, a general distinction may be drawn between the prevalent diseases of the North and the South, as well as in the different sections of the South . . . [T]hey really call for a corresponding modification of treatment. Whoever expects to see the same remedies, administered in like doses, and in apparently similar conditions of the system, produce equally beneficial effects in these various regions and sections, will find himself egregiously mistaken.[4]

Historian Martha Carolyn Mitchell bemoaned the fate of southern health in those antebellum years when Georgia, Alabama, Mississippi, and Louisiana attracted planters and populations—both free and enslaved. The mushrooming communities quickly outstripped their medical resources:

> Sickness and death and scarcity of the means to check the one and delay the other were as characteristic of the Lower South as of any other frontier. Here, as elsewhere, the very breaking of the soils seemed to loose

disease, and exposure and poor food added their part. Physicians were few or entirely lacking and medicines were as scarce as were those who had skill in administering them.[5]

It seemed that climate, still, that elusive combination of heat, humidity, and rainfall, seemed to augment the voracity of disease, especially those fevers that tended to suddenly strike victims down. It had all become a tradition based on ancient Greek philosophy as championed by the great Hippocrates. The laws of nature, Elisha Bartlett wrote, were not to be suspended or ignored. Those natural tenets of the Greeks and Romans—those capricious humors so deadly to man—must remain unfettered and part of the science and art of medicine.[6]

But how did the South lay claim to such distinctions? What in the mix of geography, sociology, and pathology lent an impression of distinctiveness to southern health? At the root lay a rapid southern migration in the early eighteenth century. Superimposed were the so-called miasmas—bizarre perturbations of nature that so adversely affected the human constitution.

America was still a new, raw, and rugged land—so different from the stale aristocracy and weary sophistication of the Old World. Scattered communities, endless expanses of lowland fields ripe for cultivation, peppered the narrow rim of seaboard that comprised the English colonies. Yet New World cities, so few in number, barely resembled the halls of academia found in London or Paris. True, Boston and Philadelphia housed centers of learning but those were almost amateurish compared to the lecture halls and laboratories across the Atlantic. As for the practice of medicine, in America, physicians spilled into the small farming communities with a bare grasp of the natural sciences and even slimmer understanding of therapeutics. Even at best, eighteenth-century medicine was far from a perfect science (if indeed yet a science at all). And in America, with no formal system for medical education, practitioners of varying quality abounded, some so pitiable as to be outright charlatans who peddled their lamentable concoctions likely to do more harm than good.

The common citizenry worried. "The History of our Diseases belongs to a Profession with which I am very little acquainted," wrote New York lawyer William Smith in 1757. "Few Physicians amongst us are eminent for their Skill. Quacks abound like Locusts in Egypt, and too many have recommended themselves to a full Practice and profitable Subsistence."[7] In fact, folks of Northampton County, Pennsylvania, petitioned the state legislature in 1775 that their county was "infested with a Set of Men" calling themselves physicians and surgeons but who were, in all reality, little better than "Empericks or Quacks" so that, in their practice, "some Persons have, in all Probability, thereby lost their Lives, and others been rendered Cripples, to the great Grievance, Loss and

Impoverishment of many Families." The petitioners pleaded with the assembly to reign in such practices by certifying the credentials of those claiming to be physicians. Despite their request, the petition was tabled.[8]

Indeed, their concerns were well grounded. By some estimates, in New York in 1750 there were over forty physicians for a population of fifteen thousand. In Williamsburg, Virginia, in 1730 there were anywhere from twenty-five to thirty physicians for a community of only thirty-seven hundred, including enslaved Africans.[9] Philadelphia physician Benjamin Rush was appalled by the state of medicine in colonial America, writing on the disastrous yellow fever epidemic of 1762 that had settled on marshy, hot Philadelphia that summer. "You may perhaps reply [speaking of the sweeping sicknesses] 'Fine times for the physicians.' Such a retort as this might only be adapted to those inhuman monsters who estimate their happiness by the miseries and infelicities of their fellow creatures."[10] Historian Richard Shryock maintained that "the degree to which regular physicians resisted quackery depended largely upon the extent to which they themselves had attained to professional standards and solidarity."[11]

Even for honest practitioners, eighteenth-century colonial medicine was a formidable proposition. The colonies of North America were quickly becoming an amalgamation of global migration. Hand in hand, too, America transformed into a gigantic melting pot of pestilence. There was an almost immediate intermingling of the ailments brought by Europeans, enslaved Africans, and befuddled Native Americans. Epidemics swept across the colonies—diphtheria, yellow fever, malaria, dysentery, and the feared smallpox. Despite the touted expertise of European physicians—whose practices many American physicians mimicked—therapeutics for the terrible ailments of mankind were largely ineffective. Cathartics, emetics, bleedings, and sudorifics were popular antidotes to restore balance of the elusive Hippocratic humors, a method labeled "heroic medicine."

Progressives—of which there were few—recognized more modern theories of philosophic empiricism and experimentation. Early discoveries in physiology, chemistry, and mechanics of the seventeenth century teased clinicians to rethink the worn theories of Galen.[12] One woman physician of the times voiced such empiricism when she described the human body as "a laboratory . . . the excretions are its refuse; they are both the result and the measure that gone on between the outside world, and our own organization."[13] Figures such as Benjamin Rush condemned reliance on the waning popularity of Hippocrates and Galen, encouraging instead principles learned from European sages such as Professor William Cullen of Edinburgh, who taught observation and examination before deriving truth.[14] Yet most still embraced his concepts of humoral disparities and tensions that, when treated by seemingly barbaric methods, often led to disastrous outcomes.[15]

Furthermore, Rush acknowledged the widely held belief that climate affected health. He was convinced that the particular American climate fostered its own manifestations of disease. Discounting the popular notion of nosology, Rush claimed that "[diseases] are all changed by time and still more by climate, and a great variety of accidental circumstances." A sickness, by virtue of its assigned name, prompted specific therapeutics, he pointed out, that could cause "the most extensive mischief" when not considering atmospheric influences and other exciting causes in its treatment. He railed at the deplorable condition of medicine still, outlining numbers of reasons for this implicating improbable theories without sufficient examination and the lack of a clear understanding of the displays of the various diseases.[16] In that sense, Rush subscribed to the broad familiarity of his mentor Cullen in being "intimately acquainted with the histories and distinctions of the diseases of all countries, ages, stations, occupations, and states of society." Perhaps he was inferring a special station to the young United States and its varied geography and peoples as separate from the Old World order.[17]

As for the colonial South, physicians of proper schooling were few. In fact, as opposed to urban centers in northern colonies, the rural South attracted scant medical care to the countryside. But the infrequent educated southern doctor suspected the sweltering climate of their colonies to be an inducement to ill health. George Milligen-Johnston, a South Carolina physician, claimed so much in his exposé written in 1761: "The great Heat, in the Summer Time, conspires with the Moisture to relax the Solids, and dispose the Humors to Putrefaction," leading to the "Epidemics" that appear sooner or later of varying duration. It was here, Milligen-Johnston implied, that the climatic forces influenced fevers and sickness in ways unique to the southern lowlands.[18]

Some had described a certain intellectual *vacuité* in the South. Even after the Revolutionary War, such attitudes had persisted. The eminent geologist Philadelphian William Barton Rogers lamented during his tenure at the University of Virginia in rural Charlottesville in 1841 that "[w]e are as dull as a mill-pond in a deep hollow where no breeze can touch it. My heart longs for the cheering impulses of society with my brothers and with the busy world."[19] Frederick Barnard, professor of mathematics and natural history at the University of Mississippi in Oxford, came full face with the inequities of scientific endeavor between his native Northland and the South. There was a distinct professional isolationism felt by scientists in the South and away from urban areas like Charleston and New Orleans. While in the sleepy burgh of Oxford, Barnard wrote that he had "been reduced to idleness and intellectual stagnation by the atmosphere of mental apathy which surrounds a devotee of science here."[20] And even in cosmopolitan Charleston the distinguished physician and botanist Alexander Garden remarked, in 1764, "[W]e are a set of the busiest, most bustling, hurrying animals imaginable . . . unless among the gentlemen planters, who are absolutely above every occupation but eating, drinking, lolling, smoking and sleeping."[21]

In the agricultural South, as for much of colonial North America, people tended to health affairs in their households. Births and deaths were rites of passage in the home, and even surgery was done on the kitchen table. For the most part, fevers raged, deliriums ranted, and bowels spewed all among family members. Often home remedies were used for common ailments, procured from local apothecaries or itinerant practitioners. Most medical information shared among the colonists came in the form of almanacs, small treatises on domestic medicine, or recipe books for folklore therapeutics. These were the handbooks of the day. Diseases such as diphtheria, rheumatism, rabies, smallpox, and syphilis were explained in the vernacular, with recipes for elaborate arrays of herbals and other bizarre *materia medica.*

Nevertheless, these periodicals, such as the *South Carolina Almanack,* served to disseminate some useful information concerning inoculations for smallpox and various dietary remedies for the ubiquitous southern flux, or dysentery. For many literate laymen, it was a staple of the home.[22] One genteel South Carolina physician commented, "The distance of physicians, the expense, difficulty, and delay in procuring their attendance, has compelled many inhabitants of the country to prescribe for their families" various tonics and even plant remedies. Even surgery might be performed by willing neighbors. On one occasion, that same physician called on a farmer whose severely mangled leg had been amputated by a fellow planter "with a common knife, carpenter's handsaw, and tongs." While far from elegant, as he described, the leg, fitted with a wooden prosthesis, was quite functional. Such were the necessities of backcountry living.[23] Or, very often it was a countryman's preference. Doctors might be so unscrupulous and poorly trained as to be more dangerous than illiterate town folk.

CHAPTER FOUR

CORRUPTED AIR, PUTREFIED EARTH

DISTEMPERS, EPIDEMICS, FLUXES, AND THE MALADIES OF COLONIAL LIFE

Sicknesses were the bane of existence in colonial America. They permeated all facets of life and, like the mythical grim reaper, stalked victims with persistent vigilance, always just in the shadows. More likely than not, death would come prematurely and in the throes of fever, rash, convulsions, jaundice, and delirium. The Old South was no different. Diseases were a visible encumbrance. Tropical climates produced so many ailments that they were unwelcome residents of every household. In an age when illness was thought an imbalance of bodily humors—phlegm, black bile, yellow bile, and blood—internal harmony was at the mercy of nature. It was the air and soil itself, most believed, putrefied in southern climates, that permeated bodies with such loathing that only the severest of treatments would help. Charleston physician Jacob de la Motta would write in 1820:

> The condition of our atmosphere at particular seasons, is very much subject to certain alterations, resulting from a greater or lesser supply of those materials, that make it innoxious [noxious] or injurious. If the exhalations from the earth, and decomposed animal and vegetable matters, are less abundant at one period than another, we are to look for an atmosphere more or less surcharged with those offensive ingredients that enter the system; pass through every vascular ramification . . . Our enquiries must lead to the origin and production of these pestiferous particles; and here we must revert to what is familiar to every one; I mean

heat and moisture, those essential agents in producing putrefaction, and a consequent elimination of those vapours, so prejudicial when respired.[1]

A foremost manifestation of disease was fever—from the Latin *febris*, meaning "heat." Eighteenth-century scientists called it distemper. Flushing of the skin, an unusual warmth to the touch, headaches, body aches, and chilling signaled its presence. The medical geographer James Lind had studied distempers and blamed them on contagions. In his opinion they were "imbibed particles by which a fever may be communicated." How were they spread? Proximity. Lind concluded that even the fetid smell of some feverish patients—a stink of vomit or stool—in and of itself, was a vector for communication.[2] More terrible, Lind observed, were those fevers of the South. By the time one reached South Carolina, sicknesses were "much more obstinate, acute and violent."[3] They resembled the fatal distempers of the Caribbean West Indies.

As for the consequences, Lind had an opinion. A weakened state often prevailed but depended heavily on one's constitution. "Many, especially women, and those of a delicate habit, and particularly during hot weather, are often reduced, by fevers, to an extreme degree of imbecility," he contended. Imbecility? Obfuscation it was. Hallucinations. Approaching doom. For those whose effluviums were of a copious or violent nature and did not respond to all the remedies known, the outlook was not good. Fevers continued. The patient seems to waste away, and "to bear the resemblance of a mere animated skeleton." If rest did not restore health, the inevitable outcome would be death.[4]

Fever showed no favorites. Planter, bondsman, adventurer, white, brown, Black, all fell victim to its maliciousness.

MALARIA

In particular, malaria—the periodic fever of antiquity—was the scourge of the South. The name itself came from the Italian term of antiquity *mal aria*—"bad air." It almost certainly did not exist in the New World prior to Columbus's voyages. Spanish colonists and the Africans they enslaved may have imported it during the sixteenth century.[5] Some theorize that it was Hernando de Soto's Spanish expedition through Florida and the American Southeast that introduced the periodic fevers. As part of his troupe, he brought a number of enslaved Africans likely infected with it.[6]

A plague of immeasurable consequence, some contend that over half the deaths of mankind have been due to it. All civilizations felt its wrath: Chinese, Assyrian, Babylonian, Egyptian, Greek, Roman. Indeed, malaria, infection with the *Plasmodium* protozoa as we know it today, has been around for millennia, perhaps contracted by humanoids in Africa from the great apes. Hippocrates mentioned it in his *Epidemics*, feeling that a particular set of atmospheric conditions were responsible for the disease. More pragmatically, though, he also noted an association with stagnant waters, felling many citizens of Greece's city-states.

Luigi Torelli in his 1882 opus *La Malaria d'Italia* contended that spread occurred from the shores of North Africa through Sicily and onto the Italian mainland by 800 BC.[7] Its signature was recurring fever—tertian fever it was called. Rigors—bone-rattling shakes—and blistering temperatures peaked every other day. The condition was often accompanied by vomiting and the rush of such a weakness that the afflicted was forced to take to bed. Julius Caesar felt its wrath, and, during the civil war with Pompey, malaria shattered his armies. Low-lying marshy areas, the Campagna region around Rome, were notorious for harboring the affliction. So consumed were they by the malady that Romans made a goddess of its fever. They called her Febris, and she was thought to confer protection on Roman citizens from the dreaded *mal aria*. According to Cicero, there was even a temple dedicated to her on the Palatine. Her mythology may have originated from the Roman god Februus, the "purifier," in that the profuse sweating as fevers "broke" was a process of purification, a purgative, a cure. In the first century CE Celsus studied the problem diligently, cataloging the periodic fevers so common in Roman citizenry and accurately described tertian fever as far more pernicious.[8] Of its cause, the ancient Roman scholar Marcus Terentius Varro prophetically wrote in his *Rerum Rusticarum*, "Precautions must also be taken in the neighborhood of swamps... because there are bred certain minute creatures, which cannot be seen by the eyes, which float in the air and enter the body through the mouth and nose and there cause serious disease."[9]

Roman agriculturist Lucius Columella was even more graphic: "[M]arshes threw up noxious steams and bred insects armed with mischievous stings, and pestilent swimming and creeping things whereby hidden diseases were often contracted."[10] However, others, equally credible, attributed the affliction to demons evoking innumerable spells and rituals. Most ancients agreed with Columella, though, that the toxic humors emanated from swampy ground and were by themselves the source of febrile maladies. The "Roman fevers," they were called, struck many invading armies after the fall of the empire. Merchants, slaves, and soldiers all contributed to the spread that occurred during the first millennium of the Common Era. No part of the world would be exempt, extending from Europe to the Caribbean to Asia. "Evil air," they claimed—*mal aria*. It was mentioned in Dante's *Inferno* and Shakespearian plays. "[H]e hath got, as I take it, an ague [English term for fever]... he's in his fit now and does not talk after the wisest," Stephano says of Caliban in *The Tempest*. His remedy: alcohol, and plenty of it, a common English relief for the vagaries of this tempestuous malady. "[I]f all the wine in my bottle will recover him, I will help his ague," Stephano blurts.[11]

Noted British physician Sir John Pringle recognized that these epidemics of autumn were of an intermittent nature. He described them as "a bad kind [of air] which, in the dampest places, and worst seasons, appears as a double tertian, remittent, continued putrid, or even an ardent fever."[12] Intermittent fevers were sentinel signs, the onset sudden: vague symptoms of ill-bearing, headache, muscle aches, and abdominal discomfort followed by shaking chills (rigors)—chills so severe they could literally shake the bed or throw a man from his horse—and then the fevers. In fact, the fevers were of a malevolent variety. The heat of internal combustion followed, inflaming the victim with such terrible aching, splitting headaches, and thoughts that death might be preferable. The illness might progress to jaundice, pulmonary edema, and kidney injury. In some cases, cerebral involvement led to coma and death.

As for true remedies, there was one. It happened that in the seventeenth century, a certain Genoese merchant by the name of Antonius Bollus, in trading with natives of the New World, had stumbled upon the bark of the cinchona tree (*Cinchona officialis*) that had remarkable medicinal properties. Natives had used it. They called it *quina-quina* bark, and it cured the fevers. They had even given it to a suffering Jesuit priest in 1600, which rid him of his misery. Whether myth or fact, the story went that in Lima, Peru, the wife of the Count of Chincon fell sick—it appeared to be tertian fever—and she languished dangerously near death. The governor, hearing of the illness of the countess, informed the viceroy of a remedy, which he strongly recommended. The countess consented and upon taking the substance—Bollus's cinchona bark—seemed to recover almost miraculously. Peruvian Jesuits took the bark to Europe in steady shipments, ground it up, called it "Jesuit Powder," and sold it. It proved to be a lucrative enterprise. Before long, the powdered bark caught the attention of scientific men who traveled to Peru and procured their own samples. In 1742 the Swedish botanist Carl Linnaeus studied the substance and conferred *Chinchona* to the genus, after the countess, but as sometimes happens, the name was transcribed in error and the tree would forever be known as *cinchona* (the native *quina-quina* tree).[13]

Shortly afterward, the Italian Francesco Torti found through his studies that the Jesuit Powder rid the afflicted of intermittent fevers: the so-called tertian (occurring every two days) or quartan fevers (occurring every three days), but not against continuous, unrelenting fevers. It would be a full century before the disease could be explained and before it was known that the active ingredient in Jesuits' bark was quinine, a substance lethal to the *Plasmodium* protozoa carried by the *Anopheles* mosquito.

Jesuits' bark became a standard in American pharmacopeias. Common wisdom of the day dictated that "when an European is taken ill of a fever, during a season of prevailing sickness . . . it is necessary . . . that the bark may be administered without delay."[14] Of course, the patient was flooded with a plethora of other concoctions not nearly so gentle—or effective. Naturalist James Lind recommended a most disagreeable adjunct. Flush the stomach and bowels. From one end, the emetic *Ipecacuanha* produced violent retching. From the other end, clysters cleaned out the colon.[15] For the daring, blistering was also available. More agreeable, wine was often beneficial during the convalescent stages of recovery—along, of course, with the "bitter of the bark," supposedly referring to the powdered cinchona.

It was the American southern colonies where malaria was especially malignant. There, sweaty bogs and swamps festered with it as if, indeed, bad air emanated and infused deep into the lungs of those who dwelt there (in fact, it would prove to be the ubiquitous mosquito that thrived in those sweaty bogs and swamps). Summer and autumn were worse. So it was that the planters of South Carolina would leave their plantations at the beginning of summer and take their families to Charleston or the Sea Islands where the breezes were brisk and the air clean. The planter might return to harvest, but only during the day. The night air, he feared, carried the dreaded miasmas arising from the ground.[16]

YELLOW FEVER

Epidemics of yellow fever swept through the South in waves. Yellow fever was a distemper named for the yellowish discoloration of skin and eyes caused by liver jaundice. It often culminated in a shattering of humoral harmony that left a wake of jaundiced, bloodied crises during which many perished. "[I]n general this distemper may be defined to be, a pestilential fever proceeding from a *contagious miasma sui generis*, which inflames the stomach and adjacent viscera, obstructs the biliary ducts, and dissolves the adipose humors; to which generally succeeds an effusion of a bilious or other yellow humor upon the external or internal surface of the body," wrote Virginian physician John Mitchell to the eminent New Yorker Cadwallader Colden, scientist and epidemiologist.[17] Mitchell described epidemics raging in Virginia in the years 1737, 1741, and 1742. There was no solution to this malady, he had observed. All the purges and emetics, all the sweating and lancing, all the laudanum (tincture of opium and alcohol) and opiates were unpredictable in their effect and many times to no avail. The deepening yellow hue amounted to a relentless death sentence.

Perhaps it was fitting punishment for the slave trade. There is little question the disease originated in the dark, mosquito-infested rainforests of Africa and followed captured Africans to the slave ports of West Africa where fresh European victims awaited.[18] The tiny virus—*Flavivirus*, it would much later prove to be—carried by the *Aedes aegypti* mosquito, traveled in the bowels of sailing ships plying the Atlantic to and from Africa's west coast. The virus, incubating in the salivary glands of the mosquito, entered man's bloodstream with a bite, and from there it began. The liver was a favorite target, turning affected individuals shades of yellow (jaundice). Africans tolerated it better, many having acquired childhood immunity. Whites were different. "Bilious fever"—another name for it—struck numbers; perhaps one in ten died.[19]

In 1648 and 1649, outbreaks suspicious for yellow fever were seen in the Caribbean—Saint Kitts, Guadeloupe, and Cuba. Some called it the "Barbados distemper." Before long, wherever in North America mosquitoes bred—lowlands, marshes, swamps—so would be yellow fever. Georgia and South Carolina were favorite spots. August through October were the prime months. The population centers of Charleston and Savannah were especially hard hit. Probably one of the first true epidemics occurred in Charleston in late 1699, described as a malignant disease and surely yellow fever. "[A] most infectious pestilential and mortal distemper . . . was brought in among us into Charles Town [Charleston] about the 28th or 29th of Aug. last . . . This distemper from the time of its beginning aforesaid to the first day of November killed in Charles Town at least 160 persons," so wrote Governor Joseph Blake.[20] The disease was still raging into 1700, of such virulence that it seemed an almost supernatural happening, described by one inhabitant as a "destroying Angel," which "slaughtered so furiously with his revenging Sword of Pestilence." Historian John Duffy estimated that as much as 6 percent of the population of Charleston perished in that first epidemic.[21]

Yellow fever returned to Charleston in 1728, a hot and dry summer. But then a hurricane blew through in August, causing massive flooding—and stagnant waters. According to contemporary chronicler Noah Webster, shortly thereafter, "the bilious plague raged in Charleston with great mortality."[22] It had been, Webster concluded, "the most deadly bilious plague that probably ever affected the people of this country [America]." It threatened the total destruction of the town.[23] The bilious fever would continue to strike in and around Charleston through the 1730s and 1740s.

Doctors were baffled to explain it. Some felt it was a contagion, spread by air seeded by noxious vapors. They speculated that the air around seaports was especially tainted. Others, such as Benjamin Rush, thought the miasmas originated from the filthy hygiene and unsanitary dwellings of waterfronts. In cane fields mosquitoes seemed to breed ravenously; the stored sugarcane juice made an excellent food source for *Aedes* larvae. Yet the mosquito as its willing vector was unsuspected. Still others blamed the ripe vegetative matter of southern lowlands—marshes and bogs—moist decomposition giving rise to mysterious fumes that seeped through the human frame and aroused harmful reactions.[24]

Treatment was equally puzzling. In many, the disease progressed so fast that there was little time to try anything. No doubt, the usual poultices, bleeding, and other vile remedies were tried without effect. "The calamity was so general," Charleston's David Ramsay noted in 1728, "that few could grant assistance to their distressed neighbors." And burial presented its own problems. "[S]o quick was the putrefaction, so offensive and infectious were the corpses, that even the nearest relations seemed averse from the necessary duty."[25] One resident observed that "from eight to twelve whites were buried in a day, beside people of color." He went on to say that "[t]he ringing of bells was forbidden, and little or no business was done."[26] In those times of pestilence, city streets emptied, windows were shuttered, and residents feared the air itself.

TYPHUS FEVER

The erudite American physician Benjamin Rush was no fan of hospitals. "Hospitals are the sinks of human life in an army . . . They robbed the United States of more citizens than the sword," he sardonically remarked.[27] Hospitals were lodgings of infirmities, not health. For those packed within their walls, a peculiar illness called "hospital fever" raged. It had been described by Thomas Sydenham the century before as an unrelenting fever characterized by raised, rose-colored skin spots rendering the victim the appearance of a leopard. He was so curious about the sickness that some would refer to it as the pestilential fever of Sydenham. The sickness began insidiously: aches, loss of appetite, restlessness. Gradually the fevers increased in intensity, victims broiled. Then the sores appeared: gangrenous, smelly lesions on fingers and toes. It was now a putrid fever; decomposition had begun. Toward the end, the bowels released fetid contents, a horrible rotting scent. And then, as the patient sank into cadaveric decay, death came. Under the best circumstances, just one in ten would die from the affliction. In conditions much worse, up to half would not survive. Sydenham also observed a certain fuzziness to the constitution—a delirium of hallucinations and fits. Sometimes it was seen to terminate in hysterical disorders, in both men and women—fits of laughing, crying, or demented behavior. Sometimes victims were listless and inattentive. For that reason, the dementing fever and rash would be called "typhus" from the Greek word τύφος, meaning "hazy," a reflection of the muddled minds of victims. Typhus fevers were also seen in jails, aboard ships, and in military camps—crowded spaces with little room for personal hygiene. But hospitals were the worst. Rush knew it. They were dank, dark hovels of sick inmates lying about, unclean, unwashed, and underfed. Men and women hobbled in such disrepair that their clothing hung in tatters, soaked in perspiration or excrement; the floors coated with even more waste. Stale, stagnant air stifled all.[28]

Treatment? "Nothing is more evident, than that blood-letting is one of the most powerful means of diminishing the activity of the whole body . . . and it must therefore be the most effectual means of moderating the violence of reaction in fevers," the eminent William Cullen of Edinburgh insisted; the ideal therapy for jail fever, as typhus was often called.[29] Cullen offered a profusion of remedies. For the racing, pounding heart, he recommended antispasmodics, neutral salts, sudorifics (agents to cause sweating), and emetics. Vomiting, Cullen pointed out, was useful in fevers. It evacuated the stomach and drained the biliary and pancreatic ducts. For the raging fevers of typhus, Cullen felt there was some benefit in chilling the patient, either applying cooling substances to the body surface or ingesting cold beverages into the stomach. For the languid, he advised stimulants such as blistering—the application of caustic agents such as cantharides to the neck, feet, legs, and shaved head.[30]

Wisely, with typhus fevers, Cullen recommended moving the patient from places of corrupted air. He urged a change of bedclothes, as the garments themselves might house contagious matter. Simple measures of cleanliness probably did more than all the blistering and bleeding. In fact, a colleague of Cullen at Edinburgh, James Gregory, made the dire observation that, without such measures, hospitalized patients had almost no chance to recover. "Sometimes they are absurdly bled, purged or sweated till their strength is entirely gone." They were prisoners of medical design.[31]

In fact, dirty garments and unsanitary conditions do contribute to typhus fever. It is known to be due to infection with *Rickettsia* bacteria transmitted to humans by the common body louse. Lice infestations are particularly likely in crowded, unhygienic conditions. Dirty clothing attracts lice, which actually jump from person to person. Congested spaces like slums, ships, camps, and hospitals were perfect repositories and the common filth of colonial life ideal conduits.[32]

TYPHOID FEVER

The distempers of colonial existence often produced similar symptoms. Constitutional complaints of fever, aches, rash, vomiting, and diarrhea were manifestations of systemic imbalance and accompanied a variety of underlying diseases, many of which, as they were of an infectious nature, seemed similar. Of a type of malady resembling typhus, seventeenth-century London physician Thomas Willis described what he felt was a new version. Willis termed his illness "Putrid Fever." He described a febrile illness of increasing intensity but characterized by periodic "cold stiffness or shivering" followed by "a Heat which is unequal" and reminiscent of the fevers of malaria. However, the intensity of fevers mounted until a crisis resulted and heat took possession of the "whole mass of Blood."[33] Even mental confusion, swooning, and convulsions were seen at this stage. Nausea and violent vomiting occurred, and invariably there was the onset of bloody diarrhea that he described as bad as the plague and that killed many. Of grave concern was the appearance of a ruddy-colored urine and a quickening and weakening of the pulse. In those cases, death often followed. To Willis, it seemed the fatal crisis was a visceral (internal) one that he attributed to a miasmatic disturbance of blood and not a putrefying erosion of viscera (as some maintained): "The cause [of death] usually is not a humor produced inwardly in the Viscera, which corrodes the intestines with its Acrimony... but some Miasm [sic] passed into the Blood, and so inwardly mixt with it, that it cannot be forced from the blood."[34]

Not until a century and a half later would the Frenchman Pierre Bretonneau establish anatomically the unique findings in typhoid fever that distinguished it from malaria or typhus. He conducted a series of autopsies on victims of typhoid fever (at times fetched through surreptitious grave robbing) and meticulously described the necrotizing lesions of the intestine, distinct from tuberculous ulceration or other forms of dysentery and that he termed *dothiénentérie* (intestinal pustules).[35] Another Frenchman, Pierre Louis, corroborated the findings of Willis and Bretonneau, combining symptoms of continual and remittent fever associated with a typhus-like rash, abdominal pain, and bloody diarrhea with a putrid evolution of intestinal lesions, often fatal.[36] Death, he surmised, was from the putrefying action on intestines causing perforation. In America, in the early nineteenth century, Philadelphian William Wood Gerhard, a former student of Louis, published his observations, concluding that the occurrence of fevers and intestinal lesions was confidently distinct from typhus, yet similar enough in symptomatology to be termed "typhoid" (typhus-like) fever. It occurred in epidemic fashion and carried a substantial mortality risk. It is likely, before this distinction was appreciated, that in colonial America many cases of typhoid fever, now known to be due to the not uncommon intestinal bacillus *Salmonella typhi* were misdiagnosed as typhus, a disease relatively common in Europe, but found eventually to be less prevalent in the New World.[37] Practically speaking, there was little value in exacting diagnosis. No treatment was available for typhoid fever—or for typhus, for that matter—and the disease was often discovered for sure only at autopsy.

SMALLPOX

There was a much grimmer affliction feared by all, even more so than the horrid bubonic plague. Smallpox. It was the Great Menace, divine retribution, the speckled monster. New England minister Cotton Mather wrote in the early

1700s: "There is a Great Plague which we call, the Small Pox, wherein the Misery of Man is great upon him."[38] It was so well recognized that the common layman had no trouble identifying it. Probably originating on the African continent millennia in the past, it was a disease of fevers and collapse followed by eruption of a distinctive speckled rash. The appearance of skin rashes differentiated the ailment from other common conditions of the day: measles and chickenpox (the term "smallpox" was used to differentiate it from the great pox, syphilis, whose rash could mimic that of smallpox). And the spread and coalescence of skin lesions correlated with the overall condition of the victim. In the worst cases, victims soon lapsed into a toxemia with dwindling pulse and consciousness, until death intervened. The contagion spread with alarming rapidity, causing epidemics that produced heaps of corpses—tragically, many of them children—awaiting burial or destruction. It had almost wiped out a number of Native American tribes in the sixteenth century with the arrival of European explorers and their unintentional cargo of smallpox virus.

A minute virus was the culprit. Of course, this was not discovered for hundreds of years. Ignorant of this, clinicians of colonial times characterized the disease topographically. "Ordinary" smallpox, seen in 90 percent of cases, was characterized by a herald fever and then, after three or four days, the appearance of the classical eruptions in the mouth, tongue, and finally skin of face, trunk, and extremities. The rash began as flat reddish spots, turned to a myriad of tiny raised papular (beady) lesions, then blisters, and finally pustules. In severe cases, the lesions coalesced, leading to a septic, delirious state and, oftentimes, death. The rash could completely consume the appearance of the patient, covering face, chest, abdomen, arms, and legs in a scarlet, spotted transformation. A second course was found mostly in children, with flat reddish lesions and extremes of fever and exhaustion. Most cases end fatally. Then there was a hemorrhagic variety. High fevers—almost unabated—racked the victim along with headache, back pains, pallor of the face, and bleeding from mouth and gums. Speckled lesions, tinier than ordinary smallpox rashes, called petechiae appeared. Affected people quickly lapsed into coma, all the while with burning fevers. Death occurred suddenly.[39] The more violent forms of the rash too often led to a "morbid state of the body" that, by definition, was a form of putrefaction—a generalized inflammatory state, today we would call it sepsis—often not survivable. A few fortunate victims were affected with a milder form that did not pose such a risk of death, with a case fatality rate of 1 percent or less.[40]

For those who did survive, the frequent consequence was the pocked scarring from pustular healing. A pockmarked face carried the stigma of social disapproval and self-imposed isolation rather than risking public ridicule. It was especially disturbing for young girls who had weathered the ailment. Even the joy of surviving the menace did not necessarily compensate.

Smallpox had been a curse for centuries. Theories of contagion abounded. The Renaissance physician Girolamo Fracastoro (1478–1553) prophetically attributed spread of illness to what he called *seminaria contagionis* (contagious seedlets) that arose either within the victim as a result of some type of humoral corruption or from the atmospheric interaction with heated air. His airborne seedlets, then, were the vehicles of transmission.[41] Others, like Thomas Sydenham, also blamed the air, somehow corrupted, as the source of the contagion. Still others, like the Dutch scientist Antonie van Leeuwenhoek and Cotton Mather, thought "animalculated business" was at play, small life particles seen only with Leeuwenhoek's bedeviling microscope, which were part of an almost invisible realm of animated matter.[42] In contrast, the great William Cullen firmly believed that the contagion of smallpox was a ferment of human fluids, transforming them into its own nature and leaking out through insensible perspiration and eruption of pustules blossoming over the entire body.[43]

As with any epidemic of the times, there was no effective treatment. Various remedies were offered. The great Sydenham, whose precepts North American doctors assiduously followed, advised bleeding "nine or ten ounces" followed by an emetic to induce vomiting. Other measures were also tried: blistering, purging, and laudanum. If these failed to improve the victim (doubtful that they did), Sydenham urged another round of bleeding—and then another.[44] Dutch physician Herman Boerhaave—whose precepts were also enormously popular in the colonies—recommended bleeding, aperients (laxatives), fomentations (compresses and poultices), acid and nitrous drinks, as well as antimonial and diuretic agents. Cullen, too, was a fan of those noxious remedies, combining proper diet, mercurial and antimonial (emetic and diaphoretic) medicines, and the ubiquitous purging. Purging, he felt, diminished the activity of the sanguiferous system (a rationale for bleeding as well) in promoting inflammation.[45] For the recalcitrant there was fresh air (reasonable) and the milk of an ass (less reasonable), a nostrum whose effectiveness is open to speculation.[46]

Smallpox came to America with the arrival of Europeans aboard ships, likely even aboard Christopher Columbus's vessels. Before long, fear of the contagion was such that ships entering port towns were quarantined until passengers were deemed free of the disease. But with smallpox there was one small ray of hope.

In England in 1721 a process of inoculation had been tried, a method of injecting pus from affected individuals into the skin of the still healthy; pus mixed with blood. A fever would rise and an illness descend but often of a mild temper. The technique had been brought by travelers from the Middle East, where it was used often. An early crusader for this "ingrafting" was the British aristocrat Lady Mary Wortley Montagu. Herself a victim (and survivor) of smallpox, she saw firsthand the method in Turkey and volunteered her three-year-old son who weathered the process unaffected. During the smallpox epidemic of 1721 in London, she inoculated her daughter in a rather public fashion, who also remained immune.

Impressed by her boldness, despite initial resistance to the technique, popularity for ingrafting quickly spread. Of almost nine hundred persons who were inoculated, seventeen had died, presumably of the inoculation, and thirteen were found later to have an "imperfect" (milder) case of smallpox. Yet the strange and worrisome procedure protected the vast majority from the disease. Physicians flaunted inoculation as "the Skill in obviating or remedying Mischiefs that would likely to happen."[47] In New England, Cotton Mather, an early proponent, had observed that "[i]t has hardly ever been seen that any after having Suffered it Once, comes to Suffer it a Second time."[48] By 1754 the College of Physicians of London had declared, "[E]xperience had refuted the arguments which had been urged against this practice; which was now held in greater esteem and was more extensively employed by the English than ever; and the college [College of Physicians] considered it highly beneficial to mankind."[49]

Nor did the southern colonies escape the wrath of the speckled monster, as it came to be known. Speckling of face, trunk, and limbs by oozing pustules created an abhorrent image, indeed almost not of this earth. According to historian David Ramsay, Charleston, South Carolina, first experienced the contagion in 1699 or 1700, which proved fatal to a large number of settlers. Another outbreak occurred in 1717 that was equally destructive.[50] In 1738 smallpox once again surfaced, likely from a shipment of enslaved Africans. This epidemic was said to infect almost half of the town's population and killed half of the neighboring Cherokee Nation.[51] Another epidemic occurred in Charleston in January 1760, thought to have been brought home by soldiers returning from the French and Indian Wars of 1754–1763. The *South Carolina Gazette* carried a poetic lament to that great epidemic, inspired by the ancient Roman poet Horace and titled "Virginibus Puerisque Canto" (I sing for maidens and boys):

> Disease malignant fills the air,
> It's noxious atoms far and near,
> Spread thro' the ambient atmosphere:
> With doubtful flight and casual wing,
> Scatt'ring their pestilential sting;
> Of thro' the Pores or Lungs they pass,
> And taint your elemental Mass . . .[52]

"A great cloud seems to hang over this province . . . a violent kind of small pox rages in Charles Town [Charleston, South Carolina] that almost puts a stop to all business," wrote Eliza Pinckney on March 15, 1760.[53] Despite quarantine of early victims, the disease spread relentlessly throughout the community. With some knowledge of the new inoculation method, the town embraced the technique, even though, with all the controversy, it was still illegal in South Carolina. Illegal or not, before the pox had run its course, six thousand people had been inoculated. By November, the contagion disappeared. Still, over six hundred people had died, half of whom were African.[54]

Alarmed by the epidemic in Charleston, residents of Savannah to the south began quarantining "ships, vessels, boats, and persons, coming from Charlestown in South-Carolina" and anywhere else that the smallpox had been seen.[55] In fact, the entire colony of Georgia stopped all entering ships, particularly slavers from Africa, to inspect and quarantine. It became standard practice, after slavery became legalized in Georgia, for arriving ships to proceed first to Tybee Island, where, in 1767, a lazaretto—pest house—had been set up for a doctor to examine for communicable diseases and, if necessary, quarantine. Once all victims had recovered (or died) the "cargo" proceeded up the Savannah River to Savannah and unloaded. One such arriving vessel, the brigantine *Gambia*, in August 1768 faced a different fortune. Stopped and boarded, inspectors found several enslaved Africans showing the smallpox. In a radical move, the governor gave permission to inoculate those aboard who had been among the victims.[56] Apparently, an epidemic was avoided and those inoculated remained protected (as did the residents of Savannah). Such progressive measures might have spared Georgia ravages of the disease that were seen elsewhere.

Throughout the southern colonies, though, it was truly a time of consternation. Farther north, in 1748, smallpox appeared in Williamsburg, Virginia. Fearful of a catastrophe (few had received the new inoculation), public officials prohibited any civic assembly and discouraged citizens from gathering in any numbers. It may have worked. Of the 687 people stricken in that epidemic of 1748, 53 died, a death rate of one in twelve, far less than the usual one-third with this disease.[57]

Yet smallpox continued to be a pestilence that haunted the colonists. As cities populated, thick with immigrants and slaves, dangers mounted. Anywhere that men and women congregated smallpox was a threat. Inoculation, while accepted, was not widely practiced until the nineteenth century. During the Revolutionary War smallpox was a primary cause of death and sickness in the Continental Army, responsible, it was said, for the collapse of the Canadian campaign of 1776. "Everything about this army is infected with the pestilence [smallpox]; the cloathes [sic], the blankets, the air and the ground," reported General Horatio Gates to General George Washington in July of that year. Only through repeated efforts at sanitation and inoculation could the disease be brought under control. For the Continental Army, such measures worked. By 1781 regimental surgeons rarely mentioned the disease.[58]

THE BLOODY FLUX

Diarrhea. Thomas Sydenham called the condition a griping, sometimes dysentery, sometimes *cholera morbus*: an exquisite torment of the bowels typified by cramping, profuse expulsions of feces, and at the extremes, mucous and blood. A condition so revolting because of the foul explosive rectal discharges that comrades—even family members—shrank in disgust. Puddles of stool from urgent movements spattered the dwellings of the afflicted. British army surgeon Sir John Pringle had seen it firsthand—the bloody flux. The most troubling of diseases in military camps, in his estimation, were those arising from the corrupted water of marshes, from human excrements lying about camp, from the rotting straw of tents, and from the breathing of hospitalized men pungent with distempers. These conditions, he knew, were at best incapacitating and at worst fatal. Some called it "dysentery," perhaps from the Greek δυσεντερία, meaning a pain or griping of the bowels. The heat and moisture of the air must be the chief cause of the dysentery, Pringle thought. It was most prevalent toward the end of summer or in autumn amid the thick heat of the seasons. Was it also a putrescent state of the blood, he wondered, exposed as it was to the constant effect of the sun in hot weather? Yet the disease proliferated also in circumstances of scant vegetable intake and a dearth of fermented liquors, both thought to exert some antiseptic properties. This is why it struck poor people and the common enlisted soldier, "who from foul air, bad diet, and nastiness are most liable to septic diseases."[59]

Some felt that the flux was entirely a southern phenomenon. Philadelphia doctor William Currie, something of an expert on yellow fever, claimed that "[r]emitting or Bilious Fevers, and Fluxes, are scarcely ever known there [northern regions] but in proceeding to the southward . . . where heat is more intense . . . and the soil more moist . . . the diseases last mentioned are very prevalent, and often fatal."[60]

That horrible dysentery began as a "bilious fever" he had observed (as also was yellow fever), accompanied by a "disorder in [the] stomach and bowels for two or three days" before the copious fecal evacuations started.[61] It was, as the great diagnostician Thomas Sydenham called it, "the fever of the season turned in upon the bowels."[62] In fact, Sydenham discoursed about the "great torment in the bowels," which frequent movements were, at first, a mixture of mucous and blood, but later blood was expelled in greater quantities until the whole mischief be terminated upon the rectum in a spasm of intense pelvic disturbances. Such urgency to defecate rendered victims unable to do any activity but squat and defecate.[63] Often a watery humor, which is always mixed with the slime was expelled. The smell of it all was disgusting. At times, "when the bowels begin to mortify," the fetor was cadaverous and intolerable. Accompanying fevers added to the misery. Hectic (high) fevers, vomiting and cramping, alteration of the countenance, weakening of the pulse, and those odiferous stools were marks of a fatal outcome. Of those who died, Pringle had found the colon black and putrid, with ulcerated linings, especially near the rectum. It was a picture of rampant gangrene, feculent access to the bloodstream, and overwhelming sepsis, as if the poor victim had decomposed from the inside out.

But what of the nature of this infection, Pringle mused. Putrid exhalations, he surmised. Some miasma or other from those stricken worked its way into the blood and from there acted as a ferment, leading to putrefaction. Did bile, that yellowish humor secreted by the liver, play a role? Surely, it must not, Pringle surmised. Despite the visceral nature of the illness, with vomiting and diarrhea, dysentery did not seem to bring on that deepening yellow of liver maladies.

At its most malignant, the flux was often labeled *cholera morbus*. Benjamin Rush, quoting Thomas Sydenham, interpreted *cholera morbus* as producing "immoderate vomiting, and a discharge of vitiated humors downwards, with great pain and difficulty—a violent pain and swelling of the abdomen and bowels . . . thirst; a quick, small, and irregular pulse . . . heat and restlessness . . . which destroy the patient in the space of twenty-four hours."[64] The illness was sudden and quite frightful. Bowel evacuations were numerous, often watery. Stomach pains wrenching, prostration severe. Victims appeared ashen, with sunken features and dry, leathery skin. Some could not recover, unable to cease their defecation and vomiting. They literally withered away in pools of rancid liquid stool.[65] This variety usually occurred in the shanties occupied by the poorest of the poor, where collections of raw sewage and putrid water lay nearby. Rats populated the areas and feasted on the garbage and excrement of those who tossed their waste from flimsy doors like so much irreverent droppings of household clutter. And the water, the slimy water that circulated among feces, was taken in as eagerly as well water.

More modern interpretations of the flux of premodern America attribute some cases to simple sanitation issues and some to what now is recognized as bacteria-specific maladies. Scientist Norman Howard-Jones points out that the diagnosis of *cholera morbus*, for example, was often confused with other gastrointestinal disorders: "[C]holera was a diagnostic label applied to diarrhea and vomiting from almost any cause and must have included *Salmonella* and *Shigella* infections, ptomaine poisoning, acute intoxication by arsenic and other minerals, and the results of an undiscriminating choice of fungi for the table."[66]

For the flux—whether camp dysentery or the treacherous *cholera morbus*—there were no cures. Despite the gastrointestinal misery, emetics and purges were standard fare. Pringle advised such, purging and bleeding, and then laudanum could be given. Some physicians—those familiar with the American variety of the flux—would recommend bleeding the afflicted if feverish. The more persistent the fever, the more bloodletting. In milder instances, laudanum alone would be sufficient. Yet even in their recovery, Pringle noted that "those men who have been sent to an hospital can be of little service for the rest of the campaign."[67] Looseness of the bowels frequently continued for an indefinite period of time, making their presence in military camps particularly disagreeable. Yet in truth, Benjamin Rush made a cogent observation when he advised that those suffering from dysenteries be moved far from the walls of the hospitals for a speedy recovery.[68]

CHAPTER FIVE

DOCTORING IN THE COLONIAL SOUTH

> Some perhaps will object, that this Country is feverish and unhealthy.
> —DAVID RAMSAY

Not everywhere could one claim a southern *vacuité*. The low country frontier settlements of the Carolinas and Georgia attracted medical men of intelligence and ambition, lured by the propensity there to abundant and exotic diseases, men who would help shape a southern medical aristocracy and lay the groundwork for a southern peculiarity not only in proclivity to illnesses but also in distinction of practice.

DAVID RAMSAY

Foremost among these educated gentlemen was David Ramsay of colonial Charleston, South Carolina. A resident of Lancaster County, Pennsylvania, Ramsay trained at the new College of Philadelphia's medical school, under the tutelage of Dr. Thomas Bond. By all measures, Ramsay was an ambitious student, that blend of intellect and will thought vital to a medical career. He graduated in 1772 with a bachelor of physic degree. While a favorite of Bond's, Ramsay connected on a deeper level with another member of the faculty, the respected Dr. Benjamin Rush, with whom he would form a lifelong association. With Rush's encouragement Ramsay continued his studies in medicine at Philadelphia's medical college and finally received his doctorate in medicine in 1780.

By intellect and appearance, Ramsay struck an impressive figure. In contemporary portraits, he looked a serious, rather intense individual with sharp angular features. Not unattractive, he spoke of bearing and refinement and was convinced of his duty to a higher purpose. Following an abortive practice on the Delmarva Peninsula in Maryland, Ramsay accompanied Irish and Scottish settlers to Charleston—initially called Charles Towne—in 1774, a lucrative settlement on the banks of the Ashley and Cooper Rivers at a place called Oyster Point. Settlers loved the place. The climate was favorable, enjoyable, invigorating. Lusty. "Men guard themselves less from the Air here," Irish physician John Brickell wrote of North Carolina in 1737, "trusting to the heat of the Climate, and [receiving] the cool of the Evenings with only a Shirt." He went on, "The Consumption [tuberculosis] we are entire Strangers to, no Country affording a better Remedy for that Distemper than the pureness of the Air; neither has the small Pox ever visited this Country." It was promoted as a literal nirvana, a refuge from the ills and harshness of northern weather—certainly a pleasant alternative to European environments.[1]

And the economy was booming. Crops—indigo, rice, cotton, corn, and tobacco—grew with vigor, ripe for hungry markets abroad. Winters were mild—a delight one could not dismiss. One visitor remarked on the great improvements made in the province, due solely to the "industry and labor of the Inhabitants" applying themselves to clear the land, cultivate, and manufacture commodities to accelerate revenue to the Crown. "If this place were duly encouraged," the author went on, "it would be the most useful to the Crown of all the Plantations upon the continent of America."[2] The area around Charles Town had become an economic force, a staple of wealth and prestige. Yet illnesses plagued the inhabitants, such sicknesses in abundance that attracted men the caliber of David Ramsay. One visitor to the place in 1765 commented, "The heats are much too severe, the water bad, the soil sandy."[3] Another wrote: "Some perhaps will object, that this Country is feverish and unhealthy, and all the Advantages which might be found in other Respects, would not make Amends for the loss of Health: Besides, that you are plagued there with several sorts of Insects, and especially with great Rattle-Snakes; so that you are in Danger of your Life every Moment."[4]

Ramsay came with exquisite credentials furnished by Rush: "[H]is abilities are not only good but great; his talents and knowledge universal . . . His manners are polished and agreeable . . . he is sound in his principles . . . severe in his morals . . . He will be an acquisition to your society."[5] Ramsay was enamored. "I never was in better health, better humor, or better spirits," he wrote Benjamin Rush that July from Charleston. Yet the economy of Carolina's low country was based on slavery. By 1790 half the population of South Carolina was enslaved.[6] And by no means was Ramsay pro-slavery. "Oh that it had been my lot to have spent my days where slavery was unknown!" Ramsay went on: "To speak as a Christian, I really fear some heavy judgment awaits us on that very score. *Culpam sana prenuit* [an appropriate cause produces the sin] comes. I have not read Granville Sharpes book [noted abolitionist] but, I am informed that he proves by instances that slavery has always proved the bane of countries that gave into that illicit practice."[7] But it was frontier territory as he soon found out:

> I have no connexion [sic] with the Doctors here, & thank God I have nothing to fear from them. Duelling [sic] has been practiced so much here that illiberal language is seldom used. Indeed I never heard one Gentleman villify [sic] the character of another in plain terms. Doctor Haly has at sundry times discovered a willingness to decide medical controversies with the sword. To this I attribute my escaping positive censure; but notwithstanding I believe the most of them are willing to treat me with silent contempt.[8]

Ramsay soon rose to prominence as a capable physician. He had studied under the best: Lord William Cullen (1710–1790), professor of the Edinburgh Medical School; the Scottish physician John Brown (1735–1788); Erasmus Darwin (1731–1802); and of course, his mentor, Benjamin Rush. Perhaps Rush held the greatest influence over Ramsay. It was Rush who had proposed a convulsive motion of the arterial system as a proximate cause of fever, and fever was commonplace in colonial South Carolina. Bloodletting, Rush maintained, was the only reasonable therapy: let loose the harmful effects of that agitated blood. And Rush did it liberally.[9]

In short order, Ramsay faced the sicknesses in this humid, marshy country. In 1790 he addressed the Medical Society of South Carolina in means of preserving health. Practices in northern climates did not apply here, he said. He cautioned against too much sleep, even in those pleasant, cool, early morning hours, that "the air which has been fouled by its perspiration through the night, and in a situation which tends to relax it nearly as much as if it was in a vapor bath." Rise early, he counseled; it was a very wholesome habit. At the same time, in those dew-covered grounds, be careful, he warned, such wet earth produced fevers. Cleanliness was paramount. Rooms should be well ventilated to avoid stale air. Destroy all harbingers of noxious vapor: "[O]ffensive and putrefying substances should be burnt up, or at least removed, so as to prevent their poisoning the air we breathe. The number of dead animals, and the quantity of putrid vegetables in our streets, is a nuisance of the most dangerous kind." Cold bathing was an excellent way to prevent diseases in this country, he advised. As for dwellings, avoid brick structures. Wooden houses were preferred in this country, he argued. They were drier and, as a result, healthier. Be careful of lying in damp rooms, or in linen not sufficiently dry; and put on dry clothes, as soon as possible, after being wet. Chilling winds, night air, and evening dews were dangerous. "The latter are more pernicious than a thorough wetting from rain." Ramsay discouraged too much inactivity. It was an evil to health, he believed. Suppression of perspiration was detrimental, even in the hot season. And of diet, he abhorred "intemperate use of animal food ... especially in summer." Worse yet was immoderate drinking of spirits," particularly in Carolinian climates. It added fuel to the summer heat. "Every evil that naturally results from an excess of heat, is aggravated by a plentiful use of ardent spirits." Yet the temperate use of "good sound wine" was an excellent antidote to fevers (perhaps his preference).[10] Antislavery in temperament, David Ramsay nevertheless noticed dissimilarities between whites and Blacks and implied this was a source of consternation for medical practitioners. In his magnum opus, *History of the American Revolution*, he pointed out:

> The stagnant waters and low lands, which are so frequent on the shores of Maryland and Virginia and on the coasts, and near the rivers in the Southern Provinces, generate diseases, which are more fatal to whites than blacks. There is a physical difference in the constitution of these varieties of the human species. The latter secret less by the kidnies [*sic*], and more by the glands of the skin than the former. This greater degree of transpiration renders the blacks more tolerant of heat, than the whites.[11]

And for the young bachelor in search of a suitable bride, no dowry connected with slavery would do. He was attracted to one particular woman whose "fortune does not consist in negroes, but is reducible to an annuity from the rent of houses and interest of money." He married Sabina Ellis in June 1776. As the local *South Carolina Gazette* described it: "Dr. David Ramsay, a young gentleman, whose abilities promise that he will rise to eminence in his profession, and be a useful member of this community, was married to Miss Sabina Ellis, eldest daughter of the late Mr. William Ellis; by which it is probable his residence will be fixed in this town."[12] It was not a year later that the young woman was dead at age nineteen. Ramsay mourned the loss of his wife in a long letter to Benjamin Rush in August 1776. He described her chronic asthmatic condition in some detail, revealing that she would often induce vomiting to forestall a bronchospastic episode. In fact, it appeared that her death was due to some type of respiratory infection (perhaps an influenza sickness) that produced fever, delirium, and cardiovascular collapse. "She was really a worthy woman," he wrote Rush, "possessed of a good understanding well cultivated by reading, a sweet natural temper, & a serious religious turn of mind."[13]

Professionally unwavering, it was his personal life that would produce turmoil. Stricken with grief at the death of his first wife, Ramsay longed for female companionship. Profoundly religious, he cared much that marriage was a God-driven union and that men and women were joined to complement, fulfilling the divine plan as set forth in Christian doctrine. Yet Ramsay had expressed heartfelt compassion, as attested by his unswerving attention to his ailing wife. In fact, after her death, he took in and cared for her youngest sister, afflicted with rheumatism. He seemed deeply concerned about the plight of young women in southern climates. He had written to Rush one year later that "[t]his climate is very fatal to women, their sex & inaction ... Should not ladies in warm countries delay marriage till the age of twenty." It may be that he blamed those mysterious climatic vapors for his own wife's death. Ramsay then disclosed that women, apparently meaning those in South Carolina, lived only an average of thirty-three years and many died in their first or second pregnancy. As it turned out, his feelings were prophetical.

In his quest for family, Ramsay remarried in 1783 to Frances Witherspoon, daughter of one of the signers of the Declaration of Independence. She died in 1784 after childbirth at age twenty-five. While he was tempted to remain celibate, he would remarry again in 1787, this time to Martha Laurens. Martha, while outwardly a prolific mate—she providing him with eleven children—was plagued by a conviction that sin had corrupted her ("Lord, deliver me from sin ... My soul longs for deliverance and rest."). That strong desperation for death ("how pleasant is the thought") hinted at a deep and abiding depression, little known to her husband until shortly before her demise at age fifty-one in 1811.[14]

Ramsay's eager professional engagement with Charleston's community soon spilled over to civic responsibilities as well. Following his exile to Saint Augustine during Charleston's occupation in the Revolutionary War, Ramsay sought and was elected to a position in the new liberated Charleston assembly. He had told Rush in 1785 of his abiding commitment to the town. "I desire to be sincerely thankful for the continuance of a life rendered dear by intrinsic worth & great obligations conferred." But his position on slavery remained unchanged. "I hope you will introduce Slavery as one principle source of vice. It appears to me that previous to the extirpation of this evil it must be made in the first instance odious in sentiment."[15]

Ramsay had become a force in a new, southern brand of medicine and a pillar of Charleston society. A prolific writer and historian, he wrote the *History of South Carolina* and the *History of the American Revolution*, both incorporating events of local medicine and illnesses. He left no doubt about the health problems of his community. Writing in his *History of South Carolina*, he remarked: "[Historian] George Chalmers ... observes that 'Charles-town was long unhealthful. From the month of June to October, the courts of justice were commonly shut up. No public business was transacted. Men fled from it as from a pestilence, and orders were given to inquire for situations more friendly to health.'"[16]

Yet on a sunny afternoon in early May 1815, as Ramsay approached his three-story home in post-Revolutionary Charleston, as was his routine, the unthinkable happened. Yes, Ramsay had been told of a disgruntled tailor whom he had examined and recommended confinement in an asylum. The deranged man had threatened to "kill the doctors who had joined in the conspiracy against him." Ramsay shrugged it off as so much nonsense. Nothing but the rantings of a mentally unstable but harmless wretch, he reasoned (the same wretch had already set upon and wounded a previous attorney some years before). But indeed, William Linnen, that very lunatic tailor, was dead serious and, for the moment, deadly insane. He now hid behind the massive alabaster pillars of Saint Michael's Church, just cattycorner to Ramsay's house. How this encounter happened at the day and hour it did was anyone's guess. Perhaps the unsuspecting Ramsay had been stalked by Linnen and now the opportunity arose. Linnen, after identifying the doctor and within sight of Ramsay's home, spun from concealment and pulled his horseman's pistol from a handkerchief. Almost point blank, he shot Ramsay three times. The first round passed harmlessly through Ramsay's coat. The second entered the hip and passed out the groin—not necessarily a fatal wound. However, the third shot entered the doctor's back near the kidneys and traversed the intestines. Ramsay dropped to the street and was at once carried back to his house. Remaining conscious, he was reported to have said, "I know not if these wounds be mortal; I am not afraid to die." Even more stirring was his willingness to forgive the gunman: "I consider the unfortunate perpetrator of this deed a lunatic, and free from guilt." His abdominal wound, though, was lethal. Ramsay lingered until morning the following day when he quietly passed away, bleeding and peritonitis the likely cause. Linnen was immediately apprehended and taken into custody. Insane, he clearly was.[17]

PETER FAYSSOUX

Southerner Peter Fayssoux (1745–1795) was the son of Huguenot *émigrés*, born and raised in Charleston. He grew up in the era of elegance in a city crowned with domed churches, theater, and assembly halls and surrounded by indigo and rice plantations. Fayssoux learned quickly, as every resident did, that epidemics were a way of life in South Carolina. In 1760 smallpox appeared in the town, killing almost a thousand people and forcing most families to so occupy themselves with protective measures that there was no time to grieve. Such brushes with death must have impressed young Fayssoux because he chose a career in medicine. Like many aspiring doctors in the colonies, he apprenticed with the more renowned of physicians, such as the local Alexander Garden. Yet before the Revolutionary War, to gain respectability as a medical practitioner—particularly one of local upbringing—training abroad was almost a necessity. The Scottish University of Edinburgh featured a number of eminent faculty, among them the great William Cullen. It was there that Fayssoux traveled. Fayssoux then returned to Charleston in 1769, diploma in hand. The now educated twenty-five-year-old, full of confidence and the latest medical theories, found the port city swarming with quacks. "It is Sufficient," he wrote acquaintance Benjamin Rush in 1770, "for a man to call himself a Doctor, & he immediately becomes one, & finds fools to employ him." Fayssoux was nothing of the kind, of course. He was a meticulous, thoughtful physician who studied his cases, much in the tradition of Edinburgh's Cullen. Only after careful reflection did he arrive at a diagnosis and treatment. Before long, Fayssoux had taken a wife and became quite comfortable in high Charleston life. "Men of Letters, & Candor ... with these only I generally associate," he wrote.[18]

There was no shortage of business. A booming slave trade enhanced by opening of rice fields farther inland brought an abundance of African contagions. Slave ships unloaded not only their human cargo but every pestilence carried aboard. During the Middle Passage, there was a steady attrition from disease. Each arriving ship with any sign of "plague or distemper" was to quarantine for ten days, during which time it would be thoroughly cleaned. Violations were punishable by steep fines. Of course, for those unable to pay or for offending enslaved individuals the punishment was much more graphic: "[N]o less than thirty-nine stripes on the bare back, in some public place," the law read.[19]

Epidemics were particularly onerous. Yellow fever and smallpox plowed through Charleston in 1699 and again in 1732, killing many, including whole families. Yellow fever came in waves with startling suddenness. As opposed to white residents, enslaved Blacks seemed relatively immune to the ailment. They were not as fortunate with smallpox. The pustular illness erupted without warning on Blacks and whites, children and adults. The skin blisters and scabs seemed to emanate from the air itself. By mid-century, many had heard of the wonders of inoculation, but not all believed and they feared it as much as the disease itself.[20] Any reputable physician, including Fayssoux, used a variety of treatments. Their pharmacopeia was replete with medicines to induce sweating (sudorifics), like sweet spirits of nitre (ethyl nitrite), and liberal use of the lancet (bloodletting). Purges and emetics were given in abundance to rid bodies of excessive humors. Most physicians followed the tenets of the popular Dutch physician Herman Boerhaave (1668–1738), who taught that diseases were ascribed to "morbific matter in the blood" and therapy directed at expelling them with liberal bleedings and other manners of bodily discharge.[21]

Nothing worked. The diseases ran their course unchecked. With smallpox, one in ten died, and the survivors often were marred with scarred, pocked skin.

It was an Eden beset with maladies. Was it a climatic element that fostered such sickness? The great English physician Thomas Sydenham (1624–1689) had revolutionized concepts of disease, theorizing a variety of sicknesses, many of which manifested similar symptoms. He also emphasized the striking effect of atmospheric conditions on the human body: "Hence, it becomes possible that the *sensible* and *appreciable* qualities of the atmosphere may produce such fevers as appear under all constitutions indifferently; but not those which are proper and peculiar to certain particular ones. Nevertheless, we must admit that even the *sensible* qualities of the atmosphere have a predisposing effect upon our bodies even in the development of epidemics."[22]

Sydenham's arguments on atmospheric distinctiveness could not have been more apropos than in the South. Marshes, swamps, humidity, and luxuriant but petulant vegetation seemed to offset the beneficial nature of the air. They exuded dangerous vapors that settled into trespassers. It all fit with the obsession about medical geography. Philadelphia physician William Currie (1754-1828) emphasized that climate and "situation" had a dramatic influence on constitution and health. Latitude (proximity to the equator) conferred special properties to the environment that affected susceptibility to certain fevers and ailments. As for the southern regions, in particular South Carolina, Currie maintained that "the strength or weakness of our bodies keeps pace with the weather" so that, as observant people perceived, "an increase or abatement of his own strength" resulted from seasonal changes providing susceptibility or resistance to the various diseases. Seasonal changes caused havoc with the constitution.[23] Europeans were certainly aware of it. Scotsman James Lind (1716-1794) wrote extensively in the mid-eighteenth century on medical geography and pointed out the distinctiveness of the southern regions of North America. That hot environment of the American South—in particular, the Carolinas—was not the same as in northern climates of Canada, Newfoundland, and New England, very similar, he felt, to the temperaments of the English Isles themselves. Beware, he seemed to admonish his readership, the maladies of the southern provinces were impenetrable and fraught with lethality. Of those "much more obstinate, acute and violent" in South Carolina, he elaborated: "In that colony, especially during the growth of the rice, in the months of July and August, the fevers which attack strangers are very anomalous, not remitting or intermitting soon, but partaking much of the nature of those distempers which are so fatal to the newly arrived Europeans in West Indian climates."[24]

South Carolinian John Lining (1708-1760), a doctor of respect despite his lack of formal medical education, carried it a step further. He made a number of weather measurements, including temperatures, rainfall, wind speeds, and even intensity of thunder. Lining was convinced that the perturbations of weather and climate were directly responsible for the behavior of epidemic diseases. "For are not these the Effects of different constitutions of the Air on human Bodies?" he wrote in 1743.[25] Such beliefs based on experimentation and measurements had taken hold. A contemporary of Lining's, Lionel Chalmers

(1715–1777), was another disciple. Chalmers argued that climate, customs, and diet defined the inhabitants. Knowledge of the "qualities of the air" was essential, he went on, to understand the perturbations of health among the men and women of South Carolina. The hot, humid weather promoted a sickly constitution. Thus, it was understandable that epidemic distempers (fevers) of South Carolina seemed predictable and even expected. All the convolutions of climatic influences coupled with the specific perturbations soil, water, and vegetation slowly gave rise to the idea of southern medical distinctiveness.[26] The relentless summer sun putrefied plants, spoiled water, and altered air, giving rise to invisible miasmas, surely the source of human suffering.

JOHN WESLEY AND *PRIMITIVE PHYSIC*

Similar illnesses would also plague the lowlands of Georgia. Georgian weather and soil, like other parts of southern coastal areas, harbored a variety of evils. Once again, the relentless sun was thought to work mischief on wetlands just like in the Carolinas, causing "emission of mephitic particles, a vitiated air must be the effect, and diseases the inevitable product," so went a report from Dr. J. E. White to the Georgia Medical Society in 1806. "[I]t is plainly a melancholy fact that from the nature of our climate, and the existence of causes riveted to it and to the soil in the vicinity of Savannah, it must ever remain unhealthy... these causes have been known to produce multiplied diseases," White continued.[27] Drawn to epidemics of ill health, practitioners of physic—legitimate and otherwise—settled throughout Georgia just as they had done in South Carolina. Some came directly from Europe; others migrated from neighboring South Carolina. They were a professional heterogeneity: charlatans among scholars.[28]

Residents of Savannah, Georgia, found that amid the sultry months of summer fluxes (dysentery) and fevers dominated, crippling efforts to deliver a profitable crop. Even in healthy times, field work was laborious and draining for white planters. The solution was, of course, slavery. By 1790, the lowlands of coastal Georgia would host 12,669 enslaved Africans and 4,179 white settlers. Enslaved Blacks would outnumber whites three to one. Georgia thrived.[29]

Even slave labor of Africans would not erase the miseries of southern health, though. Fevers, coughs, rashes, and diarrhea affected all. Questionable practices and remedies peddled by physicians failed to make an impact. Many relied on folk medicines, which became a preferred substitute for the snake oils of passing "healers." Popular among these almanacs was one titled *Primitive Physic: An Easy and Natural Method Curing Most Diseases* by a former southern preacher-turned-medic, the Reverend John Wesley. The evangelist Wesley (1703–1791), an Anglican preacher, arrived in Savannah, Georgia, from Kent, England, in

1736. The healing arts were not unfamiliar to Wesley. He had studied under the polymath Robert Boyle at Oxford and read several medical treatises. Preachers of the day might be expected to double as physicians for their congregations; his great-grandfather had done such. Wesley's exposure to the wilds of the New World had only reinforced his conviction that healing could be done by the Holy Ghost but also by common sense. He had a jaded opinion of educated physicians of the day, feeling that they had become too enamored with their lofty dabbling in the natural sciences and less interested in the practical applications of medicine to relieve ills. "[N]either the knowledge of astrology, astronomy, natural philosophy, nor even anatomy itself is absolutely necessary to the quick and effectual care of most diseases, incident to the human body," he had written.[30]

The subject of some controversy in his ministry, he eventually returned to England disenchanted with the New World. Yet his compassion for the suffering was unquestioned. Upon returning to England, Wesley and selected companions visited and cared for the sick. He carefully recorded his observations and, with the aid of an apothecary and a surgeon, published his first work in medical studies in 1745, attaching to each ailment some easily assembled medications and remedies. The culmination of his self-styled philosophy and therapeutics was the *Primitive Physic*, a publication that was a tremendous aid in the common household, a practical handbook for the ills of everyday life.[31] "For the sake of those who desire, through the blessing of God, to retain the health which they have recovered, I have added a few plain, easy rules," he wrote in the preface. Most were harmless concoctions: emetics, cathartics, aromatics, or demulcents dosed with a generous portion of religious fervor. A strange mixture of common sense and superstition, one historian noted.[32]

By 1764 his almanac had reached America. It was a ready convenience to southern planters and their families rather than risking the dubious prescriptions of untested doctors. Wesley listed over eight hundred preparations for 257 diseases and conditions. Yet even Wesley's book of instruction fell in disrepute as the colonies broke with England and matters British became distinctly unpopular.

CHAPTER SIX

REVOLUTION

The Glorious Ally of Disease

A Country as hot as the Antichambers of Hell.
—PATRIOT DOCTOR ROBERT WHARRY

What would launch the South into a dominion of both distinction and difference would be the grand—but bloody—American rebellion for independence. That indomitable southern climate and topography would sabotage British efforts to dismember the rebellious spirit of Whigs and Patriots. And much more. While the Revolutionary War was certainly not the sole instigator of slave (and hence southern) culture, it provided impetus to address the importance of plantation agrarianism to the welfare of the new United States. If nothing else, warfare and the dangers of ruination to lucrative agricultural enterprises brought into sharp focus the prominence of planter society—and, hence, slavery—to national economy. Historian Laura Sandy claims that the planter elite—whether Patriot or Loyalist—was compelled to preserve slavery at all costs, even to the detriment of allegiances to Crown or country.[1]

But it was the immediate consequence of latitude that spoke loudest. The revolt of the colonies against England and its duplicitous governance in 1775 would bring into apposition the desultory nature of southern lands. Poorly acclimatized British, out of frustration in their failure to subdue rebel elements in the North, were forced to campaign amid the cryptic ethers of the South. The strong permutations of air and its so-called putrid vapors (a product of those relentless southern suns) wrought havoc on physiognomies more suited to cooler, drier weathers. Summer months were especially abhorrent, as temperatures soared and moisture-laden air closed in. Torrential rains poured and aided in perpetuating its marshy coastal terrain. No better proof of a hostile medical geography could be found, then, than that expanse of lowlands extending southward from Virginia. Into this morass the British would march, hoping to quell a revolution of backwoodsmen and illiterate farmers. They would come face to face with the virulent distempers and epidemics waiting. It would cripple their troops even more so than ill-trained rebel militia and rearrange a fateful strategy that would eventually bring their southern army to the gates of Yorktown.

From the Declaration of Independence in 1776, Whigs and Tories, Patriots and Loyalists mingled indistinguishable in the South's lowlands and backcountry. Sentiments vacillated for liberation from British rule, yet an enchantment with immense profit crops yielded by royal markets tempered a rebellious nature. Passions seemed to waver with the oppressive humidity of southern summers and the vicissitudes of season, sickness, and security. It would be American against American, the first taste of civil war.

For the British forces, cautious of the deadly climate, the South nevertheless held strategic value. Frustrated by the elusive General Washington and his ragtag Continental Army, British eyes looked south, sensing that vast planter affluence would influence attitudes. Once Redcoats were seen, Loyalists would rise anew and join the ranks of the Crown to subdue these rebel bands. In the South, it would become America's class struggle. Nineteenth-century southern novelist and historian William Gilmore Simms saw it so. Simms underscored a conflict as immersed in "hatred, revenge, and cupidity" marked by "hideous atrocities and excesses" on both Patriot and Loyalist sides. Simms identified three caste divisions in lowland culture: the aristocracy of planters and merchants, small landowners and artisans, and then those poor whites barely able to scratch out an existence. Of course, enslaved Africans were not even considered. Simms's riveting stories of those revolutionary times brought out the rustic nature of attitudes and the keen desire to preserve and defend native soil and the enslaved laborers who toiled it.[2]

Yet the British were wary. Southern campaigning would revolve around avoiding one distinctive feature of the region—the voracious fevers and ailments that plagued travelers, especially newcomers. Many, if not most, of the European—British and German—soldiers had not previously served in the New World, either North America or the Caribbean. In contrast, resident southerners, even if only a few generations, had acquired an immunity to at least some of the more prevalent contagions. One particular patriot, Richard Hudson, remarked that a British invasion of the Southland in the hot months "would be the height of madness and folly for them to come here during the sickly season."[3]

British physicians may have known full well the dangers of venturing into hot and humid low countries. Their own Sir John Pringle (1707–1782), labeled as the Father of Military Medicine, had laid it out years before. There were diseases arising from the low countries, he noted: a certain corruption of the atmosphere spawned by an imperfect mixture and ventilation of humidity and air currents. In such flat and marshy countries, contaminated water, collected in cisterns, tended to putrefaction so that "[e]verything, therefore, in that country conspires in summer, not only to relax the solids, but to dispose the humors to putrefaction: and as the combination of heat and moisture is the great cause of the speedy corruption of all animal substances." This was the reason, he concluded, for the "fevers, and other distempers of a putrid kind."[4] Indeed, he contended, the interchange of warm and cold, damp weather checks perspiration, retaining "the more putrescent parts of the blood . . . where they produce either a fever or a flux."[5]

It was such permutations of the climate that led to cholera and dysentery—"particular determinations of the vitiated humors," often outing as diarrheal fluxes.[6] So, British strategy in the South distinctly tried to avoid those sickly times. The summer months seemed particularly dangerous. It was for that reason that British commander Colonel Archibald Campbell had been dispatched by Sir Henry Clinton, commander of His Majesty's troops in North America, in December 1778 to lay siege to the port town of Savannah. With three thousand Redcoats, he completely outmaneuvered American defensive forces and captured the town on December 29. He almost bagged Continental General Robert Howe's entire army in the process. The Crown would hold Savannah until the summer of 1782 despite attempts by Continental forces to dislodge them.[7] The following January—taking advantage of the cold season—Campbell marched out from Savannah and quickly took Augusta but, short of provisions and lacking the popular support he so counted on, beat a quick retreat back to Savannah by February, alerted to a possible approaching Patriot force.

Clinton was not done with the South. He devised a plan for another major offensive. Key in his strategy was the gem of the South, the port city of Charleston, major hub of economic vitality for the entire Southeast. In fact, in the later eighteenth century Charleston rivaled Philadelphia, Boston, and New York as capital American trade centers. South Carolina, in general, was considered the wealthiest of the thirteen colonies. Frustrated by Washington's clever tactics, Clinton looked southward. The South should present few obstacles. For one, it was not densely populated country. In 1776, roughly three hundred thousand residents lived in the Carolinas and Georgia. Almost half the population were enslaved, unlikely to offer much resistance. In fact, enslaved individuals might be allies, ready to rise against the hated plantation owners.[8]

It was seductive strategy. According to General William Moultrie (1730–1805), commander of the Continental southern army, "the British finding they could make no impression upon the northern states, reversed the proverb of 'taking the bull by the horns' and turned their thoughts on the southern states."[9] This plan would give them virtual control over rebel factions once deprived of their major seaport and commercial center. Even Georgia, a breeding ground for discontent, was in Clinton's sights. Historian Martha Searcy contended that Georgia would be a coveted base of operations because harbors there were good (Savannah the prime developed port, which they already held) and the river systems extended far into the interior. The land could become a literal "bread basket," plantations already producing large exports of rice, indigo, beef, and hides. The British Army would scavenge a fertile land, reaping ample provisions for their occupation.[10] Moultrie's only reservation was the inhospitable climate.

Patriot forces were not sitting idle, though. In the summers of 1776 and 1778 Continental expeditions attempted to invade British Florida and harass enemy troops stationed there. It was to no avail. Disease ravished the troops until the operations were aborted and the columns limped home. During the 1778 expedition, one officer, Major John Faucheraud Grimké of the Charleston Regiment of Artillery, reported that at least "one half of the number of Men we set out with are already Sick. Many of them dangerously So & that by the encreasing [sic] inclemency of the Climate, the greatest part of the Army now well, will either by Continuing here or advancing be most probably destroyed."[11]

As it happened, Clinton would have no better luck. Even before his troops departed New York that fall of 1779, a good number of men were stricken by fevers—likely malaria. Perhaps up to one-third of his soldiers took to their bed because of it. The military commander of New York, James Pattison, made the candid remark to Lord Viscount Thomas Townshend in England, "I am sorry to acquaint your Lordship of the Unhealthiness of the present Season, so Sickly a Time is not remembered in this Country." Apparently, at one time, nearly five thousand British soldiers had mustered out unfit for duty.[12] Eventually, health improved, and Clinton rounded up a formidable army: twelve regiments, four flank battalions, over two hundred cavalry, artillery, and a detachment of Hessian troops. Avoiding the hot season, he elected to leave in October, but a delay caused by the rumored presence of a French fleet sailing up the coast put off his departure until the day after Christmas. The delay worked wonders for the health of the troops. By the time of his southern voyage, only slightly more than 15 percent were infirmed—an admirable figure for the times.[13] Clinton's forces arrived off Savannah, Georgia, toward the end of January 1780. In early February, his same troops boarded transports, which took them close to Charleston, landing at Edisto Island. The British quickly took possession of other coastal islands: Johns and James Islands and Stono Ferry. By doing so, they completely surrounded the town. Artillery batteries were set up, troops readied, and an ultimatum sent to General Benjamin Lincoln, commanding the Charleston garrison. Lincoln rebuffed the offer.

Lincoln had bravado but also his share of problems. Sickness was upon him and his townspeople that fall of 1779.[14] Numbers of citizens had been plagued by an attack of smallpox. Although victims were quickly moved to the "pesthouse" to quarantine, it still was a grave concern for second-in-command William Moultrie. Mustering enough fit troops for any British attack was of paramount importance, and smallpox was a feared, highly contagious, and lethal epidemic. It alone, in the present state of war, could substantially weaken the city's defenses. So feared was the pox that Moultrie knew militias hesitated coming into town as reinforcements. They "dreaded that disorder [smallpox] more than the enemy."[15] Even by late February, militiamen in the area were reluctant to enter, apprehensive that, if they were besieged and the weather warmed, they might likely fall victim to the scourge.[16] But smallpox was not the only problem. Other ailments shadowed the inhabitants. David Ramsay had noticed a strange disorder arising in enslaved Africans. "It begins like an Anasarca in the lower extremities & gradually ascends, & under the best treatment (I suppose) upwards of 100 have died . . . I confess that I cannot account either for its universality nor its peculiarity to negroes." Was it also contagious? Would it spread to strike soldiers as well?[17] By March, Ramsay was aware of the predicament. Charleston was surrounded. "Five thousand land forces are now in sight of Charles-Town," he wrote Benjamin Rush on March 21, 1780.[18]

Clinton's move on Charleston that March of 1780 was not the first attempt to subdue the town. Charleston had been home to anti-British sentiments long before. Residents had incited the ire of the Crown by ousting then Governor Lord William Campbell in September 1775. The enraged Campbell promised the British would return with a vengeance. "Charles Town is the fountainhead from which all violence flows," wrote Campbell to then secretary of state for the colonies William Legge, Lord Dartmouth, a month later.[19] After formal onset of hostilities, there had already been one unsuccessful attempt to take Charleston in 1776, and Ramsay was fairly certain there would be another. He had written Rush in February 1779 that "[o]ur country is now invaded and we are called upon for our Southern Quota of continental blood." He feared an invasion that would turn the towns and countryside into carnage. "If the war should be continued here next summer the consequences will be fatal. The camp diseases aggravated by our climate will make . . . havoc in our army if stationed in the country." Yet he was determined to do his duty, now totally immersed in the civic workings of his adopted city.[20]

Nevertheless, between the aborted British siege of 1776 and the capture of Savannah in 1778, prosperity abounded for Charleston and Savannah. Largely ignored by His Majesty's forces during that time, trade with Europe and the

West Indies accelerated for the prized commodities of rice, tobacco, and indigo. An endless stream of fattened merchant ships sailed in and out of port, and their greedy captains payrolled Carolinian economy with lavish amounts of gold and silver. Socially, concerts, charity balls, and card games continued unabated. Women were preoccupied with fashion and finery, the latest Parisian styles quite the fad. Trappings of European royalty were hard to abandon.[21]

Still, only a fool would think the American rebellion would not again touch the South. So it was, in that spring of 1779, rumors of invasion circulated through the streets of Charleston. War had come and gaiety ceased. The town prepared for attack. The prospect of siege and casualties from sickness and injuries loomed large, prompting Moultrie to task another respected Charleston physician, David Oliphant, director-general of the Southern Hospitals, to organize an infirmary for use by "State troops, Militia, Sailors, and Negroes in the public service."[22] Just in time. That May, Major General Augustine Prévost, commander of British troops at Saint Augustine, crossed the Savannah River and marched on Charleston in a gamble to capture the city after General Benjamin Lincoln and his South Carolinians (and a sizeable force of French regulars and men-of-war) had left to retake Savannah. Moultrie and his determined militia repelled the Redcoats. Moultrie's success may have been due in part to rampant sickness that weakened Prévost's forces—and even Prévost himself, as he later relayed to Henry Clinton.[23] During the attack, Oliphant's hospital served as a convenient refuge for the sick and wounded of Charleston's militia and was put to good use. It would take on even greater importance during and following the siege of 1780.[24]

Now, in the spring of 1780 Clinton was ready. Irked by Lincoln's refusal to surrender, he unleashed his cannon and mortars on the town on April 13. The cannonading continued on a daily basis, and his disciplined infantry forayed against vulnerable outposts manned by exhausted defenders. Lincoln's troops were clearly outmanned and outgunned. Despite his early refusal of surrender, Lincoln realized the situation had turned hopeless. After several days of further negotiation with Clinton, Charleston capitulated on May 12, 1780. Lincoln surrendered over 2,500 men. The Continental troops—North and South Carolinians and Virginians—were allowed to leave after turning in their arms. Some 500 or 600 sick and wounded remained in Oliphant's Continental Hospital. David Ramsay and other doctors were declared "prisoners on parole" and allowed to roam the streets of Charleston with relative freedom. Yet for one, Ramsay's attitude toward British rule was intransient. Despite warnings and incentives, Ramsay failed to satisfactorily comply with matters of the king's service, blatantly obstinate to Royalist rules. In his words, he and like-minded patriots "resisted every temptation to resume the character of subjects." After a few months of this insolent behavior, he was arrested and taken as formal prisoner (as were other colleagues of the same mind). His capture on August

27, 1780, provided a dramatic moment for later biographers: "It was on the morning of the Lord's day, while the [C]hristian patriot, on his knees before his maker, was invoking the aid of heaven for his bleeding country, seeking consolation for himself, and in his petitions even remembering his enemies, that band of armed men burst in upon him, dragged him from his habitation like a felon, and conveyed him to the prison ship."[25]

The prisoners were taken to the guard ship *Sandwich* in Charleston Harbor and eventually shipped off to Saint Augustine on September 15. The message to others in Charleston was clear: abide by Royalist dictates or suffer exile, poverty, and ruin. Of course, enslaved persons were largely ignored. Courted by neither victor nor vanquished, they languished in their familiar servitude, immune to the consequences of war. For that matter, they proved compliant detainees. But there was no love lost for their enslavers. What small contribution they could make went to the other side, throwing "the weight of their little influence into the opposite [Royalist] scale."[26] Meanwhile, Ramsay the prisoner suffered little at Saint Augustine. During imprisonment, he and his companions were allowed to rent houses, bring their servants, and "congregate in dining areas . . . and to receive remittances and supplies from home."[27] Privilege had its benefits, even in war. He remained there until July 1781, at which time he was freed under a prisoner exchange. Once released and upon departure for Philadelphia, the "prisoners," according to one individual, were lavished with gifts from the locals: eggs, ducks, even heifers and wine. As for Ramsay, he would stay in Philadelphia and not return to Charleston until the fall of that year.[28]

And for Peter Fayssoux, now thirty-five, he volunteered for military service as soon as the rebellion began. A staunch Patriot, Fayssoux railed at Parliamentary injustices and pledged his convictions to liberty by backing the Provincial Congress of South Carolina. He was assigned to Moultrie's Southern Continental Army, and during the first assault on Charleston in June 1776, the young physician hunkered behind palmetto log barriers to care for the desperately wounded on Sullivan's Island.[29] He was part of Moultrie's detachment sent to reinforce General Robert Howe's ill-fated defenses during the siege of Savannah in December 1778. Once again, in 1779, he deployed as a member of Lincoln's expedition to retake Savannah, an attempt thwarted by Prévost's move on Charleston.

Then, with Clinton's siege of Charleston that early spring of 1780, Fayssoux sensed the community was doomed and sent his wife away; Charleston was now no place for the innocent, and sicknesses were sure to rise. Aside from the smallpox concerns of the past winter, a variety of illnesses, from distempers to rheumatism to venereal disease to worms, affected the community.[30] Fayssoux himself was soon promoted to Lincoln's surgeon general to the southern army. After Lincoln's surrender, Fayssoux, like his colleague David Ramsay, found himself a prisoner on parole and allowed to remain in the city. However, his irascible behavior matched that of his colleagues. Not intimidated by British rule, he was determined to "advance, in the most publick, and insolent manner the grossest falsehood."[31] Such attitudes had the predictable consequences: Fayssoux was arrested with the others that August and marched aboard the *Sandwich*. Unlike his compatriots, though, Fayssoux was released a few days later. His role in manning Oliphant's Continental Hospital was considered indispensable, even by his British captors, who had little inclination to provide medical service to the sick and wounded.

Worse was yet to come for Patriot forces. Shortly after Charleston's fall, Colonel Abraham Buford and his troop of Continentals met disaster farther to the north. Lincoln had summoned Buford's men to reinforce his garrison earlier in the spring. Before reaching the town, when they were near Camden, Buford received word of Lincoln's surrender and turned his force around. For some unexplained reason he chose to split his army into two separate columns. Alerted to the retreating Continental force, Clinton ordered Lieutenant Colonel Banastre Tarleton and his mounted regiment of Loyalists to track them down. He found them on May 29, 1780, near the South Carolina town of Lancaster in a wooded, hilly area known as the Waxhaws. It would prove to be a slaughter. Tarleton and his saber-wielding cavalry fell upon Buford's men with a vengeance. Unable to acknowledge a white flag waved by Buford's beleaguered troops because he was momentarily trapped under a fallen horse, Tarleton could not restrain his horsemen from continuing their attack "with the horrid yells of infuriated demons." A letter by the surgeon present, a Dr. Robert Brownfield, gave a graphic account of the consequences thereafter: "The demand for quarters, seldom refused to a vanquished foe, was at once found to be in vain; not a man was spared—and it was the concurrent testimony of all the survivors, that for fifteen minutes after every man was prostrate. They went over the ground plunging their bayonets into every one that exhibited any signs of life."[32]

Brownfield vividly described the mutilating wounds suffered at the hands of a cavalryman's saber. Some victims took as many as two dozen slashing injuries. One poor Patriot officer by the name of Captain John Stokes tried to parry sword blows with his arm, losing a finger and having his arm hacked into eight or ten pieces. Finally, the incensed slashing dragoon sliced into his head "the whole length of the crown." Still not dead, Stokes refused any quarter and asked to be finished off, which Tarleton's dragoon tried to do using his bayonet. Not enough. Stokes was still alive. This caught the attention of a nearby British officer, who compassionately stood over the young Continental. Eventually, Tarleton's surgeon roughly dressed Stokes's wounds, filling the deep head lacerations with coarse lint, a material that stuck to poor Stokes's brain for several days. Unbelievably, the irrepressible Stokes recovered and became a federal court judge after the war. Others were not so fortunate. Reports surfaced of Tarleton's men plunging bayonets into victims on the ground to finish them off. In total, Buford's company lost 112 men dead, and another 150 wounded and unable to travel. Tarleton counted only 5 men killed and 31 wounded.[33] Numbers of Continental injured filtered through the surrounding villages and settlements; simple farm people completely unfamiliar with the wounds of warfare gathered to help. One of those was a young Andrew Jackson, future war hero and United States president. His entire family sifted through the injured at their local meetinghouse. "None of the men had less than three or four, and some as many as thirteen gashes on them," Jackson later recalled.[34] So egregious was the massacre that, just like later cries of "Remember the Alamo," and "Remember Pearl Harbor," cries of "Tarleton's Quarter" and "Remember Buford" would fill Patriot rhetoric.

By mid-June, a stifling pestilence had taken its toll on inhabitants of occupied Charleston. Many were down with yellow fever without any medications to assist them. General Moultrie appealed to the British to furnish doctors and medicines to treat his sick. "The surgeons at Haddrell's-point represent to me, a number of patients under inoculation [the ships were thought riddled with smallpox]; and many down with the yellow-fever; and no medicines, or the common necessaries of life, to assist them," he wrote on June 15, 1780.[35] By November, the situation was even grimmer. Oliphant reported that "the mortality is great; by much the greater number of deaths happen to those patients from on board the prison-ships [overflow from Buford's remnants]." And suffering from "malignant putrid fever." Much of this was attributed to "jail fever," a common term for epidemic typhus, of course, particularly prevalent in overcrowded conditions.[36]

As for the victor Clinton, satisfied he had eliminated Patriot resistance throughout the state, he left for New York and turned command of his southern forces over to Earl Charles Cornwallis. But while he had outclassed Patriot tactics, he had not dampened Patriot zeal. That summer, Continental troops called forth from Maryland and Delaware began their march to South Carolina under General Horatio Gates. He naïvely hoped to clear the British out of the Carolinas and liberate Charleston. As he trekked through Virginia and North Carolina, local militia of variable skill levels reinforced his column. It all made for an arduous journey. Marching through countryside almost devoid of provisions and clean water led to outbreaks of dysentery. Diarrhea added to "[t]he heat of the season, the unhealthiness of the climate." Soldiers unaccustomed to the rigors of field duty erupted in grumbling and discontent.[37] Even veterans found it all hard to take. The head of the Sixth Maryland Regiment, Colonel Otho Williams, remarked that "the fatigue of campaigning in this country [Carolinas] is almost inconceivable." Militia soldiers were even more pitiful. As a regular Continental officer, Williams was appalled at their plight: poorly fed, clothed, and equipped. Indeed, he was no fan of the South in general—full of nothing but an ignorant bunch of tramps in his opinion.

"There are a few virtuous good men in this State [meaning the colony of South Carolina] and in Georgia, but a great majority of the people is composed of the most unprincipled, abandoned, vicious vagrants that ever inhabited the earth." They were no match for the Redcoats in discipline. Gates's force trudged along in sloppy file, many like raucous boys just off the farm. And to make matters even more interesting, Gates's men were accompanied by a good number of women ready to help with provisions and care of the sick and wounded—or simply to supply more carnal needs.[38]

Cornwallis, ensconced in Charleston, upon hearing of the approaching rebel force, hurried to Camden with reinforcements for the British garrison there. The town lay directly in the path of Gates's advancement. Southern illnesses, though, had trimmed his ranks. Disease riddled Cornwallis's army, forcing him to leave behind almost 800 ailing soldiers. "Our troops are in general sickly, the 71st [one of his crack units] so much so, that the two battalions have not more than 274 men under arms," he wrote Clinton on August 10, days before meeting Gates's forces near Camden.[39] Nevertheless, Cornwallis itched for a fight and attacked Gates on August 16, 1780. Despite a numerically superior force, Gates's army was thoroughly destroyed. That hodgepodge collection of militiamen formed up Gates's left flank, but with the advance of Redcoat bayonets, they threw down their weapons, turned, and ran. Williams's Continentals on the right flank held for a while but, seeing the stampede of the militia, knew they were in danger of being outflanked and also retreated—whether their retirement was more orderly is a matter of dispute.

Overall, it seemed a thoroughly cowardly scene. According to Tarleton, "[R]out and slaughter ensued in every quarter . . . The continentals, the state troops, and the militia, abandoned their arms, their colours, and their cannon, to seek protection in flight, or to obtain it from the clemency of the conquerors." Waggoneers of the supply train cut out their teams, grabbed horses, and galloped away—even the cries of the women and wounded did not deter them.[40] Other, more chivalrous types gave up their horses to assist in carrying off the wounded.[41] Two hundred and ninety injured Americans were taken prisoner and carried back to Camden, housed in British hospitals. After the battle, North Carolina Patriot physician Hugh Williamson toured those British hospitals containing a number of wounded and sick Continentals. Many were suffering from smallpox, thought to arise from British troops not properly inoculated. He went on to write to Thomas Benbury, speaker of the House of Commons of the Assembly of North Carolina: "That small Boys suffered most by the Flux; That the sufferings of our men were greatly increased by the want of Sugar, Tea, Coffee, Vinegar, and such other palatable antiseptic Nourishment as is best suited the Sick . . . supplies were so scanty as hardly to deserve the name, nor was anything of the kind to be purchased for Money, unless in very trifling Quantities."[42]

Many were force-marched back to Charleston. Peter Fayssoux was there to meet them. The ragged captives had been marched 120 miles "in the most sickly season of this unhealthy climate," he remembered.[43] Too many for the Continental Hospital, overflow captives were loaded aboard prison ships in the harbor, where they festered and collapsed from spoiled rations, rancid water, and epidemics of smallpox. The wretched prisoners were fed rotten salt provision without any medical aid. Their only recourse was to turncoat and enlist as British soldiers or face an indefinite stay. Few took up the offer. Many died as a result. So despairing was their circumstance that the women of Charleston came to their assistance. As recorded by historian Chalmers Davidson, "[S]everal of the ladies of Charleston, [laid] aside distinction of whig and tory . . . procuring and preparing every necessary of clothing and proper nourishment for our poor, worn-out and desponding soldiers."[44]

Fayssoux was appalled by it all and did not hesitate to sharply criticize the British. This earned the young physician no favoritism. There was worry he might be imprisoned or worse. General Moultrie tried to arrange an exchange of Fayssoux for captured British surgeons but was turned down. "They did not like him," Moultrie said of his captors, and he felt they resisted every opportunity to set him loose. (Royalists no doubt knew the petulant doctor would not go quietly.) It was not until April 1781 that Fayssoux was, in fact, exchanged. The British were right. Fayssoux did not sit still. He promptly joined Nathaniel Greene's southern army. Just in time, it seems, as the summer fevers were soon upon the troops, and Fayssoux had plenty to do in the high hills of the western Carolinas. He was not to return to his home in Charleston until March 1782.

Indeed, in the Carolinas that summer both armies had suffered from sicknesses. According to historian Louis Duncan, British surgeon Robert Jackson told of the illnesses afflicting large numbers of British troops: "The disease was of a character . . . of the remitting class, but with remissions scarcely perceptible. Two thirds of the regiment were sick; and of course, there were persons in all stages of the disease."[45] Jackson had been assigned to the First Battalion, Seventy-First Regiment, the ailing Scottish unit mentioned by Cornwallis to Clinton before Camden. Later in August and September, now camped near Camden but on the vaporous, swampy banks of the Pee Dee River, Jackson reported that "[t]he weather was . . . hot, and fevers were frequent—sometimes malignant and dangerous." That encampment proved foolhardy for the men. "In a fortnight or three weeks, the intermittent fever began to shew [sic] itself. It spread so rapidly . . . [that] before the end of July . . . few were left who had not seen its influence." Even in the fall, febrile epidemics seemed to degenerate into dysentery and dropsy so that there was a continual misery suffered by many of the unaccustomed troops.[46]

It would be called southern land fever by Hessian troops in Cornwallis's army. Veteran soldier Johann Ewald from Hesse-Kassel (present-day Germany) served in the Hessian *Jäger* (light infantry) Corps during the Carolina campaign. He himself was so wracked by the regional distemper that "I thought it would throw me from my horse." It was, he felt, an illness spawned by the southern "great heat" that caused decomposition of rich Hessian blood. Of course, he admitted that some of the complaints were from drinking contaminated water.[47] And that dirty water would corrupt the bowels. That detestable condition called the bloody flux brought all reasonable activity to a halt and soiled many a fine Hessian uniform. The eighteenth-century New England Puritan minister Cotton Mather spoke of it thusly: "The Bloody Flux, what a Nasty, Filthy, Lothesome [sic] Disease. Patient, Cry out, Lord what a loathsome Wretch am I. I Loathe myself before thee. I Abhor myself, and Repent before thee, and thy People also."[48]

Southern fevers befuddled Cornwallis, the victories at Charleston and Camden notwithstanding. He simply could not mount sustained offensives because of the number of his troops near collapse—both officers and men. He himself suffered some type of distemper, feeling so ill that, for a time, he turned over command of his army to his subordinate, Lord Rawdon. In truth, malaria may have seized him. He was so aggravated by the raging fevers that he begged forgiveness to London that summer: "This climate (except in Charleston) is so bad within one hundred miles of the coast, from the end of June until the middle of October, that troops could not be stationed among them [sic] during the period, without a certainty of their being rendered useless for some time, for military service; if not entirely lost."[49] There was no doubt.

Soon after General Gates's defeat at Camden, the health of the men plummeted, which put an end to any further military operations by the British. South Carolina was not nearly as hospitable as Cornwallis had hoped. The endless requisitioning of provisions from local planters, the abuse by Cornwallis's soldiers of the population in general—even, to some degree, local Loyalists—had set in motion a slow burn of hostility and incited guerrilla activity. Cornwallis decided to move north, perhaps to Charlotte and a climate more conducive to wellness. Yet that fall of 1780, he was disinclined to turn his army back toward North Carolina. It would be a sluggish, anguishing march. According to Tarleton, "[T]he number of sick in the hospital . . . the late addition of wounded [from Camden] . . . the deficiency of stores . . . operated with the present heat of the climate."[50] According to the legendary Continental cavalry officer Harry Lee, then raiding Redcoats throughout the Carolinas, British troops were exposed to constant rain and swampy terrain. The subsequent "chill exhalations" of the ground caused widespread sickness, Lee surmised. The only ones not so affected were local Loyalist militia, acclimatized to the environment, as were many Patriot men.[51]

Despite popular discontent, though, in 1780 the British, when they cared to, roamed with impunity across Georgia and the Carolinas, driving Patriot forces into the wilderness. The fall of Charleston and the defeat at Camden were a nadir for revolutionary aspirations. Rebels could mount only sporadic resistance, no more than guerilla activity. As for medical care, whether for battle wounds or low country maladies, help ceased to exist. After the whipping at Camden, physicians scattered, applying their trade to the victims of war only by happenstance. Few were regular members of the military anyway, and rarely found in militia groups. Perhaps no great loss. Doctors were not always held in the highest regard. Even regular regimental surgeons were suspect. Speaking of one in particular, "[h]e was often ignorant, frequently resentful ... generally averse to discipline and intent on accomplishing his personal ambitions," so wrote historian Wyndham Blanton.[52] There was a sharp dichotomy in quality. Urban physicians (few in number) were a more elite, educated group and country doctors less so. Military surgeons fell somewhere in between—sadly, more often among the barely competent. There were not nearly enough for the types of illness and injuries produced by troops on the move. Townspeople took up the slack: simple measures of balms and bandages and self-styled remedies. Battle wounds were challenging. Gashes were wrapped, bullets extracted when they could be, and fractures splinted. Shots to the chest or abdomen were grim findings. It was almost certain death. Womenfolk offered bedside comfort and laudanum and watched the poor souls anguish and die.

But resistance and rebellion still festered. Sizeable numbers of southerners hated the British, and Cornwallis would soon fall victim to insurgency. With cooling autumn temperatures, he had dispatched Major Patrick Ferguson and his hometown militia into the Carolina backcountry. Cornwallis hoped to garner more Loyalist support there. Colonel William Campbell, a rabid Patriot, took after Ferguson with his Carolina mountain men. They caught up with him within miles of the North and South Carolina border on October 7, 1780. It was near a forested rise known as King's Mountain, where Ferguson's forces had taken cover. Assault after assault finally dislodged the Loyalists, killing Ferguson in the process. Loyalist losses were heavy, and Campbell's men showed no mercy in retaliation for Tarleton's butchery at Waxhaw. Of Ferguson's militia, 250 were killed, 130 wounded, and 700 taken prisoner; Campbell lost fewer than 100 men.[53] For all the savagery of this combat, much of it hand-to-hand with knife and bayonet, there was not a single Patriot physician available. Only one surgeon of the enemy survived, a Dr. Johnson, who attended Patriot as well as Loyalist casualties. Fearing that Cornwallis would pursue them, the frontiersmen hurried off to their mountain retreats, carrying sick and wounded with them. "The softest accommodation that could be made ready [for the injured and ill] for conveyance was the fresh hides of the slaughtered cattle, fastened to two poles, these attached to two horses, one before and one behind," wrote chroniclers of the event, a technique almost certainly learned from native tribes.[54] For those dragged away, backwoods ingenuity prevailed. According to another record, "[T]he frontier people were much accustomed, from necessity, with splints, bandages, and slippery elm poultices, to treating gun-shot wounds and other disabilities."[55]

Cornwallis, now at Charlotte, was in no mood to chase. His men were ailing. "[T]he Sickness of my Army prevented moving," he later wrote to Henry Clinton.[56] Anyway, he was tiring of the Carolinas. Loyalist support was simply not sufficient to sustain an occupying force. "[T]he immense extent of this country, cut with numberless rivers and creeks, and the total want of internal navigation . . . renders it impossible for our army to remain long in the heart of the country," he wrote to Lord Germain.[57]

In December 1780 Major General Nathaniel Greene was appointed the new commander of the Continental Army in the Carolinas, replacing the nearly incompetent Horatio Gates. Greene had been a trusted member of Washington's staff in the northern campaigns and had served as his quartermaster general, a position that would be invaluable in refurbishing a decimated southern army. He was determined to clean out the British from the Carolinas. But the southern army he now commanded was hardly ready for action. Greene told Washington: "Nothing can be more wretched and distressing than the condition of the troops, starving with cold and hunger—without tents and camp equipage. Those of the Virginia line are literally naked, and a great part totally unfit for any kind of duty, and must remain so until clothing can be had from the Northward."[58] Perhaps upward of one in five soldiers was sick. Of the 2,300 men on paper, 1,482 were fit for duty and only 800 adequately equipped.[59]

Move his troops he must. There were not enough provisions in North Carolina to sustain them. His strategy was mobility—a "flying army"—sending refurbished forces throughout the Carolinas to harass British troops. For this, he divided his men into two groups. He gave command of the other wing to the veteran General Daniel Morgan. He urged Morgan on, to take his soldiers into upcountry South Carolina to forage and rally patriot spirit.[60] Cornwallis got wind of this and told Tarleton to give chase.

The two met in an area called Hannah's cow pens, a pasture for the grazing of cattle, in South Carolina on January 17, 1781, (near present-day Spartanburg).[61] Continental troops under Morgan routed Tarleton's elite legion, throwing them into a panicked retreat. "Such was the inferiority of our numbers that our success must be attributed under God, to the justice of our cause and the bravery of our Troops," Morgan wrote Greene two days later. British surgeon Robert Jackson of the Seventy-First Regiment and Patriot surgeon Richard Pindell cared for the wounded of both sides, almost 260 men. Both Pindell and Jackson appealed to Morgan to allow an interchange of wounded prisoners, some of whom were still lying in the field five days later. Morgan eventually relented, setting up a temporary infirmary in Gilbert Town, twenty miles from the battlefield.[62]

After that defeat, Cornwallis was done with the South. "The late affair [at Cowpens, as it would come to be called] has almost broken my heart," he wrote Lord Rawdon from Buffalo Creek, South Carolina, on January 21. "I was never more surrounded with difficulty & distress."[63] He decided to abandon his post at Charlotte, collect his sick and convalescing troops, and begin the journey northward. His plan to subdue the Carolinas was a failure. The strategy now was defense and one that would not draw favor in London.

In point of fact, it was southern sickness that had eroded the health of his army. A costly battle at Guilford Court House (North Carolina) in March 1781 further depleted his forces. Virginia was now his destination, the safety of New York too far away. "I had no option left," he wrote Henry Clinton in July, "such was the situation and distress of the troops, and so great were the sufferings of the sick and wounded."[64] By summer he was at Gloucester, Virginia, just across the York River from Yorktown, perhaps hoping to evacuate by sea to Charleston on Clinton's transports. Blood was in the water now, and Americans and French were readying for a feeding frenzy. To add to British misery, spring bled into summer, and the coastal climate of Virginia began to take its toll. The Hessian Johann Ewald wrote that the heat was unbearable: "The nights are especially terrible, when there is so little air that one can hardly breathe." The "torment of several billions of insects" only added to the misery.[65] "Flux" was a common trouble, likely from dirty water, but malaria and smallpox also apparently added to their troubles. In fact, Benjamin Franklin later contended that the British, in their march through Virginia, would inoculate captured Africans with smallpox and let them escape, hoping to mix with the enslaved and white population, thus spreading the illness among them.[66]

On August 15, arriving at Yorktown, wounded and sick accounted for almost 30 percent of Cornwallis's army. By September, Cornwallis knew he was bottled up. The siege had begun. French warships offshore erased all hopes of a seaborne evacuation. By mid-October, Cornwallis wrote to Clinton, "My situation here becomes very critical."[67] His numbers of infirmed mounted, and only slightly more than four thousand men were fit for duty. The Hessian officer, Ewald, recalled that toward the end, his command was spent, "nearly all plagued with fever . . . Their strength is exhausted through want and hardship." Dysentery was everywhere; the curse of cramping and explosive diarrhea incapacitated even the lion-hearted.[68] Finally, on October 17, a white flag flew. Cornwallis was finished. At his surrender, Ewald noted "the wounded and sick lying helpless without medicine, and the army melted away from 7,000 to 3,200."[69] In fact, in some of Cornwallis's units almost one-half of the men were injured or ill.[70] Estimates told of 1,500 bed-ridden British soldiers. They were moved across the York River to Gloucester, where they were cared for by British doctors.[71]

Continental soldiers were hardly in any better shape. On October 17, physician James Thatcher wrote that the troops from New England "have now become very sickly, the prevalent diseases are intermittent and remitting fevers [probably malaria], which are very prevalent in this climate during the autumnal months."[72] Thatcher also wrote (as Franklin had suspected), "The British have sent from Yorktown a large number of negroes sick with the small pox, probably for the purpose of communicating the infection to our army."[73] Smallpox among enslaved Blacks worked by the British Army was rampant, apparently, as inoculation was probably sparsely given to bonded men and women. Quartermaster General Timothy Pickering wrote to the governor of Virginia William Nelson, shortly after the surrender of Cornwallis: "On my arrival here [Yorktown] I found the American sick in a suffering condition, and I fear it will not be in my power to yield them adequate relief."[74] Indeed, military hospitals were probably no place for them. Patriot physician James Tilton remarked that those impromptu lodgings—the name "hospital" would be a stretch—servicing Patriots during the war accumulated vast numbers of the ill. "[With] the sick and wounded, flowing promiscuously without restraint into the hospital, it soon became infectious and was attended with great mortality." Anyone attending the ill would likely be stricken as well, dysentery being a ubiquitous ailment. Tilton himself caught "jail fever" (typhus) and recovered but after "a tedious illness." Nevertheless, after the British surrender Tilton began using Jesuits' bark (cinchona) for treatment of the many feverish disturbances and "languid and putrid conditions," and to the amazement of his French colleagues, it seemed to rally the ill.[75] In any event, Washington wasted no time moving his army back to the Hudson to escape the sickly Virginia locality.

The Southland, though, did not rejoice in Cornwallis's surrender. Savannah and Charleston were still in British hands. That low country would continue to cause havoc among troops sent to liberate, particularly those soldiers not yet accustomed to the South's buggy miasmas and sickly conditions. In November 1781 the First Pennsylvania Regiment was dispatched from Yorktown to join General Greene's forces in the Carolinas. The British there still needed rooting out. The march south was predictable. While pleasant and scenic enough during the winter months in North Carolina, the wetlands of low country South Carolina soon rendered foot travel almost unbearable. Doctor Robert Wharry likened the march to South Carolina as a journey through country "as hot as the Antichambers of Hell." "[N]o pure water for to drink, but sand, mud & water . . . the deuce take the country, I would not live in it for a million a year," he went on to say.[76] "[D]isagreeable," another Continental physician, William McDowell, wrote in his journal. By May the following year, McDowell himself had taken sick. By June, heat had settled in and soldiers were dying of afflictions—"a sickly time," as McDowell recounted. He had little faith in his fellow physicians, self-treating his broiling sicknesses with local teas and emetics that "almost killed me." By the end of August "[w]e are daily experiencing instances of mortality among us, soldiers dying fast." Desertions were also on the increase, whether from dissatisfaction or pure misery, one could not tell. On Sunday, September 8, McDowell counted 370 sick in the hospital "and better than half of the men sick in camp." By September 29, McDowell again was sick with fever and vomiting. He took "the Bark" (cinchona) and a few days later had improved—probably a bout of malaria.

Throughout the autumn and into winter 1782, McDowell continued to be plagued with intermittent fevers, vomiting, and a generalized weakness that almost incapacitated him. The "Bark" provided some relief, and he began taking it most days. By September, both Generals Greene and Anthony Wayne suffered from the fevers, Greene "exceedingly sick," McDowell described. By November, McDowell recorded 106 deaths from illness in his regiment. In December, his regiment turned and headed north. The British were in no mood for a fight and began deserting their posts. Under near-siege conditions, the British finally quit Savannah that July, and Charleston was evacuated in December. Still shaking from periodic fevers, McDowell finally arrived home on Saturday, December 21, 1782. The war was over, and he was bone tired. Since May 1781 he had traveled over 2,700 miles.[77]

For one, Nathaniel Greene was keen to liberate the South. Cornwallis had appointed Lord Rawdon to oppose him, but Rawdon shortly was struck ill and left for England. The less experienced Alexander Stewart then assumed command. Greene wasted no time. He pounded the British outpost at the settlement of Ninety-Six in backcountry South Carolina until they capitulated. Greene then struck out for Charleston. He was met by Stewart's troops near Eutaw Springs in a sharp clash that severely depleted Greene's forces, although he held his position on the battlefield and forced the British to retire. Neither side had enough energy to pursue the other. Stewart took his men back to Charleston, and Greene sped to the safety of South Carolina's interior.

Greene's soldiers, like many militiamen of the day, had tired of combat. The swampland had taken its toll; fatigue and exposure brought on sweeping sicknesses.[78] Desertions accelerated; men simply took their weapons and walked out of camp. For those too sick to lift from their cots, fate took another turn. That rascal Tarleton had raided Greene's hospital stores. The most basic comforts for the infirmed were now lacking. "Our sick and wounded have suffered greatly," Greene wrote. "The extent of our hospitals, the malignity of disorders, and increasing sick since the battle of Eutaw, together with the numerous wounded on hand, the little means we had to provide for them, and the great number of our physicians who fell sick in service, have left our sick and wounded in a most deplorable condition."[79] Greene hoped that colder weather would chill the southern miasmas. But the winter of 1781 and 1782 brought little relief. He wrote to General Washington in March 1782: "We are remote from support and supplies of every kind . . . Not a rag of clothing has arrived to us this winter. Indeed, our prospects are really deplorable." And summer was just around the corner.[80] Despite his eagerness to liberate Charleston before the hot weather, he simply did not have the forces, and the French were unwilling to commit their fleet for a seaward blockade. No need, as it turned out. The British had no stomach to stay. They evacuated Savannah in July and Charleston by the end of the year.[81]

ALLEVIATING THE EVILS OF WAR

The Revolutionary landscape of sickly climate and ghastly wounds often outpaced the shaky ability of doctors called to care for its fallen victims. Few physicians, even those of formal education, were acquainted with the nuances of war wounds and camp disease. The only medical text available on the subject was one written by New Yorker John Jones, entitled *Plain Concise Practical Remarks on the Treatment of Wounds and Fractures*, printed in 1775. In fact, this was the first medical text published in America. Jones carefully discussed wounds and fractures, their presentation, and implications. He minutely described management: cleansing, bandaging, and splinting. It was a practical handbook for the field surgeons unfamiliar with the carnage before them. It was so much evil, Jones claimed, and doctors must do what they can, leaving the morality to philosophers: "While speculative philosophers are disputing about the origin of evil and foundation of morals, and furious bigots contending for different modes of faith, the practical good man will endeavor to employ himself in alleviating those evils which he finds incident to human nature."[82]

Extremity wounds fared best, when broken bones could be set, gashes washed, and even amputations done for dreadful mutilation. Much less so were bullets or cannon shot to the chest and abdomen. These glassy-eyed victims languished in the throes of rampant chest hemorrhage or raging peritonitis. Probing might help but, ignorant of the bleeding within, inflammation was the most feared of consequences, very likely to kill in short order. Opening either cavity for close inspection was absurd. Without anesthesia, the whole affair would be nothing short of inhuman torture. Instead, Jones—inconceivable by today's standards—urged bleeding. Bleeding, he felt, reduced inflammation and could favorably impact the course of recovery. "The great and principal attention of the Surgeon should be directed to the prevention and diminution of inflammation," he wrote.[83] Whether the text penetrated into the South is unknown. Presumably it did. If so, regimental surgeons would have done well to follow Jones's advice scrupulously. While sorely deficient by later standards, it was state of the art at the time and at least provided a framework in which to treat injured men.

One likely disciple of Jones was southerner William Read. Read was the son of one of His Majesty's Counsellors of Georgia. Born of privilege in South Carolina, young William attended boarding school followed by a finishing school of select young gentlemen in Savannah. Read seemed drawn to apothecary, and he was sent to apprentice with local practitioners. In 1774, having demonstrated an unusual aptitude for physic (medicine), he went to Philadelphia for his formal medical education. There, he met and quartered with the eminent Dr. Benjamin Rush. He must have learned his art well from the master, for shortly afterward, the ambitious young Georgian earned his doctorate. It was this association with Dr. Rush, however, that also instilled a rebellious spirit in Read and a conviction for American independence. He surreptitiously began military training, apparently for insurgency intents. Read would become a prototypical Forrest Gump.[84] Upon returning to Savannah, he immersed himself in revolutionary ventures, including General Robert Howe's failed Floridian expedition of 1778 (General Washington had been keen on eliminating British bases in Florida, but alas, it was not to be—too much disorganization in rebel ranks). It was then that the restless Read decided to travel back north to join the Continental Army. He distinguished himself at the Battle of Monmouth in June 1778, in the care of casualties, dressing wounds and amputating limbs. He even cared for fallen British soldiers. At one point he came upon fifty or sixty of them—some dead, some alive, calling for help or pleading or water. Read and his servant hurried to provide necessary aid. It was afterward, in his visits to the hospitals, that he saw the deplorable state of the Continental wounded and witnessed the reluctance of fellow surgeons to risk life or limb in their care.

Hospitals, as they were called, were loathsome places, infested with all types of putrid fevers that swept through the rows of sick and wounded men. "Among the variety of public errors and abuses," Jones had written in his text, "there is not one perhaps which more loudly calls for speedy and effectual reformation . . . [that is,] the misapplied benevolence of Hospitals for the sick and wounded."[85] Cots were crammed into spaces of stagnant, foul air with little segregation and less ventilation. Filthy bandages and chamber pots overflowed, and pus seemed to ooze from one patient to the next. Benjamin Rush knew they were vile; he had said so much to General Washington in 1777. He claimed there were upward of five thousand sick in hospitals of the Continental Army. "There cannot be a greater calamity for a sick man than to come into our hospital at this season of the year [December]," he wrote. The men were simply too crowded together, and any contagion quickly spread from bed to bed. "[T]he *great majority* [italics his] of those who die under our hands perish with diseases caught in our hospitals," he penned.[86] Spurred by such nefarious

CHAPTER SIX

reports, Washington went to some lengths to reform hospital protocols and inspections. Still, particularly in the South, such places were considered near barbaric, where gruesome wounds would mix with spreading contagions.

It was on the eve of the British offensive in the South that, at the request of General Washington, William Read surreptitiously traveled to Charleston to reconnoiter the situation. Washington himself was reluctant to send troops southward. "Prejudices were great against the climate, and the safety of the soldiery," he had thought.[87] At the Battle of Stono Ferry, where General Lincoln's poorly trained militia attempted to ambush British retreating from their aborted assault on Charleston in 1779, he saw any number of Patriot wounded cared for by neighboring planters and visited Oliphant's new Continental Hospital in Charleston run by two itinerant doctors, Tucker Harris and Earnest Poy.[88]

His report back to Washington was a major impetus for Horatio Gates to move his army into South Carolina in 1780. Read remained with Washington for a time, opened a hospital in Trenton for smallpox inoculation, then traveled to Fort Pitt on the Ohio River to visit another hospital site.

With news of Tarleton's massacre in the Waxhaws and Gates's drubbing at Camden, Read headed back south to "throw himself into the breach."[89] He was appalled to find Gates's troops in such disarray. With some aplomb, Read managed to procure flour and butter for Gates himself and other sick and wounded officers, all donated by the good will of neighboring friends. He even managed to provide lodging for wounded and sick soldiers in private homes. Through it all—and as a sign of the times—Read had to negotiate the hostility and skepticism with which fellow Americans, Patriot and Loyalist, viewed each other, quick to suspect the other of perfidies to their respective causes.

Sickness, though, had crippled Gates's forces. "Jail fever," typhus, was now the major culprit. Read contended that typhus was the effect of "exhaustion, fatigue, and chagrin of defeat."[90] When Gates was replaced by Greene, Read did not leave, despite his affection for Gates. His ultimate loyalty was to the glorious cause, and he continued his efforts to solicit local townspeople for food, water, and medicine. In March 1781 he was at Guilford Court House, where Greene tangled with Cornwallis. It was Read who procured shelter for the injured from the battle. With no distinction of friend or foe, Read once again treated an injured enemy officer, opening his valise to dress the wound with "lint and bandages" and shared a box of pills as remedy in case of spasm.[91] He later cared for the legendary General Daniel Morgan, incapacitated by rheumatism "head to feet" (sweating was the remedy, Read insisted).

He was at Eutaw Springs that September, when Greene clashed with British forces out of Charleston. Casualties were so numerous that he found surgeons near the point of exhaustion. He himself pitched in with formidable surgical aplomb. As an example of his finesse, on one shattered leg, Read picked out fragments of bone, administered bitter fomentations, and deluged the poor soul with ample quantities of laudanum. Such was his apparent skill that other wounded sought after him, and he responded with the exclamation that he "would assist Beelzebub in the character of a wounded man" (although Read had been accused of preferentially treating southern soldiers—a claim that largely went unsubstantiated).[92] Much of his time and attention he rendered, not in infirmaries, but in the sitting rooms and bedrooms of private citizens.

As for craft surgeons in general, Read may have been the exception. Many military surgeons hardly deserved the title, short on experience and scruples and long on garish antics. Of course, the term *surgeon* itself was a rough approximation, denoting all too often more the medieval barber surgeon who surreptitiously shadowed armies across France and England rather than highly trained craftsmen. So-called surgeon assistants were even worse, with a modicum of training and slim grasp of anatomic—and humanitarian—principles. Novelist William Gilmore Simms wrote of one fictional account—no doubt based on personal anecdotes—of surgeon assistant Augustus Hillhouse. Set in the South Carolinian backcountry as the British were evacuating their fort at Ninety-Six, Lord Rawdon had sent out to find help for the wounded outlaw Tory Morton at the home of the young mistress Middleton. Help came in the manner of Hillhouse. "He could take off a leg in the twinkling of an eye," so his reputation was. And much of a lady's man to boot. Whether his surgical dexterity was grounded in sufficient training was pure speculation. Rawdon had admonished him, "Now don't make a fool of yourself, Hillhouse," to which an onlooker had replied, "It is almost the only thing that he cannot help doing." Whether Hillhouse ever benefited the bloodied man was doubtful; his machinations regarding the young maiden were more to the point, it seems. Nevertheless, Simms knew full well the sometimes-unscrupulous behavior of so-called surgeons during this time, randomly called upon to treat ugly and potentially deadly wounds. The main talent, as with Hillhouse, seemed to be their easily displayed pomp and flair.[93]

As for the more credible Dr. Read, he spent the rest of the war galloping to Virginia to join Washington's forces at Yorktown. His journeys were akin to a latter-day *Odyssey* with all the twists and turns of intrigue that must have typified the rural behavior of civilian Carolina. His journey much depended on the benevolence of inhabitants along the way for food and shelter. At one point, just on the Virginia border, he alighted to find himself in hostile territory. He was accosted, made prisoner, beaten, and threatened with execution. Only at the last moment was he saved, nursed to health, and sent on his way toward Yorktown. It was a story not terribly unusual for many southern physicians during the war, spending their time, when needed, in the service of Continentals or militia, caring for the sick and wounded of battles fought in obscure locations and finding scant accommodations for their suffering patients. The countryside of the Carolinas was a quilt work of allegiances. Spies, traitors, and snitches abounded, making any journeying for Patriot or Loyalist treacherous at best—even the impartial care provided by their healers was no redemption.

The last of the southern army had returned home by the summer of 1783. Congress agreed on peace accords in April 1783 and formally signed in Paris that September. Just in time, Greene's army was close to mutiny, so vile were the living conditions in the sultry South. It is difficult to know exactly how many Continental and militia soldiers died of wounds or died of illnesses. Even more so in the South. Many sought care among local settlers and in waystations and never entered the roles of casualties. Others, maybe up to one-half of those stricken with camp illnesses, were allowed to leave and simply return home. They seldom returned. Dr. James Thatcher, in his history of the war, estimated the number of Continental soldiers who died was "not less than seventy thousand."[94] Whether from injury or disease was unknown. Of note were the large numbers of physicians who died in the conflict. James Tilton, head of the Continental military hospitals, observed that proportionately, more surgeons died in service than officers of the line, because, he surmised, "infection is more dangerous in military life, than the weapons of war; and should be a powerful excitement, with all concerned, from motives of self preservation, as well as honorable duty, to use all possible care and diligence in warding off that greatest of all evils, the plague of infection." Physicians worked among the deadly contagions blanketing encampments, a greater threat to life than shot and shell. Overall, disease felled perhaps ten times the number killed in battle.[95] And their risk was often for naught. Doctors could provide so little effective treatment for the scourges of military living.

CHAPTER SEVEN

THE ILLS OF SLAVERY

> In a warm climate no man will labor for himself who can make another labor for him . . . Indeed I tremble for my country when I reflect that God is just; that his justice cannot sleep forever.[1]
> —THOMAS JEFFERSON, 1781

There can be no understanding of the medical idiosyncrasies of southern lands without a familiarity with that most southern of depraved institutions—slavery. For a population of individuals who composed a major proportion of southern populations, the African contributed heavily to ailments percolating through the South. Their lungs breathed the same fetid air, their mouths drank the same putrid water, and their skin was bit by the same bothersome mosquitoes as white colonists and settlers, and so the manifestations of miasmatic diseases showed on their countenances as surely as on their white enslavers'. Yet they would be perceived as separate, as if another species altogether, whose constitution presented new and unique challenges in disease management. How, though, did Africans become such a staple of southern economy and relegated to a societal place not far from domestic animals? Their story of forced migration and subjugation is a legend of tribulations as profound as original sin for America yet cannot be ignored or minimized.

It started soon after the first colonists set foot in what is now Virginia. Toward the end of August 1619 an English privateer limped up the James River in desperate need of food and water. According to planter and entrepreneur John Rolfe, a member of the Jamestown community, in a letter to Sir Edwin Sandys, one of the founders of the Virginia Company, the whole affair unfolded:

> About the latter end of August, a Dutch Man of War of the burden of a 160 tones arrived at Point-Comfort, the Commander's name Captain Jope, his Pilot for the West Indies one Mr. Marmaduke an Englishman. They met with the *Treasurer* in the West Indies, and determined to hold consort ship hitherward, but in their passage lost one the other. He brought not anything but 20 and odd Negroes.[2]

"Negroes" to be sold for "victuals" it was disclosed. Apparently, Captain Jope aboard the *White Lion* and sister ship *Treasurer* had raided the Portuguese slave ship *São João Bautista* somewhere in the Caribbean. The enslaved captives held by the *São João Bautista* had almost assuredly come directly from Africa. This transaction of human cargo was also noted by Captain John Smith in his chronicles of 1619 that a Dutch Man-of-War deposited (actually his word was "sold") 20 "Negars." The *Treasurer* arrived a few days later and deposited a few more.[3] As far as can be determined, these were the first enslaved Africans imported to Virginia. By 1624, among the 1,275 whites scattered throughout the colony's two dozen settlements, there were 22 Africans, the largest group being 11 living among the Flourdieu Hundred.[4]

By 1625 indentured servants comprised 40 percent of the total population, and even by 1670 there were still six thousand such bondsmen among forty thousand residents (and two thousand Africans—already by then a conspicuous social stratum).[5] But for the planters, indentured servitude was not a permanent solution to their labor issues. Eventually most would be liberated to purchase and work land of their own. These would become the small plot farmers who dotted the Virginia countryside. And now who to sew, reap, and cultivate the tobacco fields? Native Americans? Not likely. They proved too restless, too connected to the earth, and not durable beasts of burden, decimated and depleted by the sicknesses European settlers had sewn among them, so the reasoning went.[6] Black Africans were the answer.

And in the form of a more permanent manner of servitude: indefinite ownership—slavery. That held some attraction. Of course, such practices were not unfamiliar to Englishmen. So-called slavery long held sway in the Mediterranean, among Spaniards and Portuguese. Even by the sixteenth and seventeenth Centuries, Muslim corsairs had taken tens of thousands of Christians as slaves, perhaps as many as one hundred thousand.[7] The British themselves had partaken; their African chattel littered the Caribbean Islands, the human motor for their New World economy. Yet for English settlers in the New World to contemplate the use of fellow Englishmen as permanently owned servants was simply unconscionable.[8] Not so with Africans, it seemed. The blackness of their skins already set them apart, and their endurance under blazing Caribbean suns was impressive. As pointed out by author Winthrop Jordan, Africans—"Negroes" was the common term—looked different, acted different, were distinctly unChristian, and seemed morally divergent from European societies. Voyagers to Africa even reported a primordial tendency, some claimed to the point of cannibalism. But what might have appealed most strongly to colonial-minded Europeans was the behavior of Africans once captured, the ease with which they could be transported across the Atlantic, and their robust stamina to withstand the rigors of climate and labor—especially the crushing physical toil of field work (for those who survived the arduous Middle Passage, of course). For the most part, if fed, clothed, and housed, the genre attained a certain docility—albeit often under an enslaver's whip. And might it not be the obligation of Christian men to nourish such humans both physically and spiritually and, doing the Lord's work, expose them to the salvation of Christian faith?[9]

To the contrary, many held that practice of African slavery was ethically reprehensible to Europeans. The libertarian Alexis de Tocqueville (1805–1859) castigated American planters when he wrote in 1831, "I cannot believe that Nature has prohibited the Europeans of Georgia and the Floridas, under pain of death, from raising the means of subsistence from the soil . . . [except that] their labor would be more irksome and less productive," he said.[10] Why should not the southerner himself labor, de Tocqueville argued. Greed was the answer. The steamy, oppressive climate and the range of contagions notwithstanding, the southerner embraced the profits but scorned the labor. His tastes were those of an idle man, he continued: "[H]e covets wealth much less than pleasure and excitement." Work equates to servitude. Slavery became a must.[11] And so, southerners of the Carolinas embraced slavery as did their predecessors in the Caribbean. "Negroes [are] an heathenish brutish and an uncertain dangerous pride of people . . . created Men though without the knowledge of God in the world," so went contemporary thinking. Therefore, they were to be considered as other "goods and Chattels." Slavery henceforth was declared the normal state of Africans.[12]

So, in continental North America, manacled women and men struggled from the holds of random ships, fortuitously harbored in colonized ports. Slavery, a perfect storm of need, opportunity, prejudice, and defamation, singled out the African as a domesticated and subjugated participant in lucrative agrarian ventures. Historian Phillip Morgan contends that it arose through any number of factors: ideas borrowed from the Caribbean, experiences of British and Spanish enslavers, attitudes extrapolated from indentured servitude, opinions formed by encounters with imported Africans, and the unique exigencies of the southern colonies themselves. Soon, gone were the indentured servants to fields of their own. Vast plantations had been stripped of workers. Before long, those acres of ripening tobacco became populated by Black figures living a hapless existence. Africans seemed the ideal subjects. Already by the seventeenth century, lines of inferiority had been drawn between the white Europeans and African migrants.

Professor John Coombs has argued: "The negative perception of 'Negroes' prevalent among the English . . . had become so deeply entrenched by 1619 that the colony's government saw no reason to legislatively create a category of legal personhood . . . such 'brutis' people who were 'not Christian' could be treated as property."[13] There was little moral compunction about enforced, sometimes heartless discipline. Africans, stunned by New World customs, illiterate, inarticulate, and terrified, were an available and susceptible group. They were perceived as almost subhuman, and poorly integrated into European culture, hardly equal partners in the socioeconomics of these new colonies.[14]

Legal maneuvering soon followed as a stamp of authoritative approval. The legislative body of the Virginian colony, formed in 1619 and consisting exclusively of white men, began issuing a series of laws from 1642 on that placed a distinct barrier between white persons and persons of color—primarily Africans.[15] Although referred to as "servants" at first, bondage of Africans was deemed inheritable, figuratively chaining the African to a permanent chattel state. By 1665, the Black African was becoming synonymous with slave and heathen—few were baptized as Christians, despite a professed religious imperative to do so. "Negroes and infidels remain slaves all their lives," one French traveler observed in 1686, noting that Christians over the age of twenty-one could not be enslaved more than five years.[16] The Virginia legislators had systematically stripped Africans of civil protections and instated laws that inserted government in the regulation of slave behavior.[17]

A slow trickle of Africans continued throughout the 1680s and 1690s so that by the end of the century there were over 5,000 permanently indentured African servants/slaves in Virginia. Once the Royal African Company was reorganized, chartered to trade along the west coast of Africa, the importation of enslaved Africans exploded. According to historian William Hesseltine, by 1705 there was an annual arrival of 1,800 enslaved Africans to the colony. That same year Virginia law had clearly distinguished between servant and slave: "All servants imported and brought into this country, by sea and land, who were not Christians in their native country [Muslims excepted] shall be accounted and be slaves and as such be here bought and sold."[18] With such escalating numbers, key was the passage of colonial legislation that protected, first, the property rights of the enslaver and, second, society itself from a belligerent and rebellious element of "an alien race and savage civilization" growing rapidly in size. Not all Africans had remained docile. Whites beware.[19] As for intermingling and intermarrying, "that abominable mixture," white offenders were to be committed to prison; the Black participant likely killed.[20]

According to historian Hugh Thomas, between 1721 and 1730, the British carried more than one hundred thousand slaves to the Americas, ten thousand of whom were shipped to mainland colonies.[21] Authors Michael Byrd and Linda

Clayton contended, "Black Africans hailing from sophisticated agricultural and craft-based cultures and backgrounds in Africa worked well within New World plantation systems. They also seemed to be stronger, hardier, and more resistant to several dreaded diseases, such as malaria and yellow fever, than were Amerindians [Native Americans]."[22] It seemed the perfect solution to the need for manual labor in the vast southern expanse of planter landscapes, where toiling fertile soil could reap untold economic gains. Yet trepidation on the part of some remained. During the early decades of the eighteenth century, introduction of slave labor in the thirteen colonies could create such numbers of bonded Africans—as unruly and barbarous as they were said to be—that misfits might incite violence or even open rebellion. First targets were likely to be planters and families.[23] Still, the monetary bonanza was irresistible. By 1724 Virginia had become heavily dependent on slave labor for its tobacco crop. In a letter to the Lord Commissioners of Trade, Francis Fane argued against excessive duties on imported Africans, pointing out that "this Colony cannot Subsist or be improved without the planters are furnished with large and constant supplies of Negroes and at the Easiest Rates so it cannot be supposed that the Merchants will be so readily and freely Import them while they are clogged with Duties which raise the Value of them and discourage their sending a sufficient Number to the Colony."[24]

Similar conditions were to exist south in the Carolinas. An agricultural economy developed beyond anyone's wildest dreams. Even from first encounter, the potential was obvious. In his voyage of 1666 to Port Royal and up the Ashley River, the Barbadian explorer Robert Sanford was impressed by the "high banks richly crowned with timber of the largest size." He envisioned habitation on this land "for thousands of people with conveyances for their stock." It was marvelous territory, this Carolina. He wrote, "[W]e could see of nothing here to be wished for but good store for English Inhabitants, and that we all heartily prayed for." The fertile coastal plain was ripe for colonization. Extended five hundred miles from below Cape Fear to East Florida, there were fields that, once carved from swamps and forests, could be geared for market agriculture—primarily rice—and seemed well suited for mass production of crops worked by slave labor shown so profitable in the British Caribbean. In short, this geography could be transformed into a plantation paradise.[25]

From May 30, 1721, to September 29, 1726, a total of 3,632 Africans were imported into South Carolina. The major port of entry, of course, was Charleston, where, in one three-month span, 732 Africans arrived. By 1739, some estimated the number of Africans in South Carolina at 35,000.[26] In August 1754, Governor James Glen reported to the Board of Trade: "As Negroes are sold at higher Prices here than in any part of the King's Dominion, we have them sent from Barbadoes [sic], the Leeward Islands, Jamaica, Virginia, and New York, this I think is a plain proof that this Province is in a flourishing condition."[27] Yet the fear of violence persisted as the number of enslaved individuals rose. Here and there, a few enslaved persons were not so docile. In a letter to the Board of Trade from Lieutenant Governor William Bull in 1765, Bull wrote that "above 8,000 [Africans] have been imported this year . . . whether this sudden addition to a number already beyond a prudent proportion will be productive of unhappy consequences cannot be certainly foreseen."[28]

For a time, the situation in Georgia was different. Contrary to other southern colonies, trustees for the new colony of Georgia had explicitly forbidden slavery at its founding. Not for any moral conviction, but of a pragmatic nature—to make the colony more defensible. Georgia was a colony besieged. By not diluting the population with enslaved people who could not or would not help in defense and who might be persuaded to rebellion by Spanish just to the south, whites stood a better chance at protection. In fact, anyone caught smuggling in "Blacks" or "Negroes" would face a hefty fine and their human "possessions" forfeited.[29]

Industrious Scot and German settlers were in a quandary, however. In generating marketable timber, their staple industry in Georgia, they could not compete with their neighbors in South Carolina without slave labor. It was not long before their righteous resolve buckled, and they appealed to the trustees. "The want of the use of negroes, with proper limitations, would both occasion great numbers of white people to come here, and also render us capable to subsist ourselves, by raising provisions upon our lands, until we could make some produce fit for export," their 1738 petition read. In short, the colony would fail without Africans. Despite arguments to the contrary, mostly contending it would disadvantage poor white farmers (as had been feared in the Carolinas), economic considerations predominated. So, within two years of Georgia's founding, the tangle of woods, an unhealthy climate, and languishing economy pushed sentiments toward slavery. In 1742 and 1743, Georgian Thomas Stephens, as spokesperson for the citizenry, lobbied for slavery in front of the House of Commons. It was feared, he argued, that unless enslaved Africans were imported the colony was finished. On August 8, 1750, His Majesty acted on recommendations from the trustees and repealed the aforesaid act excluding Africans from the colony. Georgia was open to slavery.[30]

The settlers were right. By 1784, enslaved Africans had become indispensable in Georgia. The capacity to generate vast profits on the bent backs of bonded Blacks had become part of the fabric of Georgian society and affluence. "The Negro business is a great object with us, both with a View to our Interest individually, and the general prosperity of this State [Georgia, now part of the United States] and its commerce, it is to the Trade of this Country as the Soul to the Body, and without it no House can gain a proper Stability," wrote statesman and Revolutionary War veteran Joseph Clay on February 16, 1784.[31] Of course, the prime mercenary mission was tempered by that tired refrain from civilizing missionaries that, above all, they were bringing the heathens to God.[32]

⁓

In contrast to the English, whose interest was establishment of permanent agricultural-based colonies, the French were more concerned with the trading potential of interior North America. Throughout their vast Louisiana Territory, a series of fortifications had been built to facilitate exportable commerce with Native Americans and protect against the intrusion of the English and Spanish. Their footprint was mostly inland waterways, primarily along the Mississippi and Ohio Valleys.[33] As advocates of slavery, they had no qualms. Their first efforts used Chitimacha Native Americans acquired through back-country warfare in 1716. Natives proved unsatisfactory for the same reasons as the English had seen. Unreliable, restless, and volatile. Africans were different. Disoriented, disenfranchised, and usually docile, they were good field workers on the plantations along the Mississippi River. Of course, homeland France was heavy into the slave trade. According to historian Tyler Stovall, "The profitability and extent of the slave trade and the Caribbean plantation economy gave race an undeniable significance in 18th Century French life."[34]

In 1717 the Compagnie d'Occident determined that six or seven thousand enslaved Africans would be required annually and attempted to work out an arrangement with the Compagnie du Sénégal in West Africa. Such was the effort to bolster French slave trading, that bartering with the nearby Spanish—historically strong in slavery—was strictly forbidden. A few years later, in 1719 the slave ship *Duc du Maine* transported 250 Africans to Dauphine Island just outside the Bay of Mobile. Twenty of these were then sent to the inland French trading post of Natchitoches.[35] Dauphine Island proved a convenient disembarking site, and from then on sale of Africans proceeded at a steady clip. The entire process was outlined carefully in the "Minutes of the Council of Commerce of Louisiana." Arriving shipments at Dauphine Island were examined and sold to the highest bidders. Moving the merchandise was top priority. Unsold Africans—toddlers, teenagers, or flawed adults—were an economic waste and a liability. Special discounts were offered for any unsold humans. For those still remaining the future was dismal. They were left on the island, usually to fend for themselves. There was little compassion. Many died, languishing on the white sands, unable to find food or water and not prime property for touring planters. Their meager sustenance was one meal per day and nothing but brackish water. Dogs were treated better.[36]

From Dauphine Island, purchased humans were transported to New Orleans for distribution. In the year 1721 the Compagnie d'Occident brought over 1,300 enslaved Africans there. Commissioner de la Chaise remarked in 1723, "Everybody, Gentlemen, is asking for negroes in order to be able to have work done on preparing land to plant indigo for next year when the colony expects to send you some returns. It grows marvelously here and in spite of the floods that lasted until the beginning of July it has grown perfectly well."[37]

"You may be assured, gentlemen, that tobacco, rice and silk will thrive in this colony . . . but remember that without a great many negroes, you cannot expect any profit, since the white laborers can barely feed themselves," a planter wrote from Natchez in 1721.[38] The slave population grew at an astonishing rate, increasing almost tenfold from 580 in 1721 to 5,209 in 1766. Lack of finances in the struggling towns and a shortage of voluntary white labor drove the colonists to procure Africans. Only then could costs be reduced, profits optimized, and the communities provided with the necessary accouterments of civilization.[39] By mid-century, New Orleans had become a major slave port and auction. From 1763 to 1783 between 3,000 and 4,000 slaves reached Louisiana; between 1783 and 1796 another 8,000 to 9,000 arrived; and between 1800 and 1803 1,200 slaves landed at the mouth of the Mississippi. That was certainly not the end. A staggering 12,000 Africans, from Africa, the Caribbean, and America (over 1,600 from Charleston alone), were unloaded during the early American period, the first decade of the nineteenth century. Despite slavery's federal prohibition, at least fifty-five slave ships arrived at the port of New Orleans during that same timeframe.[40]

For Africans the whole process was brutal. Senegal slaves faced a particularly odious transit to the New World. As many as 450 were crowded onto ships barely able to accommodate a fraction of that number. Malnutrition, mistreatment, and disease killed as many as one in five on the voyage, sometimes almost half. The bloody flux (dysentery) and scurvy were likely culprits in finishing off weakened numbers already deficient in food and water.[41] Journeys to the inland plantations were even more arduous for the already weakened Africans. The director of the colony at Natchez wrote disparagingly in 1721 that he had ordered 30 Africans, but when they arrived, 17 were sick, so he returned them for fear of spreading disease among the healthy and kept a paltry 13.[42] On one particular arrival, from the frigate *Venus*, of the 363 survivors of the Atlantic crossing in 1729 (450 had begun the voyage in Africa), only 320 arrived upriver, and "they were so violently attacked by the scurvy that more than two-thirds of those who were sold at auction . . . have died."[43] Yet the healthier Africans seemed better suited to agricultural labor, even under a harsh sun and drenching humidity. Far better, it seemed, than Native Americans, who could not endure prolonged heavy exertion in that climate; many perished from the toil.[44] "The colour of the skin in the negro gives him a decided advantage over the white," wrote South Carolina physician and planter Philip Tidyman in 1826, "by enabling him to endure the scorching heat of the sun with less suffering; whilst he is protected by the very nature of his constitution from the unhealthiness of hot climates." In this bayou country, so abhorrent to white workers, Tidyman insisted, could be found the Black man, "working with cheerfulness and alacrity."[45]

This New South was raw, frontier country. The Delta region of the fresh state of Mississippi, that monotonous floodplain between the Mississippi and Yazoo Rivers where the soil was as rich as the luscious nutrients deposited there, had been occupied by the Choctaw Nation. A rash of Jacksonian "treaties" with the white man removed them in short order, providing token payments to the former inhabitants. The first settlers probably arrived around 1825, hewing through hardwood trees and setting up homesteads along the river itself. By 1820, over 42,000 whites had settled in Mississippi along with almost 33,000 enslaved Africans. Ten years later, more than half the population of Washington County were of African ancestry. Planters continued to populate, many from the "Old South" states of Carolina and Georgia, bringing even more enslaved Blacks so that in 1840 Africans outnumbered whites by nearly 10 to 1. By mid-century, over 290,000 whites had moved in, but Africans still exceeded the white population by 14,000.[46]

But the Delta was toxic wilderness. Its marshy, often flooded flatlands harbored a variety of unhealthy invisible miscreants. Malaria, cholera, and typhoid fever swept through the region in bouts of illness during the 1830s. If they could, planters left the area from May to October to avoid the plethora of mosquitoes, the heat, and the humidity. "This would be the most delightful country in the world if it were not for the months June, July, August, and September," one planter's wife recalled. Her baby itched and scratched to the point that she thought he would go mad, his skin pocked like smallpox. It was not just a nuisance. Shortly the small child would be dead. In another instance, a planter's family was devastated by fevers, killing his twenty-six-year-old wife and, before long, two of his six children.[47]

Life on the Mississippi was generally harsher than other parts of the South for bonded subjects. The Bohemian physician Simon Pollack, who had immigrated to the United States in 1838, saw firsthand the plight of bondsmen on his journey down the Mississippi River to New Orleans. Slaves manned fleets of steamers on the river, loading and unloading bales of cotton at such ports as Natchez and Vicksburg. "They were under strict discipline ... No play, no rest. On, on, was the ceaseless cry of the driver on shore, and the 'mate' on deck. The air was thick with profane words, blows and curses not a few." He saw one Black man rise up to beatings and, in an instant, fatally stab his white tormentor only to then jump overboard into the river and a certain death. On farms and plantations, Pollack observed, enslaved Blacks were treated well and cared for in sickness and health. However, in the field they were under the watchful eyes of drivers or "overseers"—white and Black—and there subjected to great cruelty.[48]

By 1790, with the birth of the new United States, in the Atlantic South (Virginia, North Carolina, South Carolina, and Georgia), 529,768 enslaved Africans were counted. A mere 20,106 Africans were "free," just 4 percent of the total number of African imports. Lands of the Louisiana Purchase would add substantially to that figure.[49] The practice would foster a rift between cultures—African and European—which would inevitably deepen with time until there was little doubt among most whites of the South that a basic distinction must be made between ethnicities, as if phenotypic differences spoke to species differentiation—a matter many now referred to as "race." Black and white, they reasoned, were not only different in skin color but in the very genetics of intellect and behavior. There would not be a more defining factor in interpreting the South and its distinctive cultures—medical and otherwise—than the choking pall of color, "race," superiority, and subjugation. This, in itself, seemed to alter the comportment of white Europeans as if their ancestry at some primal age diverged, and any resemblance of equality was simply no longer possible. Thus, racial differentiation was self-perpetuating and inherited from generation to generation for centuries. Even war and bloodshed would not alter it. Alexis de Tocqueville, after his lengthy tour of the American continent, wrote this cogent observation:

> The modern slave differs from his master not only in his condition, but in his origin. You may set the Negro free, but you cannot make him otherwise than an alien to the European. Nor is this all; we scarcely acknowledge the common features of mankind in this child of debasement whom slavery has brought amongst us. His physiognomy is to our eyes hideous, his understanding weak, his tastes low; and we are almost inclined to look upon him as a being intermediate between man and the brutes. The moderns, then, after they have abolished slavery, have three prejudices to contend against, which are less easy to attack, and far less easy to conquer, than the mere fact of servitude: the prejudice of the master, the prejudice of the race, and the prejudice of color.[50]

Africans proved to be a resilient people, despite their grueling journey to the New World. Of course, that trek killed or maimed not a few, and the first few years of captivity were equally hazardous. Of those who survived, though, their longevity could be comparable to their white enslavers. For example, mortality rates for Africans in Charleston were consistently better than for Philadelphia through the 1830s, the presumption being that the pervasive yellow fever was less likely to strike down Africans than whites.[51] In the Mississippi Valley, enslaved Africans held up as well as whites. The expectation of life of an enslaved twenty-year-old in Mississippi in 1850 was not much less than that of a white man of the same age.[52] Despite grim reports of high childhood mortality—historian William Dusinberre claimed that half of the children on President James Polk's Mississippi plantation died before the age of fifteen—the slave force, including Polk's, increased at a rate of from 2 to almost 15 percent per decade.[53]

Yet just as white southerners did, Africans could have a myriad of health problems. Perhaps, some whites surmised, it was the change of climate, dietary differences, the hardships of field labor, harshness of the enslaver, and even despondency and suicide. Illnesses such as smallpox, dysentery, venereal complaints, scurvy, and worms were found among enslaved populations. As whites used bondsmen for care of their livestock as well, diseases from animals, while affecting white planters and yeomen too, were found more often in enslaved Africans. Brucellosis from hogs, goats, and cattle hounded the field workers, particularly during the slaughter seasons as this was a chore usually relegated to Africans. Leptospirosis and anthrax were two other feared conditions caused by exposure to infected animals, diseases that all too often had a painful and fatal outcome.

The squalor in which many enslaved Blacks found themselves proved a major source of ailments no more or less than poor, underprivileged whites. "The principle causes of sickness upon plantations," former Mississippian Erasmus Fenner wrote in 1850, "are the use of spring, well, creek, or bayou water."[54] That was water heavily contaminated with bacteria and protozoa hostile to the intestinal tracts of man. Those epidemics of *cholera morbus*—the ravages of uncontrollable diarrhea, cramping, vomiting, prostration, and death—seemed particularly prevalent in overcrowded, poorly sanitized habitations. Great numbers of Africans perished from them. The vicious cholera epidemics of 1832 and 1833 in Louisiana and Kentucky were especially notorious, far worse for enslaved Blacks than their white owners. "There is more sickness, and consequently greater loss of life, from the decaying logs of negro houses, open floors, leaky roofs, and crowded rooms, than all other causes combined," pointed out one Mississippi planter in 1851. He provided comfortable quarters, plenty of fresh meat, rest periods, change of clothing, and even a large hospital when they were sick (a "very experienced and careful negro woman" was put in charge).

In Georgia, typhoid fever struck slave populations hard. In many cases victims dwelt in fetid conditions, with litter and filth cluttering households, dampness, dirty drinking water, close-packed quarters, family members living and sleeping almost on top of each other (some planters had noticed that exclusive use of rainwater would prevent the choleras).[55] Not far away, whites who lived in cleaner, well-ventilated homes, with proper diet and with better sources of water for bathing and drinking were hardly touched, just like freed Africans who lived in similar circumstances.[56] "Remove all the well Negroes, on the first appearance of the disease [cholera], to some remote and comfortable quarters," advised Dr. New of Mississippi. Cholera epidemics created panic among those enslaved on plantations, New argued. Separating healthy from sick hid the ravages of the illness that seemed to weaken even the unaffected. For those with the malignant diarrhea, New assaulted them with enemas and filled them with tincture of camphor, opium, sugar of lead, morphia, and dry mustard. But above all, watchful examination of all enslaved persons—and their bowel evacuations—would catch the epidemic at its inception and, by segregation, limit the spread.[57] Diseases were mostly viewed as economic wastage. To lose valuable work time—and returns on investments—rankled planters and hardly warmed them to humanitarianism for their labor force.

Certain other conditions hounded Africans. Trismus nascentium was a disorder affecting newborns. Spasms seized the tiny victims to such a degree that their backs arched in rigidity and jaws tightened shut. It was called "lock jaw," like the affliction of tetanus in adults that usually proved fatal. In infants, too, death was almost certain. Likely, the grime of unkempt cabins or even early return to field work by new mothers carrying their infants along was the cause, the fresh umbilical stumps of their babies contaminated with soil and filth and infected—as it would later be shown—by the bacterium *Clostridium tetani*.

Black children also could develop marasmus, a wasting condition most often associated with malnutrition, leading to death in infancy or early childhood. It was likely that such dietary deficiencies in infants and children were due to hard labor among pregnant women and meals lacking in vitamins and protein. Most peculiar in some adults was the syndrome called Cachexia Africana, or in the vernacular, "dirt eating." Physicians described it as a "groveling propensity" for literally eating dirt and its denizens, like earthworms. Such affected individuals often exhibited a livid, manic, and ghastly expression, leading some to think it was a moral rather than a physical disorder. "They are the sots in this species of intemperance, and exerting no control over the groveling taste, they with an awful rapidity anticipate their doom." Lack of nourishment stripped limbs of their muscle, and the cachectic victim slowly wasted away to a state of irreversible impoverishment until perishing almost a mere skeleton.[58]

Pneumonia struck Africans hard. Doctors referred to it by a variety of names: congestion of the lungs, cold plague, typhus pneumonia, or bilious pleurisy. And influenza: the Italians called the condition *influenza di freddo*, the "influence of the cold." Indeed, it was associated with cooler temperatures of autumn and winter. Too often, even in the young, it progressed to the classic signs of pneumonia. With Africans, the disease seemed especially virulent, sometimes so profound that typhus or a typhoid-like illness was suspected. The notorious Louisiana physician Samuel Cartwright leveled the bizarre claim that "[t]he negro's lungs . . . are very sensitive to the impressions of cold air."

Sleeping habits also contributed, he surmised, the African covering his or her head and face, trapping impure air "loaded with carbonic acid and aqueous vapor." This led to imperfect "atmospherization" of the blood—"one of the heaviest chains that binds the negro to slavery" (the logic obscure).[59]

Nevertheless, white or Black, pneumonia was an alarming disease. Normally airy lung tissue filled with fluid and inflammation. Breathing became labored. Oxygen levels fell, and vital organs were starved of healthy blood. Victims took on a bluish tinge. Lungs percussed a sickening solidity. Fevers soared, and patients finally lapsed into a state of troubled consciousness. There was little effective treatment, doctors fiddling with various barbaric remedies. Paramount in these inflammations, of course, was the lancet. Bleed, bleed, bleed, was the common admonition. Between blood loss and gagging instillations, many perished despite the best intentions. A particularly vicious form of pneumonia for Blacks was called typhoid pneumonia. It seemed to break out in epidemic fashion and strike "the very best negroes on plantations," sparing any white inhabitants. The condition was so malignant that many victims fell ill in hours and were dead the next day. Lungs at autopsy had the consistency of liver (called "hepatization"). Survival was infrequent. One enlightened doctor cautioned, though, that the high death rate could be due to a "rude and often careless manner in which everything pertaining to their management is conducted." The key, in his estimation, was good nursing, tending the patient at the bedside and administering any of the many available tonics and therapies early on.[60]

In those times, consumption—that mysterious disease of the lungs now called tuberculosis—was an insidious but common malady. Cheesy tubercles filled lung tissue, eating into blood vessels and producing coughs of pure blood. It was a slow but inexorable process. In Africans, so-called "Negro consumption" was a particularly odious affliction, less likely to destroy lungs but causing cutaneous eruptions termed scrofula—a great bursting to the outside of those same gummy abscesses of *Mycobacterium tuberculosis*. Tongue and gums were covered with a slimy white mucous, and respirations were labored with chronic coughs. Victims slowly wasted away. Cartwright contended it was "a disease almost unknown to medical men of the Northern states and Europe."[61] Of course, he blamed it on "dirt eating," another dubious connection. At autopsy of these individuals, the belly often contained large tumors of inflamed lymph nodes harboring more of the agents of consumption. "The frequency of the disease . . . results from the inaptitude of climate," the proclivity to diseases previously unknown in African environments. It would send "hundreds to their graves."

The scrofula indeed aroused suspicion among doctors of the day as to whether this was a unique form of tuberculosis among Blacks (it was).[62] Some less erudite speculators felt it was a condition not of the lungs, stomach, or liver but of the mind, causing consternation of the enslaver and superstition among the enslaved.

Figures from four areas of Virginia showed more Blacks died from tuberculosis at a younger age. According to historian Todd Savitt, over 70 percent of more than two hundred enslaved and free Blacks who died of tuberculosis were under the age of forty.[63] The high mortality from consumption in Blacks may simply have been those same crowded, dirty living conditions conducive to so many contagious ailments. In any event, the appearance of this emaciating illness with its proclivity to quick fatigue and shortness of breath was unsettling to planters, and affected individuals were promptly sold. In certain cases, the wretched dwellings of the affected were simply burned to the ground.

To care for their ailing enslaved workers, many planters relied on home remedies. Tidyman advised owners to have a liberal pharmacopeia at hand: snakeroots, Peruvian bark, antimonial wine, tar vapor, myrrh, honey, in addition to an endless array of readily assembled agents such as enemas of starch and laudanum, sulphate of magnesia, castor oil, rice water, purgatives, "serpentaria, milk punch, brandy toddy," garlic cataplasms, and countless other concoctions to combat the fevers and dysenteries that affected the enslaved.[64] Sometimes the enslaved Blacks themselves had shamans in their midst who gave various nostrums and herbs of African origin. While sophisticated European medicine urged a dichotomy between religion and medicine, Africans felt no such compulsion. In African culture, the art of healing was very much a religious endeavor. Africans had a rich plethora of healers as described by culturalist Beverly J. Robinson. "African-American healing is rooted in belief and thus is a religion which places folk practitioners and their art in the world of the spiritual." The healer, in slave societies, was both priest and medicine man. It often became family business. Dispensing medical care fell within the purview of mothers, fathers, grandmothers, and grandfathers. Like Native Americans, their pharmacopoeia was richly endowed with herbs, roots, leaves, and barks given in mixtures of soups, teas, tonics, and poultices. Whether remedies were gleaned from neighboring indigenous tribes is a matter of conjecture; in most cases intermingling of enslaved Blacks and indigenous people was discouraged.[65]

Many African practices were looked upon with suspicion, as European (white physician) methods such as bloodletting, emetics, and cathartics engendered little confidence and much distress. Doctor prescriptions such as tartar (an emetic), capsicum (chili peppers—good for asthma, rheumatism, coughs, and just about anything else), charcoal, calomel (a purgative), tonics, and various balms aimed at flushing out the imbalance of humors as well as what remained of the strength of the patient. As a result, much rural health care fell to wise men and women inventing their own remedies, learned by tradition or gleaned from Native American lore. As a result, physicians were not in high demand.

On larger plantations, though, enslavers built special infirmaries for those enslaved there. Such hospitals were erected on plantation grounds not out of any worry for comfort and warmth of ill Africans but more pragmatically, for the maintenance of commercial worth. For once, humanism coincided serendipitously with economics. A few were attractive structures, the genders separated, rooms well ventilated and lit, and good bedding. Such "slave hospitals" could be found in the Old South as well as new territories such as Mississippi and Alabama. Many others were simple cabins, isolated from the rest for quarantine purposes or to watch those suspected of malingering. Larger infirmaries arose in urban areas, sometimes associated with medical colleges, who used ailments of enslaved persons for teaching. Partnerships in such commercial institutions proved lucrative as enslavers were eager to pay necessary fees to preserve their investments. And the presence of clinical subjects was indispensable to the education of young students who would rarely ask for the opportunity to examine white men and women as training patients.[66]

The perception that Africans carried a different tolerance for diseases led some to question their inherent constitution. Doctor Samuel Cartwright, by then a practitioner in Mississippi and Louisiana, seemed obsessed with the subject. His seminal creation was the 1851 treatise entitled "Report on the Diseases and Physical Peculiarities of the Negro Race." It was one of the more phantasmagoric works of imagined reality devised by one who professed to be a skilled clinician. A fascination with Cartwright, this "race" of Africans, now living in such intimacy with "science and mental progress" (meaning, presumably, the white "race") deserved the utmost observation and investigation. It was imperative that southern physicians acquire a working knowledge of the idiosyncrasies, habits, and curiosities of this variety of mankind from the "wilds of Africa," more than can merely be gleaned from books or medical lectures. In Cartwright's ideation, it was as if such beings were valued livestock, worthy of indulgence, if for no other reason than economic.

Of course, it followed that there must *a priori* be an inferiority to these people, somehow manifested in differences in physiognomy and mental capacity. Without hesitation, Cartwright zeroed in on skin color. But not only skin, this went much deeper, he claimed. The membranes, muscles, tendons, and all the fluids and secretions were of a different color, too, he maintained. Even the blood was darker—and the bile as well. And then Cartwright went on to describe bizarre differences in stature, posture, pelvic tilt, and even their gait ("hopper-hipped," was an expression he used). Less amusing was his insistence that the African brain was smaller and nervous system excessively developed. In the era still of humoral medicine, Cartwright theorized that the African had a lymphatic temperament, in which the lymph, phlegm, and mucus predominated over red blood. Such alterations combined with a surfeit of peripheral nervous matter caused a debasement of the mind rendering a people "unable to take care of themselves," another puzzling non sequitur. Surely one of the most whacky of claims made by Cartwright was a disease exhibited by enslaved Africans he called drapetomania, the inclination of enslaved individuals to run away—he attributed it to a disorder of the mind. This must be quickly addressed, before they become sulky and dissatisfied—even leading to consumptive afflictions (tuberculosis). The cure? Whip it out of them, he urged. Cartwright praised planters for "whipping the devil out of them."

Cartwright also maintained that climate had an effect on Africans, that northern climates, with a denser atmosphere, were more conducive to their intellectual development—producing people bold and ungovernable, while, presumably, the low country of the south had the opposite effect: Africans there more docile, complacent, almost imbecilic. Why such erratic behavior? This is where he turned biblical. Perhaps the African is not of the same race as the white man, perhaps not even a son of the biblical Adam. More likely, Cartwright supposed, they were offspring of Noah's son Ham, doomed to be the servant of servants and exiled to Africa forevermore. Cursed as they were, they sank into the indolent existence where sometime later the white man found them. As such, Cartwright and his followers were the harbingers of that American Original Sin of slavery, reducing a proud and cultured ethnicity to barely the equal of apes.[67] Were Africans similar to whites in their susceptibility and resistance to diseases? Not hardly, Cartwright claimed. The African was no black-faced European, he penned to another medical journal in 1850: "The popular error prevalent at the North, that the negro is a white man, but, by some accident of climate or locality, painted black, requiring nothing but liberty and equality . . . to wash him white, is permitted to go uncorrected by the Northern medical schools."[68]

Even those cholera epidemics affected Africans differently. As such, Cartwright contrived special remedies for bonded Africans. He felt that, if treated like white men, Blacks would invariably die of cholera. Instead, he recommended carrying Blacks, sick and well, "back to an imitation of savage life, in the woods or open fields." Cartwright at one point corralled a few hundred enslaved Africans he considered at risk for cholera, stripped them and greased them with fat bacon, slapping on the lard with broad leather straps. It seemed to work, Cartwright surmised, driving out what he called "cholera of the mind." Such bizarre treatment would drive cholera out of their heads, reducing the slathered subjects to objects of ridicule and laughter instead of fear and veneration. In defense of this treatment, he claimed not one got sick. Treat them as the wild savages they were, Cartwright urged.[69]

Sadly, he was not alone. Even as early as 1802, the French sugar planter and recent immigrant to America Pierre-Louis Berquin Duvallon had already concluded: "Negroes are a species of beings whom nature seems to have intended for slavery; their pliancy of temper, patience under injury, and innate passiveness, all concur to justify this position." As far as their constitution, he tidily argued their most common maladies were "slight fevers in the spring, more violent ones in the summer, dysenteries in autumn, and fluxions of the breast in winter." A sturdy stock and industrious, they nevertheless loved their relaxation—and tobacco, smoking and chewing it "with great relish." While mortality was low, Duvallon incredibly surmised that "[d]eath is not so terrible in aspect to these negroes as to the whites." And their major incentive to obey? The whip, of course.[70] Some decades later, Erasmus Fenner echoed those sentiments: "Negroes have diseases peculiar to themselves; and even in the same diseases, the symptoms, etc., are different, and the treatment must also be different."[71]

And after him, physician and surgeon W. G. Ramsay pointed out, rather sharply, that, while the Black man is not by nature savage or barbarous—and despite a number of anatomic differences—he is endowed with the particular quality of laziness. "Laziness is one of the great characteristics of the negro," Ramsay detailed. And not, he argued, a product of slavery, as "we find in the Northern States of our country ... that this characteristic is the same." Proof was totally lacking, other than to make the unsupported claim that "[t]rue bravery, love of liberty, ambition, and all the higher feelings to which the soul of man is heir to, belongs to the white man." It did not seem to be a result of climate, Ramsay went on, but rather an inherent tendency to sloth that not even life among Europeans would change. "A negro, by being brought up among Europeans, may be much improved, but there will still remain a wide line of distinction between them, which is seldom crossed by the negro, and if it should be, it is recorded as a wonder." When accounting for differences in diseases between "Whites" and "Negroes," Ramsay finally posed the question, "Do these races of men spring from the same original stock?" Pure speculation, Ramsay concluded. There was no compelling evidence either way but, he was assured, that even several generations of life among "whites" will not change their color or "natural peculiarities." Wisely, Ramsay, in the end, backed off, writing that "we find ourselves wandering into regions dark and obscure, over which the torch of science sheds but a faint light, merely enough to convince us of our ignorance," a remark truly the vessel of wisdom in a sea of theory and speculation.[72]

But did Africans actually have a separate set of pathologic afflictions or was this a conjure of white efforts at supremacy? Scholar Katherine Bankole concluded that attempts to separate "slave medicine" were little more than a pseudoscientific inquiry used "to foster a bio-medical rationale for the maintenance of White supremacy and the slaveocracy in general." Physicians of the day were, by and large, conspirators in that effort. What becomes apparent in retrospect was the tendency for the impoverished, poorly educated and cared for enslaved communities to fall victim to those diseases and disorders of poverty: overcrowding, poor hygiene, inadequate nutrition, and neglected medical conditions, to which white populations, better fed, housed, and informed, were largely immune.[73]

Were they all that disadvantaged in their lifestyles compared to northerners? Some thought not. Before wholeheartedly condemning the institution of slavery, one might examine closely the plight of the northern working class. Laborers in many northern cities suffered terribly from low wages and squalid working conditions, some far worse than those suffered by the bound Africans of the South. "American society was marred by the existence of poverty and misery on a large scale ... on one side ... were the idle rich and the capitalists [presumably including the wealthy southern planters], living in a splendor derived from the poverty of many," so wrote historian Edward Pessen. In that sense the laboring class was not too dissimilar from the enslaved Africans of southern states. One might claim that their freedom set them apart, but hardly. It was a distinction without a difference. Northern laborers were bound to their work, their employer, and their landlords. There was indeed little freedom.[74] Pessen went on to say: "Evidence ... demonstrates that during the middle decades of the nineteenth century the real wages of Northern workingmen declined and their living conditions remained bleak, their job security was reduced, their skills were increasingly devalued, and in many respects their lives became more insecure and precarious."[75] "America has never had much use for its cities," wrote journalist Michael Shapiro. In the early nineteenth century, men and women flocked to cities of the industrializing North because too little money could be made on rural farms—a romanticized pursuit that often fell flat. Cities, of course, collected vast hordes of immigrants, and tenements and hovels were thick with humanity. The South was different. A lavish economy stemmed not from urbanized factories but immense swaths of fertile cotton, sugar, and indigo fields. Cities were merely waystations in the global distribution of raw material for which planters were paid handsomely. It had become a countrified South that opportunity for affluence, status, and social acceptance prevailed—not in its cities. "Cities were still regarded as dangerous places, dangerous to the body and to the soul, too. The country offered salvation," Shapiro wrote. No truer than in Christian Dixieland.[76]

With such enforced subjugation of Africans, it is no wonder that any Black physicians could be found in the southern colonies prior to the Civil War. In the North, there were isolated examples of Black practitioners. One such person was a man named Simon who had escaped from slavery and who, it was advertised in Philadelphia in 1740, was able to bleed and pull teeth and function as a doctor among his people. James McCune Smith of New York City was the first recorded Black who actually received a formal medical education at the University of Glasgow in 1835. Smith became a model citizen, developing a lucrative practice and engaging in a number of civic affairs, including devotion to his people. While rare examples of enslaved persons particularly adept at cures for various illnesses can be found in the contemporary literature, there is not recorded one Black physician—suitably educated—who practiced south of the Mason-Dixon Line. Only one southern practitioner comes close, James Derham of New Orleans, who apprenticed while enslaved with a New Orleans physician. Derham, by virtue of his servitude, worked as a British regimental surgeon during the Revolutionary War. After the war, Derham returned to New Orleans, where he was eventually freed and once again practiced medicine. So admirable was his reputation that the eminent Benjamin Rush pronounced him completely competent, quite an endorsement for a Black physician.

More commonly, no African rose above their Black community status as herbal savants, tooth pullers, barbers, bleeders, midwives, and soothsayers—and even that to the irritation of white enslavers.[77] What would be worse, the enslaver's duty to maintain health of the people they enslaved dissolved after the Civil War. Newly minted African Americans were now set adrift with no provisions for medical care. They were poor, illiterate, and by virtue of their marginalization, disease ridden. Historian Kelly Miller pointed out over a century ago: "There is no more pathetic chapter in the history of human struggle than the emergence of the smothered ambitions of this race to meet the social exigencies involved in the professional needs of the masses . . . without personal or formal fitness."[78] And authors Michael Byrd and Linda Clayton maintained that the long-sought emancipation created a cesspool of decline for Africans, throwing them into a tailspin of "illiteracy, poverty, racial segregation, exploitation, and national hostility." Once prime components of a thriving southern economy, now freed, their material role in an agrarian market was over. They were, in short, disposable.[79]

CHAPTER EIGHT

NATIVE HEALING IN COLONIAL TIMES

> What should I not have done for my recovery?
> —ANTOINE-SIMON LE PAGE DU PRATZ, 1758

The colonial South was an admixture of ethnic groups, foreign and domestic. Blacks, whites, and indigenous people lived in an amalgamation of beliefs, attitudes, customs, and tolerances. Even resident native tribes, while sharing certain philosophies, were, in part, heterogeneous clusters of communities coveting fierce individuality. Yet inevitably, those same norms and practices spilled from one circle to another. Doctoring in the Old South, then, was a blend of traditional, indigenous, and even local folk medicine. The informality of rural southern living promoted a curious exploitation of any novel medical therapy. Even with social disparities and rivalries there was a casual, if not intentional, interchange of ideas and practices. More so, perhaps, than in the North, the rural South lent itself to informal and unorthodox healing rituals.

In truth, on the surface, little love was lost among the populations inhabiting the Old South. Resentment, jealousy, and conniving were operative sentiments for all concerned. While Blacks had been corralled and subjugated, white settlers and Native Americans lived an uneasy peace in close proximity. Restless planters and farmers cared little about indigenous boundaries. That contagions brought by the settlers decimated indigenous communities was generally of little concern. More to the issue was the endless backdrop of agricultural potential, the stubborn resistance of embedded aboriginal heritage, and the alternating appeasement, deceit, and violence necessary to wrestle tribal lands away.

Yet day to day there existed some degree of harmony and cooperation. It was necessary, of course, for prosperity (fur trading was extremely lucrative), settler safety, and peace of mind. Not uncommonly, farmers and their indigenous neighbors shared crops, game, and clothing. What is more, natives possessed a rich plethora of healing practices useful in regions where sickness was prevalent and traditional physicians scarce. The exotic nature of aboriginal healing customs was seductive for those desperately ill. White or indigenous, seldom did remedies alter the inexorable progression of diseases of the times: smallpox, malaria, yellow fever, typhoid fever, and cholera. Hope was that symptoms abated—either from some mysterious property of the medication or from spiritual overtones—or that the patient languished painlessly in the throes of their fatal illness. Too often, though, neither happened. The sufferer suffered more, and the end came quicker.[1]

There was little science to it all. Whether European or Native American, both cultures incorporated healing methods based heavily on superstition and supposition. Of course, symptoms dominated management. Causation was wildly speculative—divine transgressions and retribution or some intangible malfeasance of humors. Therapy aimed at correction of perceived internal or spiritual dramas, largely a series of balancing acts: placation of an irritable god or correction of humoral imbalance. The more severe the symptom the more vigorous the incantations, purging, sweating, bleeding, or blistering.

How easily did white planters accept indigenous medicine? The contrast, sometimes, was stark. Indigenous ideas of sickness and health were distinctly different from European practices. For native people (although this varied from tribe to tribe) unseen forces, good and evil, vied for the health of mortals. Native people viewed sickness as demonic mischief or divine punishment. Rather than grappling with imbalances of bodily fluids, tribal practices focused on an invisible struggle of ghosts and mythical boogeymen. Appeasement of the spirits, then, was the primary aim—either to ward off demons or to supplicate good spirits, and special healers, imbued with divine talents, fulfilled the task. They were masters of rituals and charms. Concoctions of local plants and herbs rounded out their therapy. Some treatments may have even been truly effective, admixtures of the sublime and the ridiculous. Planters and yeoman farmers picked up on this. Not that consultation with indigenous healers was the norm, even in the agrarian South, but in dire circumstances, as remote as some villages and farms were, access to tribal areas and tribal healers was probably a good deal easier than traveling to find a traditional physician or being subject to the whims of self-styled white healers and outright charlatans.

For many frontier settlers, far removed from the larger towns and cities of reputable physicians, health issues loomed threateningly, and the sick jumped on any access to perceived expertise. As white communities were often located near native villages, there were ample opportunities to seek out indigenous shamans professing healing skills. Their brand of holistic care, involving use of various botanicals and divining methods, had some appeal to ailing homesteaders. The hint of spiritual messaging may have been particularly seductive to Christians, who prayed fervently themselves for divine intervention.

Southern lands—the Carolinas and Georgia—hosted a variety of trees, plants, and shrubs with medicinal properties, as pointed out by Native Americans and cultivated by early colonists. There was the medicinal sassafras tree, good for diseases of the blood and liver; the walnut or hickory tree, whose bark was an excellent remedy for general pains and gripes; china root, to cure bladder stones and gout, fevers, scurvy, and gonorrhea. And as for the venerable rattle snake root, "[i]n all Pestilential Distempers, as Plague, Small Pox, and Malignant Fevers, it's a Noble Specifick," one pioneer noted.[2]

Indigenous nations had a rich history in such matters. The dominant domestic people occupying southeastern North America in colonial times was the vast Cherokee Nation, inhabiting areas of backcountry North and South Carolina and Georgia. In fact, by the latter half of the eighteenth century, Cherokees claimed territory in what is now Virginia, Kentucky, Tennessee, the Carolinas, Georgia, Alabama, and Mississippi. Spread over this land in tribal communities were about twelve thousand of their number. Not that they were alone, intermingled were tribes of Creeks, Chickasaws, Tuscarora, Catawbas, and Yamasee.[3] Clashes with immigrant whites were inevitable, and hostility at European treachery rarely dormant. Of all the native nations east of the Mississippi River, only the Cherokees consistently remained friendly to the English. Among the others there seemed constant intrigue with British and French; both nations jockeyed for allegiance through trades, conspiracies, and trickery. The native tribes were equally pragmatic, switching their loyalty based on perceived advantage in European goods, particularly firearms. Such animosity and duplicity had predictable results. Settlers were easy prey for tribal violence; the South Carolina Yamasee massacres of 1715–1717 and the Natchez uprising in 1729 Louisiana were tragic examples. Even Cherokees were tempted by French provocateurs to sour on their English allies. The English tried desperately to counter this effort, offering newfound sentiments of solidarity and equality. A notable ambassador was Englishman Sir Alexander Cumming, who traveled west from Charleston in 1729 into the heart of the Cherokee Nation. He mingled convincingly with them and even convinced some to return to England with him to meet the king, a distinction empowering Native American chieftains with a certain flattery akin to royal status.[4]

As white settlers moved into the South, an allure with Native American mannerisms materialized. Always skeptical of European medicine, frontiersmen turned to their aboriginal neighbors for alternative treatment, some of it radically different and, by virtue of that, attractive. The Reverend John Clayton, pastor of the James City Parish in Virginia in the 1680s, was one such admirer. Upon visiting the local native villages, he acquainted himself with their conventions. "Nature is their great Apothecary," he discovered. They had a rich knowledge of local herbs and plants that, when duly processed, could provide a variety of responses: soothing remedies for sore throats and fevers, purgatives, emetics, and various salves for skin conditions and dropsy (edema). Natives shied from too much meddling. Bloodletting they did little of, Clayton recalled. What did impress him was their capacity to cure wounds. Their standard technique for open wounds and sores was a thorough cleansing, usually by sucking, then application of a paste of plant extract, then they bandaged the area. He described the care of one enslaved man ("a very good servant"), almost totally blind with an eye ailment. White surgeons the enslaver consulted were unable to help him. The enslaver then permitted a native doctor to try. The shaman promptly collected his special herbs, pounded them into a salve, smeared the goop onto a rag, and covered the man's eyes with it. The next day, sight was restored to one eye, and all pain had ceased. The enslaver was pleased, cure was declared, and the man returned to his labors.[5]

Such were indigenous healing practices. Shamans did much of the doctoring. They were considered almost divinely inspired and practiced their set of rituals that, in a scientific sense, had no proven merit. "They know little of the nature or reason things," Clayton was quick to conclude. Nevertheless, shamans, or medicine men as some called them, were almost sacred figures, venerated by the entire community.[6] Only they, it was believed, could communicate with the nether world and right a spiritual wrong so often thought to produce illness. They were the ones who straddled that Native American divide between the visible and invisible, who could treat the body or treat the soul. In so doing, shamans approached afflictions in two ways, then: "[T]hose in which the pain or disease is mastered and expelled directly by the shaman himself, with or without the help of his spirit guardians; and those where the shaman, become really more of a priest, carries out a more or less elaborate ceremonial, which, in virtue of its own inherent magical power, effects a cure."[7]

Yet healing was not just witchery. Tribal shamans used real concoctions as credible as those of Western medicine. Clayton wrote at length of the indigenous pharmacopoeia, including botanical medicine similar to opium and laudanum. He collected over three hundred herbal remedies with therapeutic properties, like angelica, a substance with remarkable potential: "It stops the Flux & cures it to a wonder; again it often loosens & purges the bodys [sic] of those that are bound, & have the gripes especially if it proceeds from a cold. & prevents many unhappy distempers." In fact, Clayton attributed angelica to saving his own life, caught in the miseries of the flux: "I take it to be the most sovereign remedy the world ever knew in the griping of those guts & admirable against Vapours."[8]

Such elixirs had a particular attraction for rural planters and traders. Native medicine seemed so much simpler and available. American botanist James W. Cooper wrote:

> Does it reflect honor on that kind Providence, who supplies the wants of all creatures, to suppose that the science of health, in which every child of Adam is so deeply concerned, must necessarily be the exclusive privilege of a few . . . requiring an age of study to explore and apply its principles to useful purposes? A reference to the Aborigines of our country is sufficient to refute such doctrine.[9]

There was no mystery, he implied. Schooling was irrelevant. Anyone adept at mashing, bruising, and boiling backyard plants could heal. Clayton was persuasive. It was almost a God-given right, he argued. Why use far-off European potions when so readily available was the vegetation of aboriginal America grown in the very climate that harbored the diseases they were designed to treat?

In the vast wilderness of the Louisiana Territory, European doctoring was even harder to find. Too often, there were few other options than indigenous healers. Rarely would physicians of any worth venture in. Trappers and traders were on their own, isolated, and living near tribal encampments in fidgety peace. In more friendly interludes, Native Americans and traders managed a transactional existence, including those related to health matters. Many times, whites relied heavily on shamans with their unique brand of medicine and rituals. No better example was that of French adventurer Antoine-Simon Le Page du Pratz.

Traveling up the Mississippi in 1718, du Pratz intended to develop a French concession (land grant) for his sponsor, investor Marc Hubert. The property would be known as the Saint Catherine concession, located close to the heart of the Natchez confederacy, or Grand Village. It was through two Natchez friendships, one of which was with the war chief of the village, that du Pratz was able to piece together an understanding of Natchez ethnography. What was most telling of Natchez customs was that of healing practices of local shamans, or what du Pratz called *jongleurs*.[10] Repeated attacks of sciatica brought on by the wet climate of the Mississippi had driven du Pratz eventually to the Natchez settlement in search of relief. He had tried French doctors in New Orleans whose bleedings and aromas did little good. The Natchez chief, the Grand Soleil, or "Great Sun," guaranteed a cure by his personal shaman. The shaman scarified du Pratz over the spots of his pain and applied a poultice to rid him of the evil spirits. Painful though the experience was, the next day, du Pratz felt a little relieved; the day after even more so. Eventually he fully recovered, totally enamored with the talents of his Natchez jongleur:

> What should I not have done for my recovery? In whose hands would I not have put myself, given the pains I felt? The remedy, moreover, was very simple according to the explanation given to me; it was only a question of a poultice; it was applied to the suffering part, and at the end of a week I was in a condition to go to the Fort. I was perfectly cured, since that time I have not felt it at all. What satisfaction for a young man who finds himself in good health after having been forced to remain in my house for four and a half months, without having been able to sally forth for a moment![11]

Not long afterward, du Pratz would again visit the Grand Soleil, this time for a troublesome fistula of his lacrimal duct—a painful eye condition. Again, French doctors were of no help, threatening to cauterize the eye and perhaps blind him. Suitably alarmed, du Pratz hurried to the Natchez encampment. The chief's personal shaman advised that du Pratz apply an herbal mixture and soak the eye in water daily, which du Pratz dutifully did. The fistula healed, and he never had another attack. Understandably, du Pratz was impressed with indigenous healers. He saw such cures work in others and, conversely, bungling by French doctors kill.[12] Even handling of war wounds was striking. Du Pratz witnessed healing of a gunshot to the jaw of the Great Chief of the Tunicas. French treatment for six weeks did nothing, but the Tunica shaman cured him in eight days. "There is no one in the colony who is unaware of the facts which I have just reported. These Doctors [shamans] have performed a large number of other cures, the narration of which would require a particular volume," du Pratz wrote.[13]

Jean-François-Benjamin Dumont de Montigny (1606–1760) was another Mississippi speculator whose curiosity about indigenous tribes along the way led him to mix with Native Americans and study their customs. His journeys took him to the regions of the Natchez and other lower Mississippi tribes. What captivated him was their profound belief in the spiritual impact on health. The jongleurs, as he also called them, were part healer, part sorcerer, and part priest. Devoid of any standard knowledge of anatomy or science, jongleurs artfully delivered comforting incantations and rituals that, if not curative, certainly soothed the anguish of the sufferer. At times, they produced as dramatic cures as the most skillful of French doctors. These native jongleurs blended plants and herbs, some of which produced astonishing relief of pain. Mostly, though, de Montigny considered jongleurs masters of the spiritual and healers of soul rather than body: "Besides the talent of Medicine which makes these [shamans] famous among these Peoples, they still have among them, as I said, the quality of *jongleurs*, that is to say, of Sorcerers and Diviners; and when some urgent need arises, whether private or public . . . one has recourse to these impostors, who, whatever way they go about it, seldom fail to give satisfaction to the requester."[14]

THE MANNER OF SAVAGES

In general, though, little respect for Native American practices filtered in from the hinterlands. Urbanized colonists flatly ignored reports of those like du Pratz, de Montigny, Clayton, and Cooper. More enlightened minds held indigenous people in low regard. Perhaps intriguing in an exotic way, they were clearly brutish in nature, so feelings went. "The Indians of North-America partake chiefly of the manner of savages," that paragon of American medicine Benjamin Rush announced in 1774.[15] Their "savage" manner, he explained, developed from a nomadic existence typified by fishing and hunting and overshadowed by "liberty and indolence."[16] The harshness of aboriginal lifestyle and constant exposure to the elements—the chief danger to disease, in his thinking—hardened the native from infancy to adulthood and altered response to life's infirmities. Diet was traditionally animal and vegetable, taken from the wild, and easily digestible. Their disposition was of a stoic nature; there was little complaining of pain or suffering. As far as native ailments, the only natural enemies to health, Rush had observed, were fevers, old age, casualties (accidental trauma), and war.

As for their healing practices, Rush had a special interest. Indigenous people resorted in many cases to "enchantment" as antidotes for complaints, he had heard. For such shadowy practices, Rush admitted, "[t]he influence of secrecy is well known in establishing the credit of a medicine."[17] The incantations, dances, and relics used by indigenous healers and diviners added mystery and magic to treatments and, like many traditional white methods, provided a sense of special powers to cure. Their botanical remedies, Rush believed, were completely without merit, nowhere near the equal of the science of European medicine. In terms of prescriptions, natives had little to offer Europeans, Rush claimed. They were ignorant of scientific medicine. In contrast to frontier experiences, in treating traumatic wounds, Rush thought many Native Americans surprisingly deficient. They could not set fractures and had no idea how to stop bleeding.

Yet in illness or injury, the Native American suffered well, Rush believed. "The Indian submits to his disease, without one fearful emotion from his doubtfulness of its event; and at last meets his fate, without an anxious with for futurity."[18] It is as if the Native American understood his simple role in the universe and trusted that death was only a transition from one world to another, from the seen to the unseen, of which indigenous people had a rich image. Treating sickness, then, was largely a measure of temporizing, not necessarily curing.

Many of Rush's generalizations were inaccurate. For one of such academic influence, he had not much practical experience with indigenous tribes. The great French doctor Pierre Jean Georges Cabanis (1757–1808) cautioned men like Rush when he wrote in 1798: "In medicine, everything, or almost everything depends on the glance and a fortunate instinct, certainties are to be found in the very sensations of the artist, rather than in the principles of art. He who has not seen objects has no idea of the proofs furnished by their observation; he who carries only inattentive or insensitive organs, has imperfect and deceptive ideas of them."[19] Indeed, among certain communities such as the Cherokee tribes, some healing methods were surprisingly effective.

Although they rarely resorted to surgery, when they did so, Cherokee healers could be skillful. Scarification for various conditions was practiced using sharpened animal bones or arrowheads. Fractures were aligned and immobilized by specially fashioned boards that functioned as splints. Natives knew, perhaps as even prehistoric man knew, that fractures needed rest to heal. A concoction of *tsi-yu* bark (from the tulip tree or poplar) was spread onto the fractured limb. Open wounds, like lacerations or gouges, were treated by application of that same *tsi-yu* bark. Often the shaman would sing chants over the victim. For those that bled profusely, the ligature was unheard of. Healers attempted to stop bleeding using various compressions such as plaster of buzzard's down, powdered gum, charcoal, and ashes. Some shamans could actually sew wounds together with animal sinews threaded onto crude needles. On occasion, more bizarre concoctions for healing were used, such as powdered insects or cow dung. As weird as some of these remedies seemed, remote settlers probably availed themselves of these men who probably were more accessible than physicians. Accidents of farming, foresting, and herding must have been commonplace, with their fractures and gashes demanding some type of treatment.[20] One could wonder, how many of these practices were soon adopted by white physicians who were at a loss to treat? Sadly, one might never know. What possible good would come from acknowledging a true therapeutic advantage to medicines of Benjamin Rush's "savages"?[21]

HERBALISTS, EMPIRICS, AND BOTANISTS

Regardless of their legitimacy, for the commonplace maladies of everyday life, English planters were eager to glean wisdom from the abundance of herbal and plant-based medicine the natives used. Stories of fantastic cures—frank miracles—fortified their curiosity and, in peaceful times, indigenous tribes were willing to share. For example, the Powhatan Nation that occupied coastal regions of Virginia catalogued almost ninety plants used for medicinal purposes. Tribes used root or root bark, sap, leaves, berries, buds, or whole plants for a variety of illness as purges, antidiarrheal agents, and for hemorrhoid flares. Ground plants, bark, and roots were given for menstrual distress, coughs, dyspepsia, skin conditions, and as general stimulants. Five plants were promoted for wound-curing, including herbaceous juicy extracts applied to cuts, scrapes, and bruises. A few of these were unabashedly used by whites, including angelica (laxative) and *Rubus* species (diarrhea).[22]

Catawba tribes of South Carolina, coexisting with Cherokees, shared similar healing practices, including a range of botanical and animal-derived medicine. Some of these found their way into pantries of neighboring settlers and doctors, including smell-root (*Hedeoma pulegioides*) for colds; bear root for rheumatism and fevers; holly leaves for measles; star-grass leaves (*Aletrias farinose*) for bloody dysentery—"it stops blood at once"; and yellow-root for jaundice. For common ailments such as colds, Catawba prescribed syrups of mullen root, wild plum bark, wild cherry bark, holly bark, green pine needles, catnip, life everlasting leaves, and sourwood bark, all boiled and reduced were ingested.[23] Adjacent Creek tribes of Georgia even tried honey locust for the smallpox to placate the misery of pustules, but nothing seemed to really help.[24]

Logic for their selection by natives was, perhaps, as fascinating as the substances themselves. Uncommonly were prescriptions founded on consistent observable benefit but, rather, on reputed messages to shamans from their spirit world, often via dreamlike connections. For example, concerning the cassena (*Ilex cassine*), a species of holly, American botanist Benjamin Smith Barton wrote in 1810,

> The Savages of Carolina . . . have this tea in veneration, above all the plants they are acquainted withal, and tell you, the discovery thereof was by an infirm Indian, that labored under the burden of many rugged distempers, and could not be cured by all their Doctors; so, one day, he fell asleep, and dreamt, that if he took a decoction of the tree that grew at his head, he would certainly be cured. He followed the directions of his dream, and became perfectly well.[25]

The tea was widely used as a violent emetic and purgative, forcefully expelling any number of offensive miasmas infecting victims.[26] Of course, this added to the skepticism of colonial physicians but still did not quiet their ardor for anything remotely effective.

Probably as a result, and despite stupendous anecdotes, few tribal botanicals seemed to possess genuine efficacy when scrutinized. No better ethnographer on the subject of Native botanicals and rituals was there than James Mooney (1861–1921), a figure known as the "Indian Man" who had lived among the tribes and studied their behavior. When Mooney looked at reports from the United States Dispensary done in 1877, only one-third of Cherokee plant medicine had any real effect. Academic physicians never were impressed by the botanicals. Nevertheless, settlers reached for anything in times of distress, and traditional doctors failed to offer anything better. As the French botanical surveyor Constantine Samuel Rafinesque (1783–1840) wrote in 1828: "When America was settled, the native tribes were in possession of many valuable vegetable remedies, discovered by long experience, the knowledge of which they gradually imparted to their neighbors. This knowledge partly adopted even as far as Europe, and partly rejected by medical skeptics, became scattered through our country in the hands of country practitioners, Herbalists, Empirics, and Botanists."[27] Yet not a few physicians and scientists felt that, in general, botanicals were the future of medical science. So many plants and herbs were novelties to Europeans that, in theory, there must be new medicines among them. Even as the colonies were staked out, traveling botanists scoured the countryside and snooped among indigenous communities for any herbs or plants that might hold promise. Respected colonial botanists like John Josselyn, John Bartram, and Pehr Kalm faithfully logged any number of medicinal plants and herbs, many used by native tribes for healing purposes.

John Josselyn (1638–1675) wrote of application of alder-bark as "Indians" do for cuts, bruises, and burns; water-lily roots for wounds. The bark was chewed into a gummy paste and applied to the injury. Natives also used birch bark, boiled and crushed between stones, the poultice poured into the wound. Tobacco boiled in water could also be used for burns. Watermelon was used for the "sick of fevers, and other hot diseases" with good success. Sarsaparilla had a variety of uses: for fevers, for colds, and for fluxes, even for wounds and burns. Josselyn also made note of other remedies used: tobacco for "scirrhous tumour." Natives had any number of other botanicals available for astringents, tonics, stimulants, emetics, and cathartics. In fact, nineteenth-century preacher, farmer, and physician Peter Smith—formally educated at Princeton—compiled an extensive text of herbs, roots, and other remedies learned from natives of the Southeast, primarily those of Georgia, that he titled *The Indian Doctor's Dispensatory*. His compendium offered botanical-based cures for a variety of diseases for the common man. It was a pamphlet for the literate settler populating America's frontiers. "My prescriptions," he wrote, "I must leave to speak for themselves." In terms of their societal usefulness, he spoke no clearer than references to his own loved ones. "I, however, feel a degree of satisfaction in thinking that herein I have in prospect the real benefit of my own children and of their rising, numerous progeny and my fellow men in general."[28]

John Bartram (1699–1777), a noted botanist from Pennsylvania, chronicled his extensive trip through the South in 1765 and 1766, recording with exquisite precision any number of plants and trees, some of which he described were favored by native people and cultivated in numbers of their settlements. He shipped many seeds from the New World to his home England. So famous was he that King George III conferred the title "King's Botanist for North America" on him. The Finnish explorer and botanist Pehr (Peter) Kalm (1716–1779) was a contemporary and friend of Bartram. He wrote the influential *Travels into North America*, a dossier on plantations and agriculture throughout the colonies in the 1740s, listing hundreds of species of plants, numbers of which he discovered on his journeys among indigenous societies.[29]

Fieldwork by experts such as these led to a better understanding of botanicals chosen locally as useful pharmaceuticals. Shortly, they would find their way into the pharmacopoeias of practicing colonial physicians and even the almanacs of medical opportunists. Of course, proper credit to indigenous tribes was rarely forthcoming. "The mention of the Indian by these medical botanists was not intended to praise or give credit to the Indians as much as it was to provide an additional example of what the plant was purportedly useful for," historian David L. Cowen wrote.[30] Perhaps one of the most notable examples of such medical plagiarism was the story of Samuel Thomson (1769–1843). A self-taught botanist, Thomson started a peculiar variety of botanical therapeutics, feeling that ordinary physicians were literally killing their patients with toxic chemicals like calomel (the ubiquitous mercurial compound). His botanical listings—many copied from indigenous practices—were simplified to the point that even the illiterate, of which in frontier America there were quite a few, could understand. Medicine is of paramount importance to lessen the burden of human suffering, Thomson began his 1822 pamphlet *New Guide to Health: Or, Botanic Family Physician*. Yet the queries of wise men through the ages have done little to attain this end, he went on. "Their inquiries it would seem have been directed to the investigation of visionary theories . . . to the neglect of what is of the greatest importance,—correct and useful practice by a direct application to the cause of disease." It had broad appeal to rural America, tiring of the quacks who dotted the countryside. Thomson's mismanagement and temperamental personality, though, soon killed his almanac, which slipped into the dusty shelves of obscurity.[31]

Even with scientific progress of the mid-nineteenth century, folk medicine—largely indigenous in origin—would endure. Especially in the rural South, the secessional Confederacy would depend heavily on trafficking of local herbs and plants for healing during the Civil War, and the expanding western frontiers of America following the war would once again put settlers in proximity to native tribes and far from traditional "European" medicine. Once again, backyard concoctions would find a place on the shelves of homesteaders. But as civilization progressed and urbanization of the West unfolded, systemization and regulation of pharmaceuticals would gradually render the herbs and plants of America's forebearers obsolete and untested. But with persistent frustrations toward unpredictable orthodox medicine, they would never completely disappear either.

CHAPTER NINE

SOUTHERN MEDICINE FOR SOUTHERN SICKNESS

> It is notorious, that practitioners educated northwardly, and who have even had experience there, are perfect novices with the principal diseases of our climate.
> —ANONYMOUS GEORGIA PHYSICIAN

A distinctiveness of lifestyle and economy was evolving from a distinctiveness of climate and soil. For those of the medical profession, there seemed a peculiar oddity to southern disease. Were those same climatic forces that stymied scientists and settlers also altering and even exacerbating sicknesses of everyday life? If so, might it be, then, that a knowledge of southern brands of illness best be served by education in the South? One who felt so, physician Erasmus Fenner, warned southern doctors of the dangers of their singular paradise by his stirring invocation in the inaugural issue of the new journal *Southern Medical Reports* in 1849:

> In respect to medical literature and science, our lot has been cast in a region where they have as yet been but slightly cultivated—a region vast in extent and abounding in the sources of human life and comfort—already inhabited by millions of human beings, and capable of maintaining tens of millions. But this fair and beautiful section of the globe is not supplied by the hand of Providence with its rich luxuriance of blessings and comforts, unmixed with the sources of suffering and of death. Here, as everywhere else, good and evil are remingled in the cup of life; almost every comfort and advantage is accompanied by a

corresponding danger, and man's intelligence, is his only dependence for safety and happiness.[1]

He acknowledged the educational opportunities of the North and its pipeline to Europe. Fenner admitted that many northern physicians had been preceptors and role models in the principles of medicine. Yet it alone could not supplant experience by *personal observation* that southern physicians gleaned. Physicians of the South had not taken the lead, he conceded, and as a result, "our [southern] Profession" has lost respectability and claim to legitimate domains by virtue of "indolence and neglect."[2]

Fenner might well know. One well familiar with southern life, he had practiced in the most rural of areas of Mississippi in the 1830s. Physicians who trickled into those areas were ill-prepared for the malicious afflictions they would encounter, many of whom fell victim themselves to the awful epidemics:

> It was there [Mississippi] that I first became familiar with that terrific type of malarious fever, the congestive, which consigned thousands of victims to their final doom. Amidst the rapid immigration, there was an influx of young and inexperienced physicians, fresh from the Medical Colleges, where they had been taught everything better than the nature and treatment of the very diseases they were to encounter. The consequence was, they sacrificed their own lives in great numbers whilst striving to stay the hand of death among their fellow citizens with a devotion worthy of a better fate."[3]

In fact, southern medical practices were still heavily influenced by traditional teachings of the North. Prescriptions stemming from those schools might hardly be applicable to the witnessed varieties of southern diseases. But what alternative had there been? The agrarian regions of the Carolinas, Georgia, and Louisiana had been lame facsimiles of academic medicine. In the words of historian Richard Shryock, "the lack of urban cultural centers in the South retarded the development of medical schools and other professional institutions."[4]

Not that northern medicine was all that enviable. The healing arts as a whole were in a deplorable state early in the nineteenth century. This originated in part from glaring deficiencies in standardizing medical education. Some schooling lasted not even four months. Some practitioners had received no formal instruction. The absence of hospitals (except in a few northern cities), aside from asylums, orphanages, and homes for the impoverished, well or ill, meant that much of medical education had to be didactic. Apprenticeships—following a practitioner from home to home—or attending at such public domiciles were the only way that young physicians-to-be would obtain practical knowledge. Quackery abounded with little regulation or supervision. Joseph Eve, professor at the Medical College of Georgia, called for radical reform in the education system, a system he felt was riddled with abuses and inadequacies. "The spirit of the times calls aloud for reformation," he wrote in 1836, "the rapid march of intellect—the numerous important discoveries and improvements in the arts and sciences require it now and ere long the voice of a more enlightened people will demand it."[5]

A growing sense of southern sectionalism fueled an extrapolation of Eve's argument for a separate southern medical education. The rural temperament of society in southern regions only amplified the isolationism medical professionals felt, and it forced an unbalanced attention to remedies not so much scientific as available and biased by traditional folklore and acceptance. Plain and simple, people of the South were sicker, their illnesses different, and customary therapeutics ineffective.

∽

For American medical professionals, Europe was a lure. In the nineteenth century, it was the font from which all knowledge flowed—refinements in learning a must for those able to do so. And in the early decades of that century, Americans were in love with Paris. Parisian science rose to the forefront and provided ample opportunities for American physicians, the pinnacle of formal education. Exposure to diseases was unrivaled anywhere else, certainly not in America. What captivated audiences was a revolution in thinking. Parisian clinicians were empiricists; observation replaced Hippocratic and Galenic supposition (so-called rationalism). If it could not be demonstrated or observed, despite hypotheses to the contrary, it was not to be believed. This was a new construct in medical thinking and medical therapeutics. From a practical standpoint, Paris furnished endless patients, paraded and examined before crammed auditoriums (too often indecorously). Bodies for anatomic dissection abounded. Cadavers offered chances to hone surgical technique. And professors waxed tirelessly of the human condition and its ailments. It was all enthralling, such a vigor to medical science. Such a contrast to the young United States, where no structured system of medical education, little governmental support, and bare financial backing was a plague of its own.

Yet European society did not gel with American clinicians. There was much to admire about European culture and sophistication, but much to dislike. Americans tended to favor a Jeffersonian approach to cultural independence and hastened to free themselves from the perceived corruption and anachronistic mire of ancient regimes. With medicine, similar feelings prevailed. European knowledge lacked practical application, something in which American physicians prided themselves. Continental physicians seemed more concerned about diagnoses and pathology than healing patients. Despite their pomp, Parisian therapeutic methods were felt either unnecessarily heartless or weak and ineffectual. And visiting Americans were quick to point it out. From his travels to Europe in the 1830s, New York surgeon Valentine Mott wrote, "It must strike every observer who walks in the hospitals of Paris, that the great ambition of her medical men seems too much absorbed with the desire to verify the justness of their *diagnosis* and *prognosis* by the *autopsies* and *post-mortem* examinations of their patients, rather than scrutinizing and seeking sedulously with unremitted vigilance for remedies for healing the maladies of the sick."[6]

Little value, it seems, was placed on preventing suffering or preserving life. In fact, impersonality dominated clinical behavior. As historian John Harley Warner characterized it, "Such attitudes, Americans widely maintained, enabled the French surgeons and physicians alike to regard patients as objects to be studied [good for American education but poor for ailing victims] more than as subject to be healed."[7] In fact, this behavior elevated Parisian clinicians to almost a mythical status, the image of a professionally ruthless doctor exhibiting no fear (or remorse) in embarking on decisive but brutal operations more compelling than a kinder, more hesitant healer. This was in contradistinction to the very personal nature of the American medicine of rural communities, where interactions of patients and their doctors was but one aspect of the social fabric. American physicians embraced specificity of therapy. Treatment, they felt, should be matched not only to disease but to patient individuality and even the environment. As Warner explained, "The epidemiological, meteorological, demographic, and social differences between Europe and America similarly demanded that therapeutics be adjusted for application within these different contexts."[8] French therapeutics, Americans thought, ignored such considerations and were not relevant. Too passive, many American physicians agreed, not in line with an interventionalist, active approach to patients' ills. This became particularly central to treatments in the South, where even more the rural nature of practice mandated special attention to environmental factors.

Still, any attempt at an academic unraveling of biologic mysteries had been lacking in the South. As a consequence, some believed the South hopelessly backward. The eminent Canadian Sir William Osler, in his essay "An Alabama Student," related the story of a southern doctor distressed by the lack of science and education in his native state. Young John Bassett, by his own effort and sacrifice, had visited the centers of medicine in England and France and had been taken by the industrious attitude of some of their great minds. Traveling to Paris he had an eye-opening experience on the competitiveness and drive of all Parisian physicians:

> When I look at some of the medical men by whom I am surrounded, it makes me blush for shame; old men daily may be seen mixing their white locks with boys, and pursuing their profession with the ardour of youth. Here is not a solitary great man in France that is idle, for if he was, that moment he would be out stripped; it is a race, and there are none so far ahead that they are not pressed by others; many are distanced, it is true, but there are none allowed to walk over the course.[9]

In returning to his native South, Bassett was immediately taken by a pervasive southern indolence. Physicians there had assumed an unquestioning and passive dependence on northern medical dogma, distinct obstacles to a robust scientific thinking, he felt.

What bred this lassitude that had, in Bassett's eyes, little practicality for the nuances of southern living? In the backcountry of Alabama and Mississippi there existed a breed of men who, as Bassett maintained, lived apart from wealthy planters and native tribes and who subscribed to the "mysterious economy of nature." These backwoods types were ingenious, hardy, and voracious in their appetite for gain. Physicians who served them, Bassett believed, despite their training and diplomas, were equally isolated and, "suffer themselves to grow so dull in diagnosis as to bleed a typhoid patient half an hour before death." Quackery was indigenous in such areas, "springing up like mushrooms in a spring morning." Bassett firmly held that education and more education was imperative to maintain healing skills. Exposure to the great minds of academia fostered curiosity and an abiding desire to excel. All too often, such stimulation was not present in the rural South. Trickery and charlatanism propagated far and wide, without the presence of learned men contradicting such abominations.[10]

Yet even in the urban North, academic medicine had a daunting task. Ascent to global respectability would be a laboriously slow process. From earliest colonial times few erudite institutions existed for the proper development of medical education. The first medical school in the thirteen colonies had opened in 1765, as a branch of the College of Philadelphia, a move championed by physician John Morgan. Morgan and William Shippen Jr., both graduates of the University of Edinburgh, assembled a rigorous curriculum, including a baccalaureate degree, mastery of Latin, mathematics, and natural philosophy (the baccalaureate requirement was shortly relaxed). In fact, William Shippen delivered the first set of anatomical lectures in North America. The course work was a combination of didactic teaching and bedside apprenticeship, based on European models. The College of Philadelphia was formally designated the University of Pennsylvania by charter in 1791 and became the foremost center of medical learning in the country.[11] By 1800 there were three other medical schools affiliated with established colleges: King's College, New York (1767); Harvard College near Boston (1783); and Dartmouth College in New Hampshire (1797). Without doubt, the Pennsylvania school was top-notch by American standards. The likes of scholarly teachers such as Benjamin Rush, Philip Syng Physick, and John Redman Coxe were without equal in America.

For southern students pursuing a medical career, though, Philadelphia held most interest. There seemed to be an intangible sympathy for southern temperaments. Southerners sensed a not-so-subtle antipathy to slave reform, and Philadelphians cherished their mannered aristocracy, reminiscent of southern culture. The city and its society were gateways to social respectability and access to networks, both professional and social, requisite for true American gentlemen and future cultivated icons.[12] In 1830 almost half (204/421) of its enrollees were southerners. Within the decade two-thirds of the graduates were from southern states, including Virginia, Georgia, Alabama, Mississippi, and Louisiana.[13] In contrast, at Yale and Harvard, only a rare student hailed from Dixie.[14] Within decades, the University of Pennsylvania medical school overflowed with eager students and applicants. Demand far exceeded supply. Efforts began in 1818 to establish a second medical school in Philadelphia. In 1826, the first class entered the new Jefferson Medical College. By 1840, more than two in five graduates from that school were from the South as well. By 1850, the number rose to half.[15]

One of the more famous southern physicians to attend the University of Pennsylvania was Richmond, Virginia, native Solomon Mordecai (1792–1869). Solomon was the son of the prominent Jacob Mordecai. Jacob had grown up in Philadelphia but moved south when his mother remarried Jacob Cohen from Richmond. Jacob Mordecai developed a lucrative mercantile business around Richmond and became a pillar of that society. His son Solomon benefited from the family wealth and excelled in his schoolwork. He was even a teacher at his father's private school for girls in Warrenton, North Carolina. But the restless Solomon wanted more and traveled to Philadelphia for a career in medicine. Southern medical students in Philadelphia were, for the most part, looked upon kindly. An article in the Washington newspaper the *National Intelligencer and Washington Advertiser* spoke of the generosity of Philadelphians in their hospitality and sympathy to southern students. Yet there remained a disgruntled group of northerners not so enamored. Southern students were little more than delinquent youths, more interested in drinking and carousing than serious study, so some claimed. The *New York Sun* newspaper had characterized the antebellum southern medical student as "a long-haired, lantern-jawed, verdant youth afflicted with chronic salivation and inveterate profanity," reared in the "semi-savage solitude of a remote plantation."[16]

But this was not Solomon. Instead, he launched into a determined and unquenchable pursuit of knowledge. Beyond book learning, the young Virginian put in endless hours studying patients and their illnesses as house physician at the Pennsylvania Hospital and the Philadelphia Almshouse.[17] Such a quest was the task of each medical student to do so. Requisite coursework generally consisted of two four-month terms of lectures followed by completion of a thesis and a final examination. In contrast to centers in Europe, exposure to living patients was a rare treat. Like others, Solomon had to patch his clinical education together. The lecture halls delivered little practical knowledge. They were crowded, noisy sessions, often with three to four hundred students in attendance, some so far away from any demonstrations as to be essentially absent. He wrote his sister, Ellen, from Philadelphia in 1819: "As yet my mind is not stored with sufficient knowledge to enable me to profit by what I hear and see, but I persevere in the hope of catching a ray of light to direct my efforts which now like a man whose vision is rendered obscure, falter and grope in the dark."[18] As house physician, Solomon quickly rose to senior ranks, which allowed him to learn surgical and obstetrical procedures and to handle emergencies, prescribe treatments, and perform usual bedside maneuvers such as bleeding, cupping, and leeching. By April of his second year, Mordecai was a trusted figure at the Philadelphia Almshouse, competent in his procedures and unswerving in patient care. The weight of responsibility, particularly as a senior student, showed in his letters home. "I must endeavor by observations and attention to prepare myself to discharge a duty in which the welfare of human beings and my own peace of mind will be so intimately entwined."[19] Time spent at the almshouse proved to be the most formative of his life, he later admitted. There was no richer experience than the surgery, obstetrics, and medical aid he could provide to the helpless poor. With his innate concern, his care was diligent and thoughtful. They no doubt benefitted immensely from one so devoted.

While more affluent students planned travels to Europe upon finishing, this was not to be Solomon's fate. His finances, generous as they were, were not sufficient for such dalliances. A successful medical practice in Philadelphia, prestigious though it might have been, was also elusive for a fresh graduate with no deep ties to the medical community. And so, in early 1822 Mordecai returned to his native Virginia. But even this would be disappointing. Seeing that there was an overabundance of doctors in the upper South, Mordecai reluctantly sought practice elsewhere and eventually relocated to Mobile, Alabama, in 1823, where he practiced the rest of his career. Why Solomon chose Mobile is something of a mystery, although the Mordecai family was acquainted with Samuel Myers, a Jewish merchant in Pensacola but with connections in Mobile. Jews were welcomed in Mobile, the largely Catholic community more tolerant than their Protestant counterparts. So, Myers likely influenced Solomon on the opportunities for a Jewish physician there—opportunities that rarely existed in the South.[20] Expecting that Mobile would be a temporary stop in his career, it was there that Solomon Mordecai would marry, raise a family, purchase property, and live his profession as one of Mobile's most respected Jewish members.

To southerners like Solomon Mordecai, eager for a medical career—and able to afford even a modicum of one—in the early 1800s, there was no alternative but northward. At the turn of the nineteenth century, no formal medical schooling could be found in the South. Transylvania College, in Lexington, Kentucky, just west of the Alleghenies, opened in 1800 for preceptorships but was barely in Dixie. And the countryside was sparsely populated. Without mentors, classrooms, and sufficient clinical material, young men who featured to practice medicine trudged north to Philadelphia or beyond, paid the steep tuition required, and embarked on one or two years of study and apprenticeship.

Not always did they come back. For example, by 1800, there were not one hundred practicing doctors in the state of Georgia, and even fewer formally trained with credible degrees. Urban centers such as Charleston and Savannah fared better. City living appealed to learned men like David Ramsay. Diseases ran rampant—more so, it seemed, in crowded conditions—and there was no shortage of desperately ill people. Not so in the country, where day-to-day medical care was largely the domain of mothers, midwives, and self-proclaimed folk healers, whether of indigenous or immigrant status. Rural health care was fraught with such oddities; anyone with ingenuity could formulate a botanical concoction and peddle it as a supposed cure—mostly for profit.[21] Even more reputable doctors were often only part-time practitioners, their major income derived elsewhere, many from estate agriculture. No wonder such conventions bred erratic treatments and elusive ethical principles. Lacking academic encouragement, then, any local youth wanting a medical career—unless uncommonly wealthy—latched onto a willing physician (respected or otherwise) and hoped for an apprenticeship. The more well-meaning—and well-monied—might have tried for some type of proprietary schooling, usually of an abbreviated duration (many medical "courses" were only weeks long). Educated or not, it all made little difference. Colonial therapeutics—even by the most well-intentioned—ranged from the ineffectual to the harmful. In the end, physicians' bedside comfort and hand-holding often mattered most.

Still, the stifling conditions of climate and geography bestowed on the South a brand of medical distinctiveness that would only add to a societal and economic one. Physicians could not resist the draw of disease and the fertile professional opportunities offered. That, at first, so few of any repute practiced there only whetted their appetites. And as southern lifestyle fostered a feeling of separatism from the North, so did health matters. Southern physicians began to resent their reliance on a North whose medical instruction had no bearing on the distinctive health problems of the South. Instead, let southern men learn medicine in the South. Let there be southern education for southern physicians.[22]

SOUTH CAROLINA

Efforts to educate physicians had begun early in colonial Charleston, South Carolina. By mid-eighteenth century, ambitious young Charlestonians were already serving apprenticeships under "respectable" physicians like David Ramsay, David Oliphant, and Peter Fayssoux. After five or six years as apprentices, those that could were off to Edinburgh for three or four years, returning home with their coveted degrees in medicine. It was that European exposure that imbued them with legitimacy as a learned practitioner of physic. David Ramsay, himself a product of colonial schooling, felt European voyages were expensive and wasteful. Besides, he facetiously argued, English weather was "too cold for young Carolinians." Instead, he proposed the radical idea of medical training right there in Charleston. To that end, he and friend Peter Fayssoux formed the first local medical society as a prelude. The society gathered like-minded doctors as an intellectual, political, and governing force for regulation of the profession. Their hope was to establish homogeneity, rid the field of charlatans, and lay the groundwork for formal education.[23] The Medical Society of South Carolina was thus formed in 1789, with David Ramsay elected its first president.

As for the medical school, it would be a convoluted process. Not until 1821, six years after David Ramsay's death, did Charleston physicians Henry Frost, James Ramsay (son of David Ramsay), and Samuel Dickson begin serious discussions on the project: a medical school for South Carolina. Some months later, in February 1822, Thomas Cooper, president of the liberal arts South Carolina College in Columbia, allied with the Charleston doctors and delivered an impassioned address before the Medical Board of Columbia on the merits of a medical college in South Carolina. The Medical Board was so moved by the petition that they sent it on to the Medical Society in Charleston. Instead of a site in Columbia, however, as Cooper had suggested (thinking, of course, it should be a branch of his own college), the Medical Society, mostly Charleston residents, considered it more apropos that the school should be in Charleston.[24] To that end, the society approached local Charleston College for a blending of resources. Trustees of the college refused; their school was struggling financially and had devastating property damage from the hurricane of 1822.[25] Undaunted, the Medical Society then developed a petition to the state legislature to approve the measure in principle only; funding could come later. In December 1823 the legislature, in a sweeping action of approval, agreed: "Be it therefore enacted, that from and after the passing of this act, the Medical Society of South Carolina shall be, and they are hereby authorized to organize a medical school to consist of such professorships as they may deem expedient, and to confer medical degrees upon such candidates as may qualify themselves therefor, under the regulations which they may establish."[26] But as expected, they offered no funding. Encouraged by their action, though, the Medical Society pushed ahead and named six professors for the faculty. The initial teachers were impressive men like James Ramsay and Samuel Dickson, but all required to bear the cost of their endeavor. Having no building for students, the Medical Society obtained from the City of Charleston land next to the Marine Hospital and constructed temporary housing for anatomy and chemistry. From those makeshift quarters, five students graduated on April 4, 1825.

At his oration for the commencement of the second session of 1825, Samuel Dickson offered no apologies for American medical education, claiming it was more practical than the centers in Europe. Unlike European "deeply read scholars," American young men needed to learn the necessary skills and knowledge to carry out the duties of an active professional life in the frontiers of the American wilderness. That was American medicine, meant for the people and practiced in backwoods America. No better example than the South, Dickson added: "What would it avail the young graduate to have received instruction from the lips of a Sydenham, a Boerhaave or a Cullen, if he were not taught by them the modifications necessary to be observed in the application of their principles under the variable influences of habit and climate, and of constitutions liable to be changed by both climate and habit."[27] Climate affected illness just as it did agriculture, Dickson maintained. Still, the basics were vital: anatomy and therapeutics led the list, to be taught by reputable men of the profession. There was no better group, Dickson was confident, than members of the Medical Society who first envisioned this Carolinian school. And what better way to learn medical skills than locally, in the very heart of their homeland.

By the 1827 session, enrollment had ballooned to 129 students, 101 of whom were from South Carolina. However, costs for the school were becoming onerous on the faculty. By 1830, each member had incurred several thousand dollars of debt; there arose no mean amount of grumbling. Frustrated by lack of support and other perceived ruses, the faculty resigned en masse to re-form a new medical school in 1832 they called the Medical College of the State of South Carolina. Students followed, unaware of (or unconcerned for) the political intrigues of the matter and quite fond of their teachers. Their home now was the old Charleston Theater Building. The respected James Moultrie (1793–1869), who had been part of the original faculty, accepted the position of professor of physiology. At its opening on November 10, 1834, Moultrie spoke with the force of a zealot, convinced that his vocation was divinely inspired. He was impressed with the trappings of French education: state control, faculty salaries, better pre-medical schooling, and extended courses of study. Similar changes were needed in America if physicians were to be more than rote practitioners. Critical thinking and a scientific rationale were essential—not mere bedside acrobatics. Think and analyze, he encouraged. Embrace a "spirit of inquiry." Strive for excellence to match that of England or France right here in Charleston, he urged.[28]

Where to find enough patients for study? The venerable Charleston Marine Hospital, that refuge for seafarers and destitute citizens, and the local Poor House were chosen. Their histories dated back to 1738, when a group of wealthy Charleston businessmen confronted the growing problem of derelicts who were overrunning the city. Poverty and homelessness were on the rise throughout the colonies. As for Charleston, herd them to the parish (of Saint Philips) workhouse, they decided. The workhouse was set up two years prior "for the Better Relief of and Employment of the Poor."[29] These workhouses at the time were the repository for all types of ne'er-do-wells: vagabonds, the impoverished, the insane, as well as the ill. Workhouse, of course, was a misnomer. Little work was done there. It functioned more as a simple structure for detention of undesirables. In that sense, they were forerunners of public confinements such as asylums, hospitals, orphanages, nursing homes, and even prisons. Now all indigents "and other lewd, idle and disorderly Persons" were to be corralled there. In the port city of Charleston, many of these unfortunates were destitute or sick seamen. Growing numbers of inmates dictated new facilities, which were constructed in 1768 and again in 1856.[30]

Mixing rowdy and smelly sailors with other unfortunates was apparently a bad idea as the numbers of sailors and their rancid habits quickly overwhelmed space and whatever decorum remained. To segregate them from the general indigent population, a separate Marine Hospital strictly for sailors opened in 1787.[31] The old workhouse was, at some point, renamed the Poor House. And so it came to pass that in 1831; the two institutions—the Marine Hospital and the Poor House—were taken over by the faculty of the reorganized Medical College. Two years later, a larger Marine Hospital was built adjacent to a new lecture hall for medical students. Doctor William Ramsay, then physician in charge, gave a glowing description of the structure: "The Charleston Marine Hospital . . . is a commodious and airy building . . . and has double piazzas to the north, south, and west, which are appropriated to the use of the patients . . . There are eight wards—three on the first floor, for surgical cases and five on the second floor." Ramsay emphasized that the Marine Hospital would play a pivotal role in medical education: "[I]t has been my endeavor to render this institution a source of instruction to students prosecuting their studies in this city." Enrolled students could take advantage of clinical lectures as well as opportunities to accompany physicians every morning. Ramsay felt a hospital was the best "text book" to the student. It was a cornerstone of their training.[32]

It was all received with great fanfare. The *Charleston Daily Courier* of November 14, 1837, announced the opening of the Medical and Surgical Infirmary, presumably referring to the Marine Hospital, and explicitly linked it to the Medical College of the State of South Carolina. "To the poor, who may select this as a private Hospital, every necessary and comfort will be offered," the article continued. And as for enslaved persons, an incentive to enslavers: "The masters of servants are assured that the most diligent care will be taken ... and all Medical and Surgical aid offered, without making them liable to any professional charges." The sole object, the *Courier* emphasized, was to "promote the interest of Medical education within their native State and City."[33]

By 1838, the old medical college founded by Dickson and Ramsay languished from inattention and students, finally closing its doors that same year. At that point, the Medical Society relinquished control and threw its support for the Medical College of the State of South Carolina.[34] During the demise of the old school and rise of the new one, animosity surfaced between a hostile Medical Society and a disinterested legislature. Yet by 1838 tempers had quieted and cordiality resumed. Trustees for the new school were eventually picked from lay individuals who bestowed the faculty with authority for management of the school's composition and curriculum. Samuel Dickson said of those times:

> In vain we have been assailed with all the weapons of malignant warfare; and the ultimate amount of advantage gained by the persevering hostility directed against us, has been merely to wrest from us for a time the results of the well-won munificence of the Legislature ... in behalf of my colleagues of the Faculty and of the Board of Trustees, a cordial welcome to this edifice now dedicated to science and philanthropy.[35]

It would be, Dickson foretold, a medical college in which southern youth could receive an education by southern teachers in the climate and culture of the South. Yet Moultrie's "spirit of inquiry" was slow to materialize. It took a full decade before the course of instruction was increased from four to five months, a paltry comparison to European academia. Yet the school began to demand evidence of maturation, ambition, and determination. By 1850, graduates were to be at least twenty-one years of age, of good moral character, have attended two full courses of lectures, studied medicine as an apprentice for three years, and completed an inaugural thesis.[36]

GEORGIA

For the town of Augusta, upriver from the port city of Savannah, there had been an evolution from frontier trading post to a vibrant economy centered on the tobacco market. But the agrarian lifestyle meant a dispersed population of planters and yeoman farmers. As a vital cornerstone of community, health care suffered from few physicians. Like many parts of the South, scattered legitimate practitioners in the backcountry mixed with local healers and assorted quacks and vied for patients. As Augusta's population grew, the town took on a more urban role as a hub of commerce for the frontiers. With that came a certain desire to urbanize medical care as well, and the first City Hospital was erected in 1818, ten beds for the poor and infirmed. Yet Augusta was hardly equipped as a center for medicine. Local schooling in medicine might hold the key, and that task fell to a remarkable Georgian by the name of Milton Antony (1789–1839).

His ancestors may have been the characters of fiction. According to genealogist Nancy Vashti Anthony Jacob,[37] Marcus Anthony (she spells "Anthony" not "Antony") was the son of a Genoese merchant who immigrated from Italy to Holland. The father, desiring a proper Italian education for his son, sent Marcus back to Italy. But the restless youth ran away to sea, where Algerian pirates captured him and sold him into slavery. Abused and mistreated, this supposed ancestor, Anthony, butchered his enslaver with an axe, fled through the woods to a beach, found a boat, and rowed to an anchored British vessel. He managed to convince the British captain to take him aboard. The British ship then deposited Marcus in Virginia. He was then "sold" into service as an indentured servant for three years to pay for his passage. Following his period of servitude, Anthony moved to the upper James River around 1700, where he established a mill and trading post from which he accumulated a large fortune.

Nancy Jacob claims that Milton Antony was the son of James Anthony Jr. (great grandson of Marcus Anthony) and Elizabeth Blakely.[38] It is a great story but unlikely true. James Anthony Jr. was born in 1782 and Milton *Antony* in 1789. If Milton Antony was descended from the Antony (Anthony) lineage, it is more likely he was the son of James Anthony Sr. This is also questionable. Milton Antony is never mentioned as an offspring of the senior Anthony. Furthermore, Milton's surname never appears other than "Antony" in Georgia records. Whether he was, in fact, a descendant of a wealthy Virginian merchant, servant, slave, murderer, and runaway is fascinating conjecture but a matter of some fancy.

Whatever his ancestry, Milton's early life was more mundane. His family indeed had moved from Virginia to Wilkes County, Georgia, when Milton was just two years of age. Like many immigrant settlers to Georgia backcountry, the Antony clan was near impoverished. In fact, family finances were so limited that Milton likely had but two years of formal education his entire life. Yet

Milton somehow seemed enamored with the medical field. At age sixteen, he managed an apprenticeship with a nearby physician. Three years later he ventured to Philadelphia, where he formally studied medicine at the University of Pennsylvania. As keen as his interest was, he stayed just months. Finances ran out, and Antony returned to Georgia. Apparently, he had learned enough as he soon married and settled into some type of practice in Monticello. In 1817, the family moved to New Orleans, where Milton doctored for two years but then moved back to Georgia, this time Augusta, permanently.

Antony quickly favored the surgical arts, with a dexterity and boldness to match his formidable intellect. In 1821 he chronicled what proved to be the first thoracotomy of modern record. Such an undertaking was considered cataclysmic and almost certain to kill. No such deterrent for Antony. His patient suffered terribly from a necrotizing infection of lung and pleura. Only liberation of the toxic humors would save him, Antony reasoned. So, he began the perilous adventure. He sliced opened the man's chest, dividing skin and muscle, and dived through ribs to enter the rancid space. Normally an exquisitely painful process in the era before anesthesia, his stoic patient remained motionless, although "weak and faint." Antony scooped out infected material and dead lung tissue, perhaps amounting to over one-half of his right lung. The radical operation succeeded. The patient, after a long recuperation, was healed. No one was more amazed than Antony, who admitted, "I did not believe it consistent with the powers of nature, for him to survive the immediate effects of the operation." He was quite literally dumbfounded at the body's ability to respond to such an insult.[39]

Bold as he was, Antony recognized the fine line between competence and quackery, and the South harbored both. So many charlatans and incompetents abounded that the public distrusted healers of any kind. Demonstrate competence, then, Antony thought. Build a medical school right in Augusta. While he had been impressed with the University of Pennsylvania, he admired the efforts of nearby Charlestonians to create their own medical college. In fact, so supportive was he that he acted as preceptor for a number of its students. In turn, the Medical College of the State of South Carolina honored him with a doctorate of medicine in 1825. Mere preceptorship, though, was not enough for Antony. That same year he and Joseph Eve, an Augusta graduate of the South Carolina school, began informal instructions in Augusta for students at the new City Hospital. At the same time, he and his colleagues formed the Medical Board of Georgia with the expressed intent, like David Ramsay had done in Charleston, of regulating medical practice and abolishing quackery. Antony was the first president.

But lectures at City Hospital and formation of his Medical Board were not enough. Antony had still larger aspirations. He petitioned the legislature to charter Georgia's own medical college. Using the rising tide of southern sectionalism, he argued for a southern, not northern, medical education. Soon the press conspired as well, printing editorials in the *Augusta Chronicle*. One peculiar piece appeared in 1822, from an alleged anonymous source:

> It is notorious, that practitioners educated northwardly, and who have even had experience there, are perfect novices with the principal diseases of our climate, until they are drilled into a knowledge of them by many years' experience . . . those who intend exercising their professional talents in the South, should be educated here . . . It is believed that an increase of medical talents within this State would tend greatly to subserve the purposes of humanity, and prevent, or relieve much of the misery necessarily attendant on disease.[40]

The "latent genius" of Georgia will come to the forefront, the author proclaimed. A medical college and general hospital, the writer concluded, would afford the opportunity for students of medicine to access teachers and patients who could demonstrate skills, whether in examination, surgery, or obstetrics, at affordable expense and close to home. Could it have been a surreptitiously clever Antony?

In any event, the State of Georgia finally agreed. While southern medical distinctiveness was the byline, a prime mover for medical education in Augusta was a legitimate southern claim to medical academia. Equally seductive was affordability for locals. Appropriations for a one-year course of instruction for the new Medical Academy of Georgia were granted in 1828. "The graduates of the medical academy shall be allowed to practice medicine and surgery in this state, in the same manner as they would have been had they been examined and licensed" by the board of examining physicians for the State of Georgia, the charter read.

Antony was elected to the executive committee and installed as professor of institutes and practice of medicine. In 1833 the legislature expanded the medical school charter to two full years, granting a formal doctorate in medicine. As a scholarly corollary, Augusta physicians—including Antony—put together and published the *Southern Medical and Surgical Journal*. It was only proper, the editors argued at the start, that southern ailments and southern therapies be thus showcased and local medical education justified: "[T]he profession at the South have long regarded and anticipated, as a most desirable object, the establishment of a Journal that should collect and preserve the valuable discoveries and improvements of Southern practitioners relative to the nature and treatment of diseases incident to Southern climates."[41] Georgia's physicians applauded. The logical conclusion was that proper education must follow. In August 1836 physician Edward Delony from Talbotton, Georgia, delivered a compelling letter to the editors of the *Southern Medical and Surgical Journal*. Delony was convinced southern diseases demanded a southern focus. Only in the South could medical students learn firsthand ramifications of local ailments. Northern remedies, he claimed, would have little effect in Georgia, Alabama, or Louisiana. Distinct to Dixie were Asiatic cholera, pleurisy, rheumatism, and typhus fever. "The profession at the south," he went on, "[is] too much in the habit of looking to the north for medical light and knowledge." It was imperative, Delony concluded, that medical information—and by inference, medical education—be aimed at the maladies which immediately affected southern people. Northern medicine, as erudite as it was, simply had no place in the South.[42]

The school would now be renamed the Medical College of Georgia. The legislature appropriated $10,000 and sold fifty lots of the Augusta town common to fund its school. Construction was completed in 1836. Even prior to its completion, the building was an impressive monument to medical education. On October 24, 1835, the *Augusta Chronicle* announced: "The large, beautiful, and classic edifice of this institution is now, we perceive, nearly finished, and will soon be one of the finest architectural ornaments of our city, while the institution to which it belongs, will be one of the most brilliant ornaments of the State."[43] With its six massive Doric columns and distinctive central dome, many thought the structure was one of the best examples of Greek revival architecture in the South. Inside was space for several laboratories, lecture halls, and a library. Milton Antony, it was commonly thought, was the prime mover for this initiative and was also instrumental in sending fellow physician Louis Dugas to Europe in 1834 for books and anatomic specimens to fill the new library space. Antony had recruited the respected Dugas, a graduate of the University of Pennsylvania, to bolster his school's reputation. Dugas was an inveterate academician and would join Antony's faculty only if his curriculum matched that of established centers in the North. Apparently, Antony had convinced him.[44]

Antony was still not done. He now wanted to reach nationally to reform medical education across the country. He modestly suggested lengthening formal didactics from four to six months.[45] No way, his alma mater, the University of Pennsylvania declared. "[T]he Georgia College found it impossible to compete successfully with the popularity of a short and cheap course with students," the Philadelphia trustees responded. A "ridiculous and disgraceful practice" they continued. The whole matter was a clever marketing ploy, used to advertise "the small amount of money required for attending a course with them."[46] The snobbish North had once again belittled southern initiative.

But then more pressing matters surfaced for Antony. Yellow fever struck Augusta. By the summer of 1839, its presence was unmistakable. Such distress arose for the community that a panel of physicians convened to investigate. Not a contagion, they surmised, citing various contradictory observations. More likely—almost certainly—it was bad air. Yellow fever seemed to obey "most of the laws which govern other miasmatic diseases. It has usually commenced its ravages during the heat of summer" and remits as the temperature decreases below a certain point. Yes, even a site for the miasmatic transformation was identified. A heap of trash, rubbish—including collected dead animals—and other filth between Elbert and Lincoln Streets, called the "Upper Trash Wharf," was the source. The beating sun invigorated this offal and manufactured the evil. No doubt, the committee concluded, it was "the source of those pestiferous exhalations that hovered, like the angel of death, over our devoted city." Physicians themselves were not immune. Four doctors died in the process, one of those being Augusta's prominent citizen. On September 26, 1839, the *Georgia Constitutionalist* reported that, in Augusta, "the fever still rages . . . To our absent friends we will still say, keep away." And in the long list of the deceased from the malady that followed was "Dr. Milton Antony, Resident."[47]

VIRGINIA

It was the statesman Thomas Jefferson (1743–1826), with his vision of higher education, who spearheaded the formation of the University of Virginia in his dear home of Charlottesville. Jefferson hoped to provide education in all the noble sciences—medicine included. Like other southerners, he chafed at the elite schools of the North and the failure to fund education in Virginia. "The mass of education in Virginia, before the revolution, placed her with the foremost of her sister colonies," he wrote to his dear friend Joseph Cabell in 1820. "What is her education now? Where is it? The little we have, we import like beggars."[48] Now in his waning years, Jefferson felt it imperative to direct efforts in centralizing higher learning, not in the capital Richmond, as some would desire, but in his Charlottesville, located ideally, in his mind, for the mingling of the brightest of professors and students. It happened that in 1817 the legislature acted to establish a university "wherein all the branches of useful science shall be taught."[49] The site chosen was that of Central College in Albemarle County (present-day Charlottesville). Jefferson envisioned an academic village—a commune of learning—outlined in the Rockfish Gap report of August 4, 1818, a blueprint for his university. He was its prime mover. The Virginia General Assembly agreed and formally established the University of Virginia at Charlottesville on January 25, 1819. A Board of Visitors oversaw development and management and approved medical studies in the curriculum. Medical science would be taught by a single professor "with a history and explanations of all its successive theories . . . [enabling the student] to estimate with satisfaction, the extent and limits of the aid to human life and health." It was their intent, moreover, to provide a foundation for students, that the finishing courses for clinical experience would be done, for the meantime, elsewhere.[50]

Jefferson's eclectic intellect drifted toward the healing arts. He dabbled in medicinals and the curiosities of doctoring. It was no wonder he wanted his university to offer didactics in physic and the natural sciences. Yes, Charlottesville would be the preferred site, he thought. Richmond, though, as the state capital, presented keen competition. Wealthy benefactors had a vision for a new medical school there, hoping to bolster a sagging William and Mary College in nearby Williamsburg. Jefferson was not in favor, even though William and Mary was his alma mater. The state of Virginia need not have two medical institutions, he argued, and Richmond held no gain over Charlottesville. Classwork was just as easy at Charlottesville as Richmond, and anyway, proper facilities were already in place. "[A]n anatomical theatre ... is indispensable to the school of anatomy. There cannot be a single dissection until a proper theatre is prepared, giving an advantageous view of the operation to those within."[51]

As for clinical experience, could Richmond offer a wide spectrum of material? Much sickness spills from seafarers. Public asylums were full of them. Richmond was no more a port city than Charlottesville. Were there other homeless, penniless drifters in Richmond who might seek the asylum of hospitals? Not many. Richmond was a haven for enslaved people. And sick enslaved people were treated at the whim of their enslavers, rarely in public infirmaries. As for the upper classes, Jefferson argued:

> [H]ow many families in Richmond would send their husbands, wives, or children to a hospital, in sickness? To be attended by nurses hardened by habit against the feelings of pity, to lie in public rooms, harassed by the cries and sufferings of disease under every form, alarmed by the groans of the dying, exposed as corpse, to be lectured over by a clinical professor, to be crowded and handled by his students.[52]

It was poverty, Jefferson went on, that filled the wards of hospitals.[53] Had Richmond paupers enough? He did not think so. Of course, neither did Charlottesville. Jefferson's solution was to use the United States Marine Hospital, dedicated in 1801, in Norfolk County for that purpose. The city of Norfolk, a seaport with "climate and Pontine country" of a notoriously sickly nature and noted for numbers of wretched maladies and wretched human beings, could furnish the clinical material.[54] Local physicians there had some interest in education as well. In fact, three had proposed a course of lectures some years before; they even submitted a petition to the legislature. Yet that part of Jefferson's ingenious plan could not carry and stalled. Not enough enthusiasm in Norfolk, but fertile ground it remained.[55]

Competition between Richmond and Jefferson's Charlottesville intensified. Momentum to move William and Mary College to Richmond and add a medical school grew. John Augustine Smith, then president of William and Mary, welcomed the transition and dangled a medical school as an added incentive to the legislature to salvage his failing college. "It is as impossible to make doctors at the University of Virginia as it is to have ships without sails or waves," he blustered.[56] It was all for naught. Jefferson's influence and Cabell's rhetoric carried the day. Movement of medical studies to Richmond was soundly defeated by the legislature. Medical training, at least classroom work, would stay in Charlottesville under the auspices of the University of Virginia.

Two professors were chosen to teach medical topics. Englishman Robley Dunglison (1798–1869) was of distinguished academic accomplishments. Raised among the privileged classes, he was slated for the West Indies as a planter but his sponsor and uncle died, leaving him adrift in plans for his career. Between medicine and law, he chose the former. He attended the University of Edinburgh and the École de *Médecine* in Paris and shortly became a member of the Royal College of Surgeons. In 1824 he was approached by law professor Francis Gilmer, one of the University of Virginia Visitors, and offered a professorship at the new medical school in Charlottesville. As are many decisions in life, his was shaped by an "ardent" attachment to one Harriette Leadam, whom he could marry forthwith if he took her to the New World. The decision was irresistible. He was off to America with his new bride. After a rather grueling voyage of several weeks across the Atlantic, the young couple arrived in Norfolk the evening of February 10, 1825. Jefferson was almost at wits end, expecting them much earlier and holding the start of the school year until his distinguished professor was on site. Dunglison's long overland journey to Charlottesville culminated in a rustic lodging experience, where they put up in accommodations "of the most inferior kind." Nevertheless, Jefferson found them permanent housing that was much more agreeable, even better than they had expected for the wilderness of rural Virginia. Dunglison was immediately taken with Jefferson. Particularly impressive in his mind was Jefferson's architectural obsession with the design of the university's rotunda and pavilions, including Dunglison's anatomic theater. Dunglison wasted no time in promoting an ambitious curriculum in anatomy, physiology, obstetrics, medical jurisprudence, and even surgery. As for his relationship with Jefferson, the two became pleasant companions, and Dunglison, Jefferson's personal physician.[57]

Not all were so enamored with the youthful Dunglison. Post-Revolution patriotic fervor had seized the new United States, encouraging homegrown talent. Gone was the enchantment with Old World aristocracy. True to form, Nathaniel Chapman, faculty member at the University of Pennsylvania, disparaged American medicine for its embrace of foreign refinement. He singled out Jefferson's hypocrisy in hiring Europeans for his new faculty, citing the statesman's prior stance: "The failure of almost all the great scientific or literary undertakings of

Americans, is to be attributed to their employment of foreigners, instead of calling into exercise the talents of their own citizens." The sponsoring of Dunglison, Chapman went on, "has excited a feeling of more general indignation among American physicians than any circumstance that has occurred within our recollection."[58] The chagrined Dunglison, nevertheless, soldiered on, true genius that he was, and, in short order, was vindicated when he received an honorary doctor of medicine degree from that citadel of Yankee schooling, Yale University.

The second professor was a man of comparable youth and vitality. John Patten Emmet (1796–1842) was born in Dublin, Ireland.[59] He came from a long line of rebellious Irish partisans. His uncle had been executed for treason against the Crown and his father incarcerated for several years following the 1798 Irish uprising against British rule. Father and older children sailed to America in 1804; John and his two younger siblings followed one year later. John, as it turned out, weathered a sequence of near-fatal diseases before he left: smallpox, measles, and whooping cough. Though he survived, the ailments permanently weakened his constitution, so much so that fragile health forced an early departure from the Military Academy at West Point. Not to be deterred, he found his way into the College of Physicians and Surgeons in New York. From graduation, he departed for work in Charleston, fearful that the southern climate might do him in. On the contrary, it seemed to invigorate him.

Viewed now as a Yankee, despite his heritage, he felt the swelling resentment of southerners for men from the North and their dalliances in matters of romance: "It is considered a very lucky hit when Northern gentlemen marry in the South, for there is great jealousy towards them notwithstanding that they generally, in a year or two, rid the good people here of the presence both of themselves and their wives."[60] When Thomas Cooper vacated the chair of Chemistry at South Carolina's Medical College for Jefferson's University of Virginia, Emmet snatched the position, buoyed by recommendations from his mentors in New York. It was all for naught. Cooper soon reneged on his commitment in Charlottesville and returned to Charleston. It took little time to elbow out Emmet for his former spot. By then, though, Emmet had quite a following and, in turn, attracted Jefferson's attention as a promising faculty member. Aware of Emmet's superb performance, Jefferson offered him the chair of the School of Natural History. "The board of Visitors of the University of Virginia . . . unanimously nominated you to the chair [of Natural History]," Jefferson wrote to Emmet in March 1825. Natural History was an entrée to a delicious variety of topics from botany to zoology, even touching on the healing arts.[61]

"I can safely say that the Virginia University will be ranked among the very first in this country," Emmet wrote his sister from Charlottesville in May 1825.[62] The work was prodigious, though, time consumed with writing and lecturing and little left over for idleness. He "toiled like an Irishman," he said and, if not for the honor of his professorship, doubted that he would stay for the weariness it caused.[63] Botany, though, enthralled him, spurring horticultural experimentation and an abiding interest in *materia medica*.

Dunglison and Emmet were the core of the university's natural science curriculum. They delivered riveting courses in physiology, pathology, anatomy, and pharmaceuticals. Students were well prepared with the knowledge necessary for medical practice. Yet clinical material was lacking. Once again, attention turned to Norfolk and its Marine Hospital, and once again, arrangements broke down. Following Jefferson's death (1826), there was talk again of moving the school to Richmond with its meager but real supply of disease-susceptible vagrants. Proponents of the plan voiced concern over bedside experience for students in Charlottesville. Even though a die-hard Virginian, Alfred Magill, the replacement for Robley Dunglison in 1832 after the dynamic professor had moved on to the University of Maryland, was outspoken in his reasoning for the move. "No amount of closet study, no book learning can qualify a man to contend with disease," he maintained.[64]

Jefferson's influence still reigned. The move failed. Yet by 1837 the topic again surfaced, this time in earnest. Should there be a second Virginian medical college? Again, pushback from the Board of Visitors. Perhaps adding more professors would help, or expanding classroom work from four to ten months. Give students time to listen, read, and learn, the reasoning went—more of an Aristotelian method. Education is an unhurried passage. In keeping with Jeffersonian philosophy, allow students to discourse, debate, and experiment. Besides, an expansive anatomic and pathologic museum rivaled any academic center, and a limited clinical experience was available at a newly founded infirmary nearby. Parenthetically, faculty pointed out, Charlottesville retained a socially healthier climate, remote as it was from cities that might tempt dissipation and self-indulgence—and it was far cheaper than its northern counterparts.[65]

Richmond saw it differently. As the capital city, its citizens deserved the finest, including a medical college, they felt. Ignoring protests from Charlottesville and now that Jefferson was gone, plans proceeded full throttle. Hampden-Sydney College in Richmond was to be the site. Alumni were thrilled. One such spokesperson was the distinguished lawyer Jesse Burton Harrison, who lobbied for higher education throughout Virginia, including Richmond, where physicians could be found "who will love to seek into the history of disease."[66] Informal medical training had been going on for years. In October 1835 the *Richmond Enquirer* had announced that a "Richmond Medical School" would begin lectures "upon the various branches of Medical Science." The faculty consisted of physicians Thomas Johnson, James Beale, Robert Briggs, and Robert Haxall. Complete chemical apparatus and anatomic models had been purchased in Europe and would be ready for instruction. Dissecting rooms were to be available, furnishing opportunities to perform "all chirurgical operations." "The anatomic facilities of Richmond and its vicinity are inferior to none in the U.S.," the article went on. The Richmond Almshouse would be available to students for "feeling the pulse, applying the stethoscope ... and making such other examinations of patients as the attending physician may deem expedient to be instituted."[67]

But it fell to physician Augustus Lockman Warner (1807–1847) to lead a serious effort. Warner was an educator at heart. He had taught anatomy in a private dissecting hall near the University of Maryland alongside his busy practice, starting in 1829. This caught the eye of Visitors at the University of Virginia, and in 1834, he moved to Charlottesville for his appointment as professor of anatomy, surgery, and physiology. Yet the lack of anatomic material in Charlottesville—despite a rash of grave robbing—prompted Warner to move to Richmond in 1837, a place, he had long contended, better suited for medical education than Charlottesville. "As medicine is a practical science ... no scheme of instruction could be esteemed perfect, which did not embrace ... attendance upon hospital practice," he later wrote. Charlottesville was simply inadequate.[68] He wasted no time, lecturing students like a scholastic zealot. Anatomic dissections and surgical demonstrations enthralled his audience. But like one obsessed, it was not enough. Richmond deserved a proper commitment to medical scholarship. He bartered with Hampden-Sydney College, a tempting target for his initiative. Warner was impossible to discount. He was a man of presence, "exceedingly handsome," some contended, with graceful manners and a pleasing voice. His prowess as physician and surgeon was unequaled, they said, and his operations soon earned him recognition in Richmond periodicals.[69]

In October 1837 Warner presented his petition to the president, Daniel Lynn Carroll, and trustees of Hampden-Sydney College. Warner pointed out that most Virginians who wanted medical training were leaving the state. Charlottesville was not enough, Warner claimed. Students needed clinical material—and in abundance. "The number of negroes employed in our factories will furnish materials for the support of an extensive hospital and afford the student that great desideratum—clinical instruction"—apparently a convenient solution to the need for educational material.[70]

And so, before the end of the year, the Medical Department of Hampden-Sydney College received its charter. Doors opened on November 5, 1838, at the old Union Hotel, an aging four-story structure now converted to lecture halls, dissecting rooms, and even an infirmary. Warner served as the inaugural dean. The first catalogue was issued in 1839, congratulating all supporters who were "well-wishers, to the prosperity and independence of the South" in establishing in Virginia "a Medical School adequate to her wants, and capable, at once, of contrasting favorably in all the appliances for instruction, with the oldest Medical institutions of the country." A glorious undertaking and crowning accomplishment for Richmond, the notice implied, providing an "abundant supply of subjects for dissection and surgical operations on the *dead* body," as well as ample supplies of patients from an infirmary within the building itself ("[t]he diseases, moreover, which are here daily presented, being many of them peculiar to the South"), the city almshouse, the Richmond City Hospital, and the nearby penitentiary.[71] Forty-six students attended the first session, all but six from Virginia.[72] As for subjects on which to practice, Black Africans were the target. Enslavers and employers were urged to refer their laborers—bonded and freed, all for the benefit of medical education.[73] As for Warner and his band, there were accolades a plenty: "[T]oo much praise cannot be bestowed upon individual enterprise, perseverance and energy, which have already achieved for it a character of stability and usefulness not surpassed by older institutions."[74] As functional as the Union Hotel proved to be, it was not a structure much amenable to medical education. Through donations, then, from the Commonwealth of Virginia and the City of Richmond itself, the board of Hampden-Sydney College approved the building of a massive monument to Richmond medical education. Noted Philadelphia architect Thomas S. Stewart was chosen. His design mimicked an Egyptian Revival style and would eventually be called "the Egyptian Building." Lecture halls, laboratories, dissection rooms, and even medical and surgical beds for teaching filled the interior. In its basement in 1852, the noted neurologist Charles-Édouard Brown-Séquard, recruited to the faculty, conducted some of his neurological experiments. In 1854 the Medical Department split from Hampden-Sydney College and continued as a privately funded medical school. Perilously close to insolvency from dwindling tuitions, the college became a state-sponsored school in 1860, renamed the Medical College of Virginia. The Egyptian Building would still stand and remain a cherished icon of the Virginia Commonwealth University (as the Medical College of Virginia was eventually to be named).[75]

LOUISIANA

New Orleans bordered on the hinterlands of young America. A port city of growing importance to the United States, the Crescent City funneled commerce and forced labor far upriver to the fertile lands spreading from the Mississippi River. Its populations of ethnicities, though, sweltered under heat and humidity, and its subtropical climate brought misery in the forms of epidemic yellow fever and dysentery. New Orleans proved a cauldron of distempers worthy of the finest of medical care, yet far removed from centers of academics of even the Atlantic South. It was such a place that only the vigorous, the intrepid, and the adventurous sought refuge. The sick, on the other hand, languished in hovels and dens of filth. The Hôpital des Pauvres de la Charité, expanded and relocated farther west to the border of the Vieux Carré, had been utterly destroyed by the hurricane of 1779. The wealthy Don Andreas de Almonester y Roxas, a nobleman of the now Spanish New Orleans, rose to the occasion. Of a philanthropic sentiment, Don Andreas had been affected by the suffering of New Orleans's poor. He donated the sizeable sum of $114,000 to rebuild and maintain the Charity Hospital. He also endowed the entire endeavor with a perpetual revenue of $1,500 per year.[76] After consent by King Charles III of Spain, the new hospital, now called Hopital San Carlos (in honor of the Spanish King), was completed in 1786 on the same site as the old and once again became home to the destitute of New Orleans. American journalist John Pope wrote of the hospital in his travels to New Orleans toward the end of the eighteenth century: "The Hospital is situate [sic] in the Western Edge of the City, where Nothing interrupts its Ventilation from the East, South and North; but unfortunately, as if intended to banish Chearfulness [sic] from its Mansions, the Priests have laid off a Burial Ground, which is enclosed on one Side by the Front Wall of the Building."[77] While an asylum for the needy was a benevolent gesture, extremes of pestilence and sanitation abounded throughout the town. Death rates continued to soar. For the year 1796 there was recorded almost one death for every fourteen inhabitants.[78] Burial of the deceased presented particularly unsavory issues. The cemetery then was located in the center of the town and emitted a distinctly rancid smell. So fetid was the odor that waves of dysentery and "putrid and deadly fevers" were blamed on it. Surely, the public outcry went, that the burgeoning numbers of dead decaying there saturated grounds already harboring putrefaction.[79]

However, fire completely destroyed the San Carlos Hospital the night of September 23, 1809. Once again, scores of destitute patients were force out and had to relocate to various places around town, including the Cabildo center-city and the Jourdan Plantation outside of the city. At the plantation, horrible conditions prevailed, and the refugees almost starved to death. Conditions were little better when some were moved to the La Vergne residence, where inattention and misery continued. A new hospital, its name now Americanized to Charity Hospital, was not completed until 1815. Located on Canal Street, Charity Hospital was an impressive structure with a surgical hall, fever wards, and even a dysentery ward. "The building is a proud illustration of Louisiana liberality" so proclaimed the Board of Administrators in 1832, noting its architectural style and sound construction.[80]

Before long, the expanding population of New Orleans and the epidemic surges of pestilence soon overwhelmed the new hospital as well. Yet another hospital was begun in 1831 and completed in 1833. It was advertised as a marvel of the age, especially suited to the New Orleans climate: high ceilings, wide halls, and spacious verandas allowing clean, cooling air to circulate. On the lower floor, there was even room for a lecture hall and library. Adjacent was the Lunatic Asylum and not too far away the "Dead House," a place for storing corpses and performing autopsies: "Well lighted—well ventilated, a hydrant of clear gushing water, and plenty of fresh subjects—what more could be desired," so the commentary went.[81] For the living, Sisters of Charity provided care to the suffering, chastising their doctors in turn, as only nuns can, to see patients daily or more, particularly in those horrid times of epidemics.

Physicians flocked to New Orleans, eager to investigate the mysteries of resident illnesses. One such individual was Warren Stone (1808–1872). Stone was born in Saint Albans, Vermont, on February 3, 1808.[82] His medical career began modestly enough under the tutelage of a Dr. Amos Twichell in nearby Keene, New Hampshire. An accomplished surgeon, Twichell imbued the young Stone with a fondness for the craft. Following his apprenticeship, Stone entered the medical school in Pittsfield, Massachusetts, and graduated in December 1831. Stone himself was an imposing figure, a giant of a man, his features more rugged than handsome, his intellect and heart just as commanding. His first practice was in West Troy, New York, where he encountered the ravages of cholera. Such suddenness of onset and the profuse fecal expulsions brought agony to victims, so dissipated by the illness that half would die. The usual platitudes of calomel, opium, and camphor did little to forestall progression. Stone, though, paid less attention to those concoctions than to the human spirit. What mattered most was compassion. Regarding one victim of the disease, he was to have said, "As he was destitute, I obtained an outhouse of the landlord and had him conveyed to it, and stayed with him the greater part of the time for twenty-four hours, administering his medicines, and even injecting a saline mixture into a vein in his arm."[83]

Still, Stone, the scientist, must have reveled in it all. Like many physicians of the day, he welcomed the perplexities of miasmatic sicknesses, intent on somehow unraveling their obscurities. And that extreme dysentery, *cholera morbus*, seemed endemic to New Orleans. Why else would he embark on passage to a place where contagions lurked in every gutter and garbage heap? In October 1832 he set sail on the brig *Amelia* from New York harbor. During the journey, storms crowded steerage passengers below decks, and hatches latched to prevent swamping. On the third day of bad weather, a foray into the stinking hold found one person dead and twenty-five others suffering from cholera. Nineteen more would die before the brig reached Charleston. *Amelia*, already damaged by the storm, beached on Folly Island off Charleston on November 3, 1832. Passengers stumbled off and quarantined locally; the ship and its unhealthy cargo were torched to the water line.

Stone, oblivious to any personal danger, unselfishly cared for his miserable fellow travelers. Struck by the man's dedication, Thomas Hunt, a Charleston physician and supervisor of sanitation, joined in. In the course of this labor of crisis, the two became fast friends, Hunt impressed by the professional care Stone rendered and by his compassionate bedside manner. Stone and Hunt got little rest in the process. Of those shipwrecked on Folly Island, forty-two more fell victim and fifteen died. Stone himself fell ill to the disease, nursed back to health by his new friend Hunt.

Thomas Hunt (1808–1867) was of southern aristocracy. His father was a prominent lawyer in Charleston and member of the South Carolina Legislature, his mother, Louisa, of the distinguished Gaillard family of Carolina. Hunt had been carefully groomed: proper education and a focus on the classics. Medicine his chosen pursuit, he graduated from the University of Pennsylvania in 1829 and, like many privileged of his day, took leisure time to study with the masters in Paris. He had just returned to Charleston when the *Amelia* disgorged its human cargo on Folly Island, and he, charged with maintaining some degree of sanitation, had been sent forth to contain the suffering.

A rejuvenated Stone continued his voyage, arriving in New Orleans in December 1833. As it turned out, Hunt, too, was on a parallel course, newly appointed as house surgeon for the Charity Hospital there. They met up again. Hunt, his Charleston legacy preceding him, fit effortlessly into his new role at the Charity Hospital. So enamored was he with Stone that he offered him a position as assistant house surgeon. Stone accepted and, on June 30, 1835, was duly registered as legitimate by the *Registre du Comité Médical de La Nouvelle Orléans*.[84] This symbiotic friendship soon crystallized a dream for the future. Like other physicians, they had both been wooed by the exotic adventure of the place, its vitality, splendor, and opportunities. In all its decadence, though, New Orleans festered with diseases. Drifters and vagrants filled the alleyways and shelters, nursing their neglected plagues. In their midst were unscrupulous practitioners who preyed upon them. Both knew medical reform was needed. Why not offer New Orleans exceptional health care? Why not train doctors themselves, right in the city itself? Stone and Hunt shortly enlisted two other new arrivals in their scheme. First was the volatile but talented Charles Luzenberg (1805–1848). Likened to a prima donna by historian John Duffy,[85] the well-travelled Luzenberg was born in Italy (but apparently of Austrian descent) and fluent in Italian, German, and French. The beneficiary of patrician luxuries and learning, Luzenberg immigrated with his father to Philadelphia in 1819. He schooled at Jefferson Medical College and traveled back to Europe, apprenticing with the great Dupuytren at the Hôtel Dieu in Paris. But he soon returned to America and to the Crescent City in 1834.

His European dabblings earned him quick recognition there, and in November, he was licensed by the same *Registre du Comité Médical*.[86] An inveterate entrepreneur, Luzenberg understood the desire for care of the sick apart from public almshouses. In 1835 he opened the Franklin Infirmary. Private rooms for white clientele adorned the first floor, wards for whites the second, and the third floor for enslaved Blacks at the behest of their enslavers. All beds were for profit. During the course of all this, Luzenberg and Stone became acquainted. In fact, so taken was Stone by Luzenberg's initiative that he would open his own private hospital in 1839, called the Maison de Santé ("House of Health").[87] Luzenberg, though, was not just an opportunist, he was a brilliant surgeon in his own right. Philadelphian Samuel Gross considered him an expert operator, "his feats with the knife have associated his name with the history of surgery in this country," Gross wrote. To wit, among Luzenberg's many accomplishments were total removal of the parotid gland, ligation of an iliac artery aneurysm, and removal of a length of small intestine—remarkable achievements, done as they were without the aid of general anesthesia.[88]

But Luzenberg was also something of a curmudgeon. His pomposity and greediness for the spotlight earned him not a few enemies. Such was the animosity that his medical ethics were, at times, called into question. On one occasion, at a hearing before the Physico Medical Society of New Orleans in 1838, he would be categorized as "abrupt in speech; uncouth in manners, irritable and petulant in temper, and arrogant and overbearing in his demeanor."[89] Yet Luzenberg had energy and a portentous vision for New Orleans. His manic undertakings directed him toward medical education. In that, Hunt and Stone had found a confederate.

And then there was the diminutive, soft-spoken physician John Harrison. Harrison was from Washington, DC, of a prominent Maryland family, his father a respected surgeon. John had served an apprenticeship under his uncle and eventually graduated from the University of Maryland. He struck quite a contrast when accompanied by Stone, one a modest, slender figure, the other a colossus of a man. In good humor, Stone referred to Harrison as his "walking-stick."[90] They also became close friends. The scholarly Harrison would succeed Hunt as house surgeon for the Charity Hospital. So, it became Stone, Hunt, Luzenberg, and Harrison; the core of the faculty of their new medical school. The four clinicians, as unversed as they were about academic affairs, would somehow organize lecture material, classrooms, and demonstrations of anatomy and pathology. On September 29, 1834, the New Orleans *Bee* excitedly reported: "We are highly gratified to notice the establishment in this city of a medical college. The gentlemen who fill the chairs of professorship are men of skill and experience . . . Messrs. Hunt, Ingalls and Luzenberg . . . the former two have been officiating in a like capacity in similar institutions, and the latter [Luzenberg] has established a reputation of the highest degree as a surgeon."[91] What followed in the *Bee* was a carefully detailed prospectus for the school—and justification for its founding.

"Health is a primary and essential source of human happiness," the article read. The authors (likely Stone, Hunt, Luzenberg, and Harrison) were quoted as saying that "want of scientific medical knowledge" in Louisiana and the total lack of medical education in the region could not meet that need. The supreme goal was to remove "the danger of death and the apprehension of disease." Prosperity and profitability were sure to follow in the wake of a healthy citizenry. Why New Orleans, the authors posited? It was the largest and most populous city in the South(west), its hospitals were the most expansive and equipped. Besides, the authors claimed, even though New Orleans was "so healthy" eight months of the year, the range of diseases and injuries was unparalleled in providing clinical and anatomic preparation for students. Lastly, they proposed their expected pitch for southern medicine. Travel to the North, particularly from New Orleans, was expensive and time consuming. These, the authors noted, were formidable obstacles giving rise to home-grown practitioners of such incompetence as to be labeled "Quack Doctors, to the destruction of human life."[92]

The announcement produced a raging furor. Established doctors—many of French origin—rankled at the suggestion that foreign, English-speaking physicians had usurped their authority and privilege by unilaterally deciding on such a significant mission without even a nod from the state legislature. Such controversy sparked a lively debate in the press. One such physician complainant—thought to be French despite a good command of English—wrote to the *Bee* anonymously that October, voicing opposition to the lack of governmental oversight or university appointments and to the lack of "Creole or European" born (meaning non-English and presumably alluding to exclusion of any Frenchmen) physicians on the faculty. (It was signed "An American Physician").[93] That New Orleans endured any number of endemic and epidemic outbreaks they had no doubt. But French doctors, accustomed to medical education linked to university settings, felt it inconceivable that a freestanding medical college could deliver the academic environment for proper training. Furthermore, opponents conceded that local medical training was needed. "The diseases of Louisiana are different than those of the North and of Europe," one editorial in *L'Abeille*, the French edition of the *Bee*, insisted. Yes, the inhabitants of this city fall prey to ill-trained charlatans, the writer went on to say. And yes, what is needed is a local medical college—but one of true academic standing—that will train men by instruction at the foot of the sickbed. Whether there would be enough qualified students to enroll and whether this college would be on par with the best centers of medical instruction were matters of grave concern. One opponent penned to *L'Abeille*—and arguably so—that lack of proper preparation for medical studies would handicap suitable learning for the clinical sciences. Instead, one should search for institutions around New Orleans to provide premedical courses. The state legislature must help, he contended. "Such a serious undertaking demands all the necessary precautions," he concluded.[94] Stone's college simply did not fill the bill. The insolence of these young mavericks (in truth, the oldest of Stone's cadre was not yet thirty)![95]

Undeterred by such criticisms, the founders pushed on. Younger, more Americanized practitioners of the community received the entire effort with more enthusiasm and predicted a bright future. They named their school the Medical College of Louisiana. Thomas Hunt, assuming the dean's role, resigned his position as house surgeon at the Charity Hospital and picked John Harrison as his successor. Under Hunt's leadership, the first course of lectures for the medical college began on January 5, 1835, at the Strangers Unitarian Church. Eleven students attended. As dean, Hunt gave the introductory lecture. No longer a matter of metaphysics, medicine was now on the level of more exacting sciences, Hunt argued. Physiology, anatomy, and pathology have placed the art on "the solid foundation of a rational and scientific theory," he went on. This was the voice of a new profession, not based on rationalism but empiricism, a profession of a younger, enlightened generation.[96]

Following Hunt that day on the podium was faculty member Edward Barton. "Climate and Salubrity," he thematically presented. Diseases of New Orleans are different, distinct, a product of climate and geography: "If diseased action then is modified by climate, it is only an extension of the same principle to say, that remedial agents are modified also in their influence on the system by the same cause." "The great mass of our mortality proceed from fevers of various grades and characters, nearly all of which are peculiar to the climate," he continued. As a result, "[s]outhern practitioners must be taught in the south; if they do not learn their education here, they will have to learn from a severe experience."[97] And so the indoctrination began.

It was now called the Medical College of Louisiana. The first course of lectures concluded on April 27, 1835. Such an accomplishment, the *Bee* noted on April 29, that "[t]his is an auspicious commencement of the college. The experiment was rather hazardous as the establishment of a medical school was viewed with jealousy if not suspicion. But the zeal and prudence of the gentlemen who had united to form the faculty nobly braved and conquered all difficulties."[98] Their accomplishment would continue to stir controversy.

Even though the state legislature granted a charter earlier that April, bickering would not stop. The rivalry was ethnic in nature. French elements had attempted to form their own medical school, the Medical College of New Orleans, a maneuver that, even though a charter was given, never materialized.[99] As for the Medical College of Louisiana, quarreling and dissent developed. More problems followed. Dean Hunt abruptly resigned in May, replaced by Luzenberg and, shortly thereafter, by Edward Barton. Deprived of his stature, the arrogant Luzenberg seethed. Further trouble and misunderstanding with Warren Stone led to his total resignation in late 1836. Nevertheless, enrollment slowly increased and lectures continued. By 1842 the faculty sensed enough public and professional support that they petitioned the legislature for funds for a building to house the college. It was completed in late 1843, an edifice adorned in Greek architecture with ornate Corinthian columns. Now there would be lecture halls, a surgical amphitheater, a museum, and dissecting rooms. New Orleans had its medical school, for the South, another emblem of southern medical distinction.

Antebellum New Orleans was not finished with medical education, though. Enter Erasmus Darwin Fenner. Dr. Fenner had moved to New Orleans in the spring of 1840. A former country practitioner in Clinton, Mississippi, the death of his wife and the sole responsibility of his small son prompted relocation to a more urban environment. A man of frugal means, he had a heart for the poor. Coming from the extremes of wealth and poverty in Mississippi, he knew full well the incumbent hardships and despair of the less fortunate. In New Orleans, Fenner saw even more destitution, ragged men and women literally dying in the streets amid their own excrement. Yes, there was a level of sophistication in the town, but abject indigence and smoldering disease were only steps away. For these wretched souls, health care was an outrage. Few had the means to seek out physicians, and even charity housing was in short supply. Fenner's first mission was to inform his medical community of the horrible conditions affecting inhabitants of the city. He had broader aims also: to provide the entire South with reputable information on medical science—and "to free the South from the era of medical darkness."[100] He found a compatriot in Abner Hester, who also had migrated to New Orleans from Mississippi. Together they solicited influential patrons with little success. Finally, they located a down-and-out French publisher who agreed to print the initial editions. In May 1844 the first edition of the *New Orleans Medical and Surgical Journal* appeared, featuring a lead article by J. F. Beugnot, "An Essay on Yellow Fever." Fenner would encourage more submissions by southern physicians "of whatever nation and tongue." Soon it became the most influential medical publication in the South(west), sought after by prospective authors not only in Louisiana but also Mississippi and Alabama. Even physicians in the North vied for publication of their work.

But Fenner's ultimate vision for the miserable plight of New Orleans's poor was a second medical school. He knew full well that Stone's successful Medical College of Louisiana was near capacity, yet Louisiana clearly needed more educated physicians—a tour of the alleyways told him that. His school would be finer, more demanding of its students, more scientific, and more representative of an academic South. He would design it and choose the faculty. His new medical journal would back his school, and he would get another local medical publication, the long-serving *New Orleans Medical News and Hospital Gazette*, to endorse it as well. The *Gazette* showered Fenner's new medical school with accolades and, at the same time, championed the strength of southern learning:

> At the present moment, when so much jealousy and harsh feelings exist between the two great sections of our country, the motive which naturally prompts one to be proud of the advantages of his locality is apt to be misconstrued by our brethren abroad into the disreputable feeling of sectionalism . . . this shall not deter us from urging on the attention of the student of medicine the advantages which are offered him by home institutions.

He named it the New Orleans School of Medicine. His vision had materialized. Facilities were ostentatious; "Most beautiful lecture rooms," reported the *New Orleans Medical News*, and there were two, each seating 300 students. Also to be found were "the finest dissecting room in the country—well supplied with gas and pure cistern water," and a splendidly outfitted medical museum. His hand-picked faculty were young and enthusiastic. "Young Medicine" it was called. Fenner himself was forty-nine, Warren Brickell was thirty-two, Cornelius Beard twenty-eight, and Samuel Choppin twenty-eight. As Fenner had designed, his curriculum almost radical, the studies demanding. Five months of lecture and daily instruction in medicine and surgery at the bedside. Anatomy and physiology were vital and drilled into students. Graduates were to be exceptionally well versed in the sciences as well as the practicalities of the art of medicine.[101] Fenner's faculty emphasized that physic—the practice of medicine—was no mean undertaking, that firm foundations in the sciences and skillful bedside behavior were absolutely essential to proper care of the sick. By the second session, 1857–1858, 126 students enrolled and 33 graduated. One year later, 164 enrolled and 36 graduated.[102] Fenner's New Orleans School of Medicine had become a rival to Stone's and a landmark in southern medical education.

So, by 1840 there was ample opportunity for young southern gentlemen to study and apprentice in the medical sciences without venturing north. Medical training in southern regions had its advantages in terms of travel and expense. But sectionalism? Was health such a unique challenge in the South? Was that such a viable argument?

The idea rankled academicians in the North. Regarding sectionalism: "We know that the thoroughly educated medical man can adapt himself to the diseases of different latitudes with as much facility as he can his wearing apparel." Southerners stubbornly disagreed. "It is the 'manifest destiny' of the South to become each year more and more independent in all that relates to educating her youth." Sentiments of the kind echoed from New Orleans to Augusta to Charleston.[103] "We are no sectionalist," another editor wrote in comparing North and South. "[C]andor will force you to admit that nature alone is the sectionalist, and we are but her humble interpreter."[104] "Medicine is only successfully learned by practical and personal experience. Surgery is likewise learned by the use of the knife," so wrote the editors of the *Georgia Blister and Critic* in that inflammatory editorial of 1854, again referring to the peculiar maladies of the South.[105]

No, it was not the intent that the South should be independent of the North, but to make the South independent within the Union, Rev. C. K. Marshall of Mississippi expressed. Send sons and daughters of the South northward and risk exposing them to elements "dangerous to our interests, and damning to our peace." Marshall said. Northern education would be particularly "pernicious to southern minds." He went on to warn, "Our sons and daughters return to us [from northern schools and colleges] with their minds poisoned by fanatical teachings and influences against the institution of slavery." There it was, the cornerstone of southern culture. Then he offered the rhetorical question: "Shall we educate our children abroad or at home?" Educate our own teachers, and then educate southern youth, Marshall believed. And as for slavery itself, Marshall proclaimed it had "contributed to the glory in arts and science . . . forming part of the patriarchal system of government established by God himself."[106] And so, North and South drifted apart, medicine just one excuse in a widening gulf of beliefs and practices.

CHAPTER TEN

SECESSION'S VULGAR SCOURGES

> The South has been swept as by a whirlwind, and like one of
> its native pines, scathed and blasted by the lightnings of war,
> its inherent powers of reproduction are almost limitless.
> —FRANCIS PEYRE PORCHER

On May 6, 1861, Howell Cobb, then president of the Confederate Congress, issued the following statement, approved and sanctioned by Confederate president Jefferson Davis: "Whereas, the earnest efforts made by this Government to establish friendly relations between the Government of the United States and the Confederate States . . . have proved unavailing by reason of the refusal of the Government of the United States . . . war exists between the Confederate States and the Government of the United States."[1] It had come to this: armed conflict. For the South it was a war of secession and of independence. Theirs was now a nation apart—no longer within the Union but truly separate from it. For the North it was insurrection, pure and simple. The War of the Rebellion, as it was to be called by the victors—and Southerners themselves enjoyed the label "rebels"—uprooted the South. Every aspect of society, commerce, and ordinary affairs would be radically altered during the four years of warfare. Health care was no exception. Doctors would be yanked from small towns and cities alike to serve soldiers of the Confederacy, and hundreds would be killed and maimed. It all began, of course, on Friday, April 12, 1861, as two secessionist siege mortars positioned on James Island, South Carolina, fired on Fort Sumter in Charleston Harbor. So began the bloody conflict of American against American that would dig a vast chasm between North and South and, for decades to come, instill a sense of confederacy in those southern states, despite their loss in the fight for independence and preservation of their beloved slavery.

The Confederate States of America came together on February 8, 1861, with the secession and subsequent confederation of seven slave states: South Carolina, Mississippi, Alabama, Florida, Georgia, Louisiana, and Texas. Mississippian Jefferson Davis was elected president and inaugurated on February 18, 1861. Following initiation of hostilities in April, four other states joined in: Virginia, North Carolina, Tennessee, and Arkansas.

Open combat of some sort with Union elements was a predictable consequence of secession. In that vein, health care seemed high priority for the Confederacy. Musters of troops meant camp illnesses; battle portended massive injuries. Davis and his cabinet organized a Medical Department of the Confederate States on February 26, 1861, which was to consist of one surgeon general, four surgeons, and six assistant surgeons. The Department of War was to find additional surgeons to carry out their mandates.[2]

The Medical Department fell under the direction of South Carolinian Samuel Preston Moore (1813–1889), appointed as acting surgeon general.[3] Moore was a true southerner. He had received his medical education at the Medical School of the State of South Carolina and was awarded a Doctor of Medicine degree in 1834. His was a Charleston lineage extending for generations. An ancestor, Mordecai Moore, also a physician, accompanied Charles Calvert, Lord Baltimore, on his journeys to the New World in 1632 when Charles I granted him the tract of land north of the Potomac River now recognized as Maryland. Descendants later migrated to the Carolinas and eventually to Charleston. Samuel Moore then served in the United States Army in various posts west of the Mississippi, many in the wild frontiers of the Kansas Territory. Transferred back to New Orleans as medical purveyor, he resigned his commission in December 1860 when South Carolina seceded. With his military bearing and experience, he was shortly named surgeon general by President Davis in November 1861. Moore was a military man through and through. Tall and handsome, he strode almost as if at attention, ramrod straight and purpose driven. His cadre of surgeons shared little of his demeanor and discipline, though. A meager few had any prior military exposure.[4]

Despite Moore's experience, the South lacked manpower. Moore's Medical Department was woefully short of physicians and surgeons. For example, in 1860 South Carolina recorded an estimated 1,000 physicians of any training and practice. Only a quarter of those were recruited. When other "unofficial" or part-time doctors were included, the number still fell under 500. Historian Wyndham Blanton eventually calculated the number of physicians serving in all the Confederate armies at 834 surgeons and 1,668 assistant surgeons.[5]

Military life baffled most. It was a radical departure from civilian practice. Author Joseph Waring found that almost all Confederate doctors at the start of the war were general practitioners (as were almost all doctors). They had few surgical skills and little concept of field sanitation. Pay was modest, perhaps $200 per month ($6,400 in 2022 dollars). Uniforms were at their own expense and precisely spelled out by Congress: an officer's tunic of cadet gray cloth, trousers of dark blue, boots, white gloves, and a green silk sash. Not many were able to comply.[6] Field service was a revelation. Sanitation early on in the camps was appalling. Most recruits came from those rural areas where exposure to common contagion (measles, yellow fever, dysentery, etc.) was minimal. Once encamped, these diseases spread like wildfire. Such was the picture portrayed in the *Confederate Medical and Surgical Journal* of January 1864:

> The medical men of the South have had their part to play in the terrible drama. To them have been intrusted [*sic*] the health and well-being of our brave soldiers. Fierce epidemics, spreading fast through crowds of raw recruits, hastily collected, but half prepared for the exposures of camp, and wholly ignorant of the precautions needed to resist disease, have been combatted; an almost total neglect of the laws of hygiene and oftentimes defective nutrition, resulting from improper and badly cooked food, or even a scarcity of the proper articles of diet, have sapped the constitution of the strongest.[7]

One Confederate physician, Herbert Nash, saw the effect of camp life on raw recruits. In 1862 he witnessed hundreds of militiamen enlisted from around Norfolk, Virginia, stricken with measles. When coupled with homesick conditions, the drama soon turned fatal. Just as dangerous were jaundice and erysipelas. He noticed that "a yellow tinge would first appear on the forehead, soon spreading over the face and followed by the blistering of erysipelas." He also saw the effects of malarial fever and dysentery as troops marched through the marshes and rivers like the Chickahominy in eastern Virginia. Camp doctors, unversed in such illnesses, were ill prepared and overwhelmed. Feeling that lethargy and homesickness weakened the constitution, Nash used a different approach. He first separated the sick from the well. Then he brought in band concerts, milk toddies, and inspiring soliloquies—all psychological remedies. In his camp, death rate plummeted. His "psychic therapeutics" were wonder agents.[8]

Others had a different experience. F.E. Daniel from Jackson, Mississippi, thought it all great fun at first, as the troops assembled on a parade ground, waiting for orders. "We just ate and flirted and drilled and played soldier," Daniel recalled. Every soldier was a hero, or so the girls thought. As for dress, "I took along a sole-leather valise with me, full of broadcloth suits, patent leather shoes, linen shirt, fancy socks and ties," Daniel wrote.[9] Once afoot and on the march, all changed. He discarded most of his comfortable luggage. Whatever he could fit into a knapsack was what he would wear and use—including cooking utensils (although Black "servants" cooked most meals). But Daniel was in far better shape than the common soldier. As the war dragged on, "[m]any of the soldiers were barefooted . . . It was painful to see the boys, some of them, hobbling along with sore and bleeding feet over stony mountain roads," he wrote. Food dwindled. During his march through the Cumberland Gap in 1863, shelled corn was their only meal for breakfast and supper.[10]

That first large-scale engagement near the Virginia town of Manassas on July 21, 1861, awakened Confederate surgeons. The messy defeat of Union General Irvin McDowell's poorly trained troops was costly. Without a doubt, if this battle was any portent, the conflict was to be a bloody one. The effects of antiquated tactics and improved firepower were sure to generate casualties heretofore unknown. Future combat was likely to be just as grisly. Evacuating injured from the battlefield and treating them behind the front lines would become formidable challenges. Medical officers would be faced with the daunting task of addressing wounds of head, chest, abdomen, and limbs that required the utmost in surgical judgment and expertise. Few possessed such talents at the onset of hostilities. And where to care for them?

At the front lines, field care lacked resources, the mayhem near Manassas showed. The ambulance system was atrocious. Evacuating the wounded from the expanse of battlefield bordered on the inhumane. For one thing, the Medical Department of the Confederacy was never supplied with proper vehicles. In May 1861 for the entire Army of Virginia, only six four-wheeled wagons could be found. To move the thousands of wounded campaigns generated, this was nothing short of foolhardy. In months to come, Confederates rummaged through Union spoils of battle when they could. Top priority were ambulance wagons. Simple carriages were the rule, many not even sprung, so the ride over rough roads was torture—especially for those with broken arms and legs. Soldiers must have dreaded the travel. In many cases, private enterprise came to the rescue. Volunteer ambulance groups formed, such as the Richmond (Virginia) Ambulance Corps.[11] Other paid contractors were not so benevolent. Some chose to leave the wounded where they lay and simply abscond with the medicinal liquor supplies instead.[12] Even railroads were an improvement, although not enough coaches could be found. Wounded were often crammed into cattle cars on straw with little else for comfort.

Behind the lines, the throngs of wounded from Manassas—1,500 Confederate soldiers alone—brought back to Richmond overwhelmed any existing facility. What infirmaries already stood were a trivial help and soon swamped. Citizens began outfitting public buildings and hotels with beds and bedding. An English visitor witnessed the chaotic scene there weeks after the battle. He counted twelve makeshift hospitals in operation. Yet they held just a fraction of the casualties. "There was scarcely a gentleman in or about Richmond who had not from one to four patients in his house, upon whom the utmost attention was bestowed."[13]

The specter of a medical disaster was on the horizon. It took only months for the full effect of battle, disease, and marginal health care to make its appearance—poorly trained practitioners had filtered into the ranks. Yet President Davis simply had little money left for the Medical Department to recruit more qualified doctors. In August 1861 he pointed out, "I am aware that there have been causes of complaint in relation to neglect of our sick and wounded soldiers ... not so much from an insufficiency in the number of the surgeons and assistant surgeons as from inattention or want of qualification." His solution was a Board of Examiners, trusted medical officers who would oversee selection and conduct of physicians. As for ability to treat the numbers of infirmed soldiers, the Medical Department faced a dearth of hospital beds. Of those available, overcrowding soon bred more pestilence and misery. Much more was needed. The secessionist Congress under Davis passed laws carefully outlining the necessity for speedy transport by rail of hospital provisions and the adequate supply of clean clothing, rations, supervision of hospital economy, and enough nurses. In September 1862 the Confederate Congress passed "An Act to Better Provide for the Sick and Wounded of the Army in Hospitals." This measure allowed for assignment of sick and wounded to hospitals near the front (mostly in Virginia) representing their home states. Each hospital of a particular state was to be numbered accordingly.[14] So, after 1862 hospitals across the Confederacy would be designated by state and number, their staffs hometown doctors, nurses, and matrons familiar with culture and kinfolk of their patients.

Indeed, the war would bring about a revolution in hospital care.

In the antebellum South, what hospitals existed were primarily designed for the destitute and poor (and enslaved). Most private citizens received their health care—and even surgery—in their own homes. Now, with a conflagration of enormous breadth, it fell to each state to confront the inadequacies of medical care. Confederate General Joseph Johnston informed Surgeon General Moore that at least 9,000 hospital beds would be needed in Virginia alone. Moore could locate only a fraction, 2,500 beds, but he chose Richmond as the site for expansion. Richmond lay directly in the path of evacuation routes from northern Virginia into the South—and of course, was the capital of the Confederacy. He recruited a prominent local doctor, James McCaw, to locate a place near town for a large hospital complex. McCaw found a site on Chimborazo Hill, a broad plateau of almost forty acres overlooking but separated from the city by Bloody Run Creek. Moore had in mind a new concept in hospital construction. Compact, single-story wooden huts would serve as hospital wards, holding 40 to 60 beds. Well-lighted and ventilated, they were the answer to the bad air many thought responsible for rampant hospital infections.[15]

Moore built 150 of his huts on the Chimborazo plain, arranged in five orderly divisions like a checkerboard. Virginia, Georgia, Alabama, North Carolina, and South Carolina each controlled a division, headed by their own surgeons and nursing teams. There was also a convalescent section of one hundred Sibley tents, each to house up to ten recovering patients. A dedicated water supply furnished clean water for drinking, cooking, and bathing. There were five large icehouses, a large bakery able to produce seven thousand to ten thousand loaves daily, a Russian bathhouse, and a jerry-rigged sewage system that effectively removed wastes. A generous and patriotic citizen, Franklin Stearns, lent the hospital his nearby farm of Tree Hill for the pasturage of two hundred cows and five hundred goats. Adjacent tobacco factories were converted to manufacture soup and furnish seasoned wood used for making beds and furniture. Even beer was available; as many as four hundred kegs were filled at any one time and stored in caves or cellars at the eastern end of the hill.

Moore might have grasped the hut concept from European activists like Florence Nightingale. In her experience during the Crimean War (1853–1856), Nightingale witnessed the deplorable condition of hospitals and the grimy living conditions forced on ill men. No wonder evil spirits inhabited such places and infected their inmates. Nightingale knew that the French seemed to have remedied the situation at the Hôpital Lariboisière in Paris in the 1840s to combat cholera. They erected pavilions, limiting the numbers of patients residing within and providing an extreme measure of airiness and cleanliness. She would do the same. Wards should hold not more than forty patients each, she felt. "The first principle of hospital construction is to divide the sick among separate pavilions," she wrote in 1863 of her experiences then. Ventilation was key, of course, stale air a carrier of pernicious vapors, she thought. Instead, circulating breezes should not diffuse from one ward to another but be speedily vented to the outside. She even went into detail regarding bathrooms, toilets, water closets, sinks, water supply, and sewage disposal.[16]

And Moore had magnificently done the same. For his Richmond complex, now named Chimborazo Hospital, Moore appointed McCaw as superintendent. McCaw himself was a loyal southerner, born in Richmond in 1823. He came from a long line of physicians: his great-grandfather, emigrating from Scotland in 1771, grandfather, and father were all practitioners. McCaw had schooled in New York City. He returned to Richmond, where he catered to his patients and all the entanglements of civil service. Military historian Edgar Erskine Hume identified McCaw as an indispensable and influential contact in Moore's effort to ramp up Richmond's hospital capacity. "'Towering physically and mentally above his associates,' says one of his admirers, 'princely Dr.

James B. McCaw, sweet, gentle, tender and true, and brave, generous and loyal, he was just, honorable, and upright, an exemplar worthy of emulation.'"[17] No sooner had it opened in early 1862, McCaw's Chimborazo filled with two thousand patients. During its three and a half years of operation, almost seventy-seven thousand patients would pass through. Enforced sanitary measures kept the death rates relatively low, below 10 percent.[18]

Thanks to efforts such as McCaw's, within two weeks, Moore had six thousand beds available. Chimborazo Hospital became the premier medical facility of the South, taking in patients from Maryland, Tennessee, Kentucky, and Missouri, but it was not the only hospital in and around Richmond. By the end of 1863, there were twenty others built to service the Confederacy.[19] The city transformed into the major medical destination for tens of thousands of sick and injured troops, a collecting point for Robert E. Lee's Army of Northern Virginia. Anywhere from one thousand to sixteen thousand infirmed were housed across the city, sometimes overwhelming even Richmond's hospital system.

One North Carolina soldier marching through Richmond in 1862 came upon the main thoroughfare: "There the scene was awful to behold. The street was filled with wagons hauling the wounded; the sidewalk was almost impossible, the wounded standing and lying in every direction." Appeals then rang out again to open private homes for the lodging and care of the wounded. Once again, women of Richmond set to work gathering foodstuffs, bedding, and nursing the afflicted. This was often vexing to misogynist surgeons, who, as true southerners, felt a woman's place *was not* in the hospital and that many of the volunteers were woefully lacking in nursing and hospital skills. Not true, of course. Richmond's women were quite capable of dressing changes, bathing, and simple hygienic functions.[20] They were the glue—if not the spirit—that held together a fragmented arrangement of health care.

It would get even worse. As the war dragged on, Richmond's hardships became more glaring. Cutting of rail lines by advancing Yankees soon interrupted timely delivery of sustenance and items of comfort for all hospitals. One nurse at Chimborazo, Phoebe Yates Pember, began to realize that war had intruded even on the mercy necessary for its suffering victims: "Now, for the first time, began to be felt what was really meant by 'war'; for privations had to be endured, which tried the temper and patience. A growing want of confidence was constantly forced upon the mind, and with doubts which, though unexpressed, were felt as to the ultimate success of our cause, came into play the antagonistic qualities of many around us."[21] Food scarcities were particularly alarming. Pantries emptied; the simplest of fares became delicacies. Even vermin suffered. Hungry rats turned into voracious visitors, seemingly oblivious to humans and intent on rummaging at will, even nibbling on the raw wounds of patients. And then Richmond itself came under attack, and the sound of booming cannons resonated through Chimborazo's pavilions. This generated hordes of wounded men who crowded the complex, vying for scant resources. So great then was the shortage of supplies that women like nurse Pember would scour the neighborhoods, ring doorbells, and ask for items as basic as soap, rags, and wash basins.

> The horrors that attended, in other and past times, the bombardment of a city, were experienced to a great degree in Richmond during the fighting around us. The close proximity to the scenes of strife; the din of battle, the bursting of shells, the fresh wounds of the men hourly brought in, were daily occurrences. Walking home after the duties of the Hospital were over, often when evening had well set in, during this time, the pavement around the railroad depot would be lined with wounded men, laid there to wait for ambulances to take them to the receiving hospital.[22]

Despite the anxieties of overworked doctors, Pember and her nurses provided most of the care. Administrative duties occupied too much of the surgeons' time, and surgeon assistants ranged in quality from frankly incompetent to barely tolerable. Bickering between surgeons (surgeon assistants) and nurses ran constant at times, creating petty disturbances that did nothing but distract from professional attitudes and comfort to patients. As admissions mounted and stores ebbed, the stress reached breaking points, and all sought some respite outside of the wards. But there was little to enjoy. Richmond had become a town under siege. Blackened buildings and rubble-filled streets were a sober backdrop to the misery of thousands of citizens and soldiers.

Elsewhere, in Charlottesville, at the direction of the Confederate Medical Inspector Dr. J. P. Smith, University of Virginia buildings were converted to military hospitals the summer of 1862. Dormitories, even apartments in the Rotunda and public hall, filled with the wounded from nearby battles. The faculty railed at such maneuvering, feeling passionate that space should be preserved for education and not proprietary assistance, even to the Confederacy. The Board of Visitors agreed in principle. It was their "positive duty to preserve University buildings for the exclusive purpose for which they were erected." Yet the deluge of casualties would not stop. The war's floodgates had opened, seeding university space, dorm rooms, and any available dwelling with blood and gore and germs. The entire campus had become distinctly unhealthy. Still, the Board of Visitors did not waver. Education must continue. The university would not close. While student enrollment and faculty shrank, they did not disappear. Lecture space was found and teachers willingly stayed at their posts "in the face of the severest sacrifices and privations." Medical training continued as well, graduating fifty-two during the war years.[23]

In South Carolina, Roper Hospital, Marine Hospital, and the Almshouse, all in Charleston (there was a state hospital for the insane in Columbia) soon emptied their inmates and prepared for the onslaught. Patients flooded in, filling the beds, and doctors clamored for more. Trustees for Roper Hospital protested, but no one listened. Out with the lunatics and the poor, in with sons of the Confederacy. Some sick were assigned to private homes, churches, hotels, and courthouses. Charleston made ready eleven structures to house the injured and ill.

By January 1862, a depot designed for use by the South Carolina Railroad Company was donated as a reception area to hold trainloads of ill coming in. These would soon be known as Wayside Homes, places of temporary respite for evacuated casualties. Many arrived hungry, fatigued, sick, and faint. Englishwoman Catherine Hopley, touring the war-torn South, described the scene on one train: "There they were, lying on sopping straw, or what was used for such ... There they had been all night in that pouring rain ... sick and dying soldiers, too feeble even to move themselves." There were desperate pleas to the community for volunteers as waiters, nurses, and cooks.[24] Wayside Homes sprang up along railroad lines, dwellings that could furnish rations and shelter to sick and wounded soldiers discharged or furloughed. The Wayside Home in Charleston, for example, accommodated, at one time, more than one thousand men.

The railroad depot in Columbia, South Carolina, was used as a Wayside Home. At first, this amounted to just one room, a former ticket office. Like elsewhere, many of these men arrived in deplorable shape, feverish, with filthy bandages. Dysentery plagued not a few. Columbia's women, distressed by the plight of their brave young men, took action. They found unused buildings at the fairgrounds and converted them into hospitals. The women, who by then had formed their own hospital committee, personally purchased cots, bedding, and crockery. Hundreds of beds were made ready and filled quickly.

That first winter of 1861 and 1862 in Columbia, forty patients died of pneumonia and typhoid fever in the makeshift fairgrounds hospital, despite care by what was now called the "Young Ladies' Hospital Association." By October 1862 one thousand men had passed through, and in the following year, the women managed to enlarge the hospital space to receive three times the number of sick and wounded. By the following summer, the Confederate government had taken over, and some of the more critical patients were moved to the South Carolina College buildings. But the intrepid ladies of Columbia were not finished. Still needing a larger space to accommodate arriving soldiers, they persuaded a factory owner to donate his ice depository as a Wayside Home. At year's end, 1862 Columbia now hosted buildings designated as General Hospital No. 1, No. 2, and No. 3. Even the governor turned over his mansion for the care of the infirmed.[25]

North Carolina made every effort to care for its troops, as it would give more men to the Confederacy than any other state. But it had few hospitals to offer.

There was a mental hospital near Raleigh and the usual "Marine Hospitals" along the coast. Besides, sick and injured North Carolina soldiers remained near the Confederate Army camps in Virginia. Yet care in parts of Virginia was an abomination. Drs. John Bellamy and William Hunter described a scene "sickening to contemplate." Over two hundred North Carolinians alone were in the hospital, "suffering for the want of proper attention."[26] One visitor sadly related her observations: "The floors of the hospital . . . have not been swept for weeks; and the dirty bandages which have been taken from their wounded limbs are thrown aside near the bed, rendering the rooms so offensive it is disagreeable to go in them."[27] The author of the letter to Governor John Ellis in July 1861, probably a nurse herself, pleaded with the governor to "authorize ladies of your state to endeavor to get others to enlist as 'sisters of mercy' for the relief of the sick at York [Virginia]."[28] It appears that shortly afterward, there was a movement to set up state hospitals in Virginia.

Surgeon Edward Warren appealed for a North Carolina hospital to be outfitted in Charlottesville, Virginia. South Carolina and Alabama had already done such for their recruits, he noted. In October 1861 the state officially opened a hospital in Petersburg, Virginia, touted as "one of the most convenient and comfortable Military Hospitals in the country." The building was three stories, divided into wards, heated, ventilated, and lighted by gas. Location was ideal, close to rail lines to facilitate transport of patients arriving by train. The governor of North Carolina would directly manage the hospital. He recruited one chief surgeon, two or three assistant surgeons, one apothecary, and as many nurses, cooks, and washers as may be needed. In fact, medical students were encouraged to participate as part of their medical training. The first chief surgeon, Dr. Peter Hines, required his two assistant surgeons to remain in the hospital day and night for the care of patients, who were never to be left unattended.[29] North Carolina's civilian participation was essential for nursing care but also to provide provisions not forthcoming from a strapped Confederate government. Troops were in dire need of sustenance, bedsheets, and clothing. The public was asked to help. Newspapers solicited for money, domestic wines, jellies, dried fruits, rice, arrowroots, sage, red pepper, cornstarch, soaps, blankets, socks, shirts, sheets, and old linens.[30]

Another North Carolina hospital was set up in Richmond in 1862, named Moore Hospital (also called General Hospital No. 24), formerly Harwood's Tobacco Factory, a three-story, flat-roofed brick structure. Of course, to outfit the hospital required total dependence on civilian donation of bedding, blankets, pillows, towels, and bandages. Even then, provisions were scarce, and newspapers frequently solicited the North Carolina public for fruit, eggs, potatoes, and butter. Women—wives, widows, mothers, and daughters—collected, packaged, and shipped items northward. Some even volunteered to travel to Virginia and staff those hospitals. In North Carolina, too, Wayside Homes opened to provide comfort. One such Wayside Home was in Salisbury, midway between Charlotte and Greensboro and a major trade route between. Solicitations rang out for assistance. "While on their way home they need places where they can obtain rest and refreshment without charge," notices read. "[G]ive him food and fire, in exchange for the blood he has shed for you." The Salisbury Home housed over 1,200 sick and wounded soldiers over a year's time.[31]

Within the state itself, the City of Raleigh took the lead as a hospital center. The state surgeon general, Dr. Charles Johnson, constructed the first hospital, known as the Fair Grounds Hospital in early 1861. He appointed a resident surgeon, Dr. Edmund Burke Haywood, as its supervisor. Haywood was another stolid southerner. Trained at the University of Pennsylvania, he had earned the respect of his colleagues for his mild, even-tempered demeanor and surgical skill. The expansive Fair Grounds Hospital was transformative, admitting over 4,700 patients, returning 4,200 to duty, and losing (only) 170. Other hospitals followed. In 1864, Haywood was given command of the new Pettigrew Hospital (also known as General Hospital No. 13). This hospital resembled the Chimborazo complex in Richmond, built around one-story pavilions and huts. Offices, a dispensary, commissary, laundry, bathhouse, wells, and furnaces complemented the patient areas. Four hundred beds housed the ill and battle casualties. Still, there was the same chronic shortage of nurses, matrons, and cooks as well as medical supplies so detrimental to the Confederate hospital system. Despite those scarcities, Confederate inspectors felt "they were the best Hospitals and better conducted than in any other Hospital District in the Confederate States."[32]

Farther to the south, New Orleans, a vital port for the Confederacy, fell in April 1862. Union troops promptly occupied the city under the command of a pompous, balding Major General Benjamin Butler. Butler, no friend of the South, quickly instituted a rather brutal martial law and policed the city in such a heavy-handed manner that he soon incurred the wrath of the common citizen. His aim, he later declared, was to take from the rich and give to the poor, as he saw the war a struggle between the impoverished and middle classes against the wealthy. At his command, federal authorities requisitioned both medical schools then in operation. Now seized, both closed to further classes. The faculty and students who could fled New Orleans to serve in various parts of the Confederacy. Yet in accordance with his philosophy, Butler managed to lavishly fund the Charity Hospital and forbade the trustees from closing it. He went to great lengths to feed the poor—he claimed the city was on the verge of starvation when he arrived—clean the streets, and attempt to rid the city of epidemics like yellow fever.[33]

One doctor who did not leave New Orleans was that bigger-than-life surgeon Warren Stone, now fifty-four. Such was his reputation (and force of character) that, even during the war, northern medical professionals regarded Stone with respect, celebrated for his talented surgical skill, "greatness of heart, independence of character and devotion to the South." This admiration apparently did not extend to newly garrisoned federal troops. Stone did not conceal his contempt for Northern incursion. After being arrested by the despised General Butler, charged as being a dangerous "rebel," Stone reportedly hissed, "I glory in being a rebel" and insolently invited the general to send him to prison. As for the general himself, Stone went on, looking him square in the face, might he "be damned."[34]

Inland, border towns like Nashville and Vicksburg suffered immensely. General Ulysses Grant's Army of the Tennessee rolled over Confederate forces at Forts Donelson and Henry and occupied the Confederate city of Nashville in February 1862. Citizens of the town panicked at the advancing Union forces, and many evacuated as refugees. The plight of sick and wounded was especially tragic. Hurriedly loaded on railroad cars and shipped to Chattanooga, they arrived in pathetic shape. Confederate surgeon Major Charles Anderson reported from there: "When the first train arrived with some three hundred on board, they were in a most pitiable condition. They had been stowed away in box and cattle cars for eighteen hours, without fire, and without any attention other than such as they were able to render to each other . . . so chilled and benumbed that a majority of them were helpless."[35] The fortunes of the wounded were grim indeed. Immediate care of battle casualties was shameful. Beyond delivering the rudiments of first aid, field hospitalization and extended treatment were unlikely. Most injured were amputated, bandaged, loaded on trains, and transported away.

Nearby towns of relative safety offered some hope of solace and healing. Arriving in Corinth, Mississippi, on the heels of the Battle of Shiloh just across the border in Tennessee, in April 1862, volunteer nurse Kate Cumming encountered Confederate wounded transported by train from the Shiloh battlefield. She was immediately struck by the awful plight of casualties several days following the battle. With no decent hospital in which to house the patients, they were funneled to private homes. Fine sofas, beds, and couches were befouled by the pus and gore of open wounds—and even those were quickly occupied. Cumming described the scene in one particular residence: "The men are lying all over the house, on their blankets, just as they were brought from the battlefield. They are in the hall, on the gallery, and crowded into very small recesses. The foul air from this mass of human beings at first made me giddy and sick, but I soon got over it."[36] Cots and beds were unavailable. Any attention to the wounded required women to kneel in blood and water and tend to filthy bandages in dim candlelight. At night, Cumming heard the constant moans of the men. Many were hungry, having had nothing to eat for days. The women gathered what water, biscuits, and meat they could. It was a mere token of care. Soldiers beyond help mostly died in silence. "I daily witness the same sad scenes—men dying all around me. I do not know who they are, nor have

I time to learn," Cumming remarked. While nursing care fell to some nuns recruited from as far away as New Orleans, local womenfolk, moved by the numbers of horribly mangled troops in desperate need of attention, took on the lion's share (much to the chagrin of army surgeons).[37]

Hardships mounted. Grant's siege of Vicksburg, Mississippi, in the spring of 1863 cast great peril on its citizens and the defending Confederate troops. Makeshift hospitals sprang up around town, but many were merely clusters of tents, caves, or even private homes. Each one flew a yellow flag, the precursor to the Red Cross emblem, but that hardly made them immune to the pounding of Grant's huge siege cannon. Rations ran short, rats plentiful, and sanitation barely tolerable. Dysentery and malaria plagued both Union and Confederate camps, and for the Confederates accounted for about one-half of the sick and wounded. At any one time, about five thousand of the thirty-thousand-man Rebel army were bedded in the various hospitals. One chaplain of a Mississippi regiment, on visiting a larger Vicksburg hospital, noticed that the ill seemed well cared for but the wounded were relegated to tents in valleys and hollows. As he entered one of those dilapidated infirmaries, "a most horrible spectacle greeted my eyes. Every tent was filled with wounded and dying. There they lay, poor, helpless sufferers; some groaning from excessive pain, others pale and silent through loss of blood."[38]

Even worse was to come. Sherman's march to the sea from Atlanta to Savannah in the autumn of 1864 had disastrous consequences for medical care in Georgia, and even South Carolina. Federal troops fanned out on a broad path of destruction, looting and murdering and completely disrupting attempts to care for the swelling count of injured and ill. Homespun remedies were often the answer, delivered by numbers of housewives and matrons. For the common ills, local blackberries seemed to help diarrhea. Painkillers were made from jimsonweed, and heart stimulants, for those pale from blood loss, squeezed out of wild cherry and bloodroot. Nothing much of an official nature was available. The Union blockade had seen to that.[39]

It was a scorched-earth policy Sherman followed. His intent was clear: to burn out and pillage any hope of Confederate subsistence on the land. Local physician Joseph Le Conte (1823–1901) witnessed it all. Le Conte had been born on "Woodmanston" plantation in Liberty County, Georgia, and educated in New York at the College of Physicians and Surgeons. He had returned to the South, taking up a practice in Columbia, South Carolina, as a professor at the South Carolina College. Sherman's march from Atlanta caught him out of South Carolina, and only by the most strenuous of efforts did he arrive back in Columbia just before the Union Army appeared—and the Confederate troops fled. He saw the condition of the wounded and the lack of care. The scene in Columbia was terrifying. Thousands of riotous soldiers filled the streets, houses were burning, and wounded seemed everywhere. "The beautiful city, the pride of the State, sat desolate and in ashes," he recalled. The college buildings had been converted to hospitals in 1862, now called, in the aggregate, College Hospital. But they themselves were under attack by plundering Union soldiers. As a precaution, all patients—both Union and Confederate—were moved out of the buildings (for fear of their destruction) and placed in an open area of campus. The ordeal of moving critically ill men was so traumatic, Le Conte recounted, that over twenty died as a result of fright and exposure.[40]

In the path of Sherman's campaign, plagues of dysentery and diarrhea followed, affecting both Union and retreating Confederate troops. Disorderly soldiers, lack of camp sanitation, and likely contaminated water sources were the cause, but southern climates may have played a role. Northern troops were less "acclimatized" to those southern miasmas—at least Southerners might have hoped. In reality, each side seemed equally affected. One of every five troopers—Union or Confederate—at one time or another dropped from the ranks because of sickness.[41]

There was perhaps no better witness to the destructiveness of the Civil War than Confederate physician Joseph Jones. Jones (1833–1896) was a true man of the South. Born in Georgia, he attended the University of South Carolina and then matriculated at Princeton College in New Jersey. Choosing medicine as a profession, he earned his degree at the University of Pennsylvania in 1855, in the course of which he numbered several distinguished professors among his mentors. But Jones had little interest in mundane clinical practice. His thrill was a life of experimentation and teaching. He had been recruited by the new Savannah (Georgia) Medical College as the chair of Chemistry, a position he eagerly accepted.[42] Sagging enrollment and elusive promises contributed to financial woes for the young physician, who struggled to maintain a sustainable clinical practice on the side. Yet his lecturing attracted notoriety, and before long, he was invited for a faculty position at the University of Georgia in Athens. Barely had he arrived when another offer came to fill the professorship in chemistry and pharmacy at the Medical College of Georgia in Augusta. Even though his father counseled otherwise, Jones quickly accepted the Augusta position and began teaching there in 1858.

Jones was fascinated by southern fevers—the common harbingers of disease. Victims burned inside as if the blood itself boiled in response to inflammation. The skin flushed, muscles ached, the head pounded, and bed beckoned. Prostration lingered until the fever passed. What was it about southern climates that gave rise to these varieties of illnesses so characteristic of southern living, Jones wondered? Research should provide the answers, and he launched into relentless analyses of topography and weather. With historical accuracy, he applied methodological research involving death records and census figures, hoping to add statistical validity to his interpretation of likely causes. His exhaustive work on malaria (as a common form of periodic fever) and the use of medical technology such as the microscope, thermometer, and even examination of blood samples resulted in voluminous publications and some celebrity, such as one in the prestigious *Southern Medical and Surgical Journal* in August 1861. "The climate of the rich low plain, clothed with a luxuriant sub-tropical vegetation . . . and which is intersected with numerous swamps . . . is necessarily hostile to the white man. To the pestilential exhalation of stagnant swamps and rich river deposits, excited and disseminated by the burning rays of the sun . . . no process of acclimation has ever accustomed the white man."[43]

Malaria was the nastiest of his "climatorial fevers." Typified by recurring distempers and bone-rattling chills, malaria toppled its victims in bed-ridden spells of total incapacity. Sometimes there was no recovery; the patient lapsed into coma, never to awaken. It must arise, Jones felt, from those morbid emanations of soil, sun, and moisture found only in the South. Hot and humid weather, rancid vegetation, and vapors of the swamps riddled communities with periodic fevers. Remedies? Jesuits' bark—quinine—held promise, and he would use it in abundance for his suffering Confederate soldiers.

But for the time, financial woes continued to follow him. Declining enrollment at the Medical College of Georgia for the 1860–1861 session meant a cut in salary, and various odd jobs Jones had picked up failed to pay the bills. He idled in fits of worry, boredom, and futility.

Secession rescued him. Lincoln had declared war on the South, and Jones responded. General Beauregard's trashing of Union troops near Manassas provided an added incentive. He enlisted in the Confederate Army in October 1861, a private in the local Liberty Independent Troop. From the start, Jones had been angered by Northern assault on Southern principles, particularly that of slavery. He had heard rumors of Northern incursion into the South, intent on brainwashing Blacks into the irrational cause of their liberty. His first assignment was the cavalry where, as an unofficial camp physician, he came full face with the spectrum of camp diseases; soldiers, slaves, and family members stricken with relentless contagions: measles, rheumatism—probably rheumatic fever—and malaria the most common offenders. Jones figured at any one time, a quarter of his unit was sick.[44] Dysentery of course was ubiquitous. Almost everyone got it; one in ten would die from it.[45] What seemed most tragic to Jones was the number of Southerners, mostly yeoman farmers, who bivouacked near disease-ridden swamps and marshes (and, likely, too near latrines), awaiting what they were promised was a quick Confederate victory. Rarely did they see combat and more often died of miserable sicknesses far from home—and far from the heroes they aspired to be.

Inertia, disease, and the unfixable lassitude of the Liberty Independent Troop soured him to military life. Completing his term of service and again desperate for money, Jones applied for and received an appointment as house surgeon for the Augusta General Hospital. As a contract surgeon, a civilian volunteer in the service of the government, pay was better, and he still contributed to the Confederacy. There, he saw, too, the epidemics of field armies, but also the consequences of combat. Tetanus was a particularly ugly problem in neglected wounds. Once begun, the ailment spasmed and contorted its victim in excruciating fitful configurations; even the jaws themselves seized in a morbid grimace that observers called "lockjaw." The outcome was invariably fatal. Typical of victims, Jones observed in one patient "[with] a shrill, piercing cry, the head and neck are drawn back and downwards towards the heels, whilst the lower extremities are drawn in like manner backwards towards the head with great violence."[46] From the grime of pulped tissue, an animal toxin, he surmised, was the cause. "The greater tendency of penetrating and closed wounds to cause Tetanus, has been suggestive of the action of some subtle animal poison, which, like that of the mad dog and serpent's fangs, is the more deadly the less the blood flows."[47] Fevers in the injured likely "caused by animal effluvia, contradistinguished from those produced by vegetable exhalations, or malaria," started the process, he concluded.[48]

Then there was that smelly, repulsive condition called hospital gangrene. It seemed to surface in overcrowded spaces where men lay unattended with filthy, pus-soaked dressings. Open gashes in legs and arms began to smell and drip a watery discharge, then turn a sickly green that literally rotted the flesh and fomented sepsis. In some areas, Jones saw so many men crammed together that "[n]ot a single wounded soldier escaped gangrene." The stench was nauseating. Covering the nose did not even help, and nurses could not stand it for long. It was all spread by polluted air, Jones felt, contaminated by the breath of sick men. The sourness drifted from one to another, as if looming corruption, and saturated men already weakened and fatigued. This agent—he called it a material agent—acted as a "gangrenous poison upon the general system," causing a "feeble, rapid action of the heart . . . great changes of temperature, the depressed enfeebled nervous and muscular forces, the trembling hands and the low muttering delirium."[49] The whole fetid process sapped victims even further. Surgeons amputated those dreadful, greenish limbs, but one in six died anyway.

Amputation itself was a dirty process. Even amputated stumps turned gangrenous. How could it not be otherwise? Union surgeon William Williams Keen spoke of the disgusting process used by surgeons both North and South: "We operated in old blood-stained and often pus-stained coats . . . We used undisinfected instruments from undisinfected plush-lined cases, and, still worse, used marine sponges which had been used in prior pus cases and had been only washed in tap water . . . We dressed the wounds with clean but undisinfected sheets, shirts, tablecloths, or other old soft linen rescued from the family ragbag."[50] Hospital gangrene was indeed the nemesis of injured men, particularly in the Confederacy with short supply of anything clean and with the congestion of Southern hospitals. Malnutrition, camp disease, and fatigue even before wounding made it all worse. And at least in the early days of the war, surgeons in their filthy garb lopped off arms and legs at a frantic pace, seeding fresh surgical wounds with the same contagion.

But mixed with combat wounds, camp epidemics still raged, dropping more than from battle. Keen came face to face with the typhus-like illness called typhoid fever. Alongside profuse diarrhea would come extreme abdominal pain that proved a sure herald of death. Sometimes there appeared that peculiar rash seen in typhus; other symptoms—fever, muscle aches, headaches—were the same. Jones likened it to typhus, but onset was different and the abdominal pain distinct. It was not "jail fever," he concluded even though sanitation was deplorable. Typhus and this typhus-like affliction were different. In fact, in his survey of Confederate camps and prisons, "no case of true typhus fever came under my observation during the war."[51] Furthermore, he wrote: "[N]either typhoid or typhus fevers can be generated by animal exhalations from putrefying excrements or bodies; but that these diseases are propagated by a special poison emitted by the living body, either directly or through the excretions and secretions."[52] Excrements from sickly bowels of typhoid victims were responsible for spreading the disease, he felt, much like the poisonous substances from the scabs of smallpox patients. As it turned out, he would be correct. Infectious organisms, *Salmonella typhi*, were shed in stool and passed from patient to patient as opposed to the rickettsia of typhus, transmitted by body lice jumping from victim to victim.

Sanitation was the key. Jones convinced Samuel Moore of the need for hygiene reform. In turn, Moore issued a circular on July 6, 1863, outlining changes in hospital care. Abiding by newer concepts of cleanliness, Moore declared that contagion wards were to be segregated from the general population. Walls and ceilings were to be frequently whitewashed, bedding aired and changed often. Each hospital bed was to have eight hundred cubic feet of private space with screens available for isolation. Medicine distribution was to be carefully regulated, and nurses were tasked with distribution of the proper kind and amounts of food. It is doubtful his dictates were ever followed. Moore was impressed with Jones's work, his praise effusive. A communiqué from the surgeon general's office July 16, 1863, read: "For the zeal, untiring energy, patient and laborious industry therein displayed, you are entitled to and are hereby tendered the thanks of this department." Signed, S. P. Moore.[53] As a result of that endorsement, Jones was interviewed by the Army Medical Board and accepted a commission as a surgeon-officer in the Confederate forces.

But battles generated their own brand of urgency and complexity. At the start of the war, few surgeons knew how to manage war wounds. Most subscribed to the Eurocentric principle of minimalism. Avoid too much probing and meddling. Dress wounds simply. Surgery was discouraged. Of course, there were those occasions when amputation was unavoidable: mangled extremities or creeping hospital gangrene. But keep away from bullet holes and saber slashes. Meddling in those wounds—recalling Keen's observations—was bound to cause gangrene. And stay out of the belly or chest. For someone so foolish as to enter those cavities, disaster awaited. Opening the chest often asphyxiated the victim from collapse of lung or quickly exsanguinated them. Liberated feces from bowel injuries spread swifter and death came faster.

Of wounded who survived the battlefield, the most common injuries were those to arms or legs—and there were tens of thousands. The so-called conical Minié ball and shell fragments tore through skin, muscle, and bone, leaving an extremity the consistency of pulped watermelon. Amputation was the only choice, and surgeons soon severed limbs with understandable eagerness.[54] To decline was to invite gangrene, they feared. Open fractures with exposed bone, so frequent from gunshot or artillery blasts, were sure to infect, and as Jones had witnessed, creeping gangrene pounced on victims with a viciousness of purple rot, inflaming nerve fibers and driving men mad with anguish until coma and death took over. As a result, piles of discarded arms and legs adorned operating tents. Surgeons sawed and crunched damaged limbs at the slightest inclination, a decision made despite the pleas of young boys to save them from a life of disability.

Might there be more humane solutions? Confederate surgeon John Julian Chisolm (1830–1903) thought so. A Charlestonian by birth, he was educated at the Medical College of the State of South Carolina. Of capable financial means, he traveled to Paris and visited military hospitals in Milan, Italy, where he saw firsthand the ravages of the Franco-Italian War of 1859. It was there that he witnessed the effects of gunshot and artillery wounds. He saw the gambits of surgeons to cleanse wounds, avoid amputations, and salvage limbs—with some astounding successes. Just as Florence Nightingale found, it all was based on cleanliness.

After bombardment of Fort Sumter in April 1861 Chisolm volunteered. His European experience with war wounds caught the attention of the Confederate Medical Department. A glaring issue facing so many Confederate surgeons was their ignorance of war surgery. They needed quick guidance, and Moore knew a handbook—text and diagrams—would be instrumental. Up to that time, Samuel Gross's *A Manual of Military Surgery*, published in 1861, was the only one available. Moore's Confederate colleagues had managed to pirate copies from the J. B. Lippincott publishers in Philadelphia, smuggle them southward, and reprint them illegally in Richmond in 1862. Gross based his book on treatments of battle wounds from the recent Crimean War but could not address the now firmly believed peculiarities of southern medicine.[55] Not good enough, Moore felt. Confederates needed their own source from someone familiar with the South—and someone equally familiar with current military medicine. He chose Chisolm to write a Southern version. Within that year Chisolm produced it, titled *Manuel of Surgery for the Use of Surgeons in the Confederate Army*.

The central theme throughout his book, as he had seen in Italy, was sanitation and cleanliness. He first addressed basic military medical doctrine. Infections, epidemics, and contagions clearly dominated military life, both in camps and on the battlefield. He focused on practical measures to contain them, emphasizing hygiene and camp sanitation. Assemblies of country boys literally fresh off the farm spelled misery from any number of maladies. Food, shelter, and waste management were key. He stressed physical conditioning, proper clothing, and protection from weather. Warm, dry, and well-feed troops were better able to maintain stamina and morale. Important, too, was regular bathing with soap and water—not always done on the farm—to protect against "fevers and bowel complaints in warm climates." Food was to be kept far from latrines and properly prepared, Chisolm wrote. "The entire health of troops depends upon the quality, quantity, variety, and the regularity with which the provisions are supplied," he said.[56] Camp life was vital to maintaining health, he knew. Combat actually consumed very little of the soldier's time (one day in twenty, he claimed) while disease, weariness, and malnutrition caused many more days of ill health, disability, and even death.

But health in his Confederate armies was far from ideal. As the war went on and deprivations mounted, Chisolm saw camp discipline—and morale of the men—decline. Raw recruits could not maintain the strict sanitation he demanded. "[T]his sudden change from civil to military life constitutes a physiological and moral crisis," he wrote in his third edition, and was likely to cause even more deaths from disease. Indeed, by 1864 Confederate bivouacs had turned into the antithesis of cleanliness. "[C]ontinued exposure and fatigue, bad and insufficient food, salt meat, indifferent clothing, want of cleanliness, poor shelter, exposure at night to sudden changes in temperature, [and] infected tents and camps," were more than ample explanation for the glum condition of the men. A sense of hunger, hopelessness, and abandonment were physical and psychological factors that contributed to death rates in camps, he was convinced.[57]

Perhaps the true genius of his surgical manual, though, was his management of battle wounds. The Minié ball produced horrific injuries. While those to head, chest, or abdomen were usually fatal, injuries to the extremities could be survivable. Yet surgeons were fearful of the awful gangrene that developed with too much prying—European surgeons had warned against it. The consequence of abstention, however, was so frequently amputation. Chisolm advised differently. For survivable wounds, he urged surgeons to probe carefully, excise judiciously, and examine diligently. His focus was on minute surgical management. He made every effort to save arms and legs—and compulsive care was crucial. Yet he understood the limits of surgical ability. Wounds of chest were too often lethal; "perhaps the most fatal of gunshot wounds," Chisolm wrote. And of the abdomen, he had no doubt. "[A]ll who have received wounds of the large abdominal viscera die," he bluntly said. Surgery for such injuries was foolhardy, he stressed, for all those horrible reasons surgeons knew well.[58]

Chisolm's work was based on experience, not conjecture. He was most comfortable at the bedside. His surgical skills were beyond par, and he reveled in the challenges battle trauma generated. But Moore had other ideas for him. Considering the drastic state of health affairs in the Confederacy, he assigned Chisolm—equally adept, it seems, in organizational skills—to administrative roles in hospitals around Richmond and in the pharmaceutical laboratory in Columbia, South Carolina. Still, his book and illustrations would be immensely helpful for rank-and-file surgeons who manned the dingy tents of field hospitals and tended to the flood of casualties spawned by the war. Chisolm might have pined to be among them, but his true value was in the manual he produced.[59]

༄

Before long, military health issues would become a matter of public concern.

The war would turn a theoretical southern medical distinctiveness into reality as medical information and medical material from the North dwindled. As for the therapeutics of medicine and surgery, the South was now on its own. Union blockades stifled delivery of important medical supplies to the Confederacy. According to Confederate physician Herbert Nash,[60] until the later part of 1863 supplies of vital drugs like quinine, chloroform, and ether were sufficient. It was only after Union ships effectively suppressed blockade-running that pharmaceuticals diminished, and Confederate sick began to suffer. Even the precious anesthetic agent chloroform was in short supply.

As the deficit of medicines grew, Surgeon General Moore encouraged the development of alternative resources indigenous to the South and independent of foreign supply. "It is the policy of all nations," he wrote on April 2, 1862, "at all times, especially such as at present exists in our Confederacy, to make every effort to develop its internal resources, and to diminish its tribute to foreigners by supplying its necessities from the productions of its own soil."[61] To this end, Moore selected Francis Peyre Porcher (1824–1895), a noted botanist and fellow alumnus of the Medical College of the State of South Carolina, to survey medicinal usefulness of plants of the South. Porcher had a strong background in botanicals, stemming from a childhood interest in gardening. His thesis in medical school was "A Medico Botanical Catalogue of the Plants and Ferns of St. John's Berkeley, S.C.," a forerunner of a number of books and presentations on botanical therapeutics unique to the South. Following Moore's appointment, Porcher developed and published his influential work *Resources of the Southern Fields and Forests*, a text that southern physicians could use to employ a variety of local horticultural substitutes as medicine:

> It is intended as a repertory of scientific and popular knowledge as regards the medicinal, economical, and useful properties of the trees, plants, and shrubs found within the limits of the Confederate States, whether employed in the arts, for manufacturing purposes, or in domestic economy, to supply a present as well as a future want. Treating specially of our medicinal plants and of the best substitutes for foreign articles of vegetable origin.[62]

Porcher's writings did not go unheeded. In fact, his wide-ranging text would become an imperative in Confederate medicine as imports withered.

Even before Porcher's publication, Moore had established laboratories east and west of the Mississippi River where pharmaceutical extracts would be manufactured. These laboratories first appeared in Richmond in early 1862, in anticipation of Northern blockade. Moore shortly issued a directive instructing medical purveyors—officers in charge of procuring medical supplies—to inventory and collect plants of potential medical use. These were then forwarded to laboratories in Columbia, Atlanta, Augusta, Macon, Charlotte, Mobile, Jackson, and Montgomery. West of the Mississippi, a laboratory appeared as far away as Tyler, Texas—now part of the Confederacy. Apothecaries, chemists, and even geologists worked tirelessly to extract, purify, and prepare antidotes. "A most gratifying progress has ... been made in the manufacture of chemicals within our own limits ... Manufactories and laboratories are rising up in every direction under the wise supervision of our medical chief," the editors of the *Confederate Medical and Surgical Journal* reported in July 1864. They then listed ninety-two plant-based pharmaceuticals available for the Medical Field Service.[63] Medical historians Guy Hasegawa and Terry Hambrecht found that enormous quantities of analeptics came out of these laboratories. For example, the Columbia facility produced over a ton of mercurial-pill mass, and the Macon laboratory prepared almost two million doses of tulip tree powder (a soothing and sustaining type of tonic, said to be both comforting and stimulating).[64]

Moore's laboratories saved the Confederacy from total medical destitution. Local botanicals eased the desperation of practitioners and patients at a time when Union ships had a stranglehold on Southern ports. President Jefferson Davis, fully aware of the health hazards posed by blockade, lavished accolades on Moore and Porcher for their initiatives:

> To supply medicines which were declared by the enemy to be contraband of war, our medical department had to seek in the forest for substitutes, and to add surgical instruments and appliances to the small stock on hand as best they could. It would be quite beyond my power to do justice to the skill and knowledge with which the medical corps performed their arduous task . . . as well in regard to their humanity [and] to their professional skill.[65]

One herbal that could be grown almost anywhere in the South, even in backyard gardens, was the poppy plant, *Papaver somniferum*. From incisions in the green poppy seedpods, a juicy substance exuded that, when collected and dissolved in alcohol, rendered opium. Opium—sometimes called laudanum—provided numbing respite from suffering and was one of the few truly beneficial therapies for the sick and injured. In fact, the surgeon general's office appealed to private citizens to grow "the Garden Poppy" as an essential service for the Confederacy. Instructions were provided to process the ornamental plant, which "thrives well in our climate." "The juice which exudes from the incised capsules or pods, when sufficiently hardened should be collected, carefully put up, and forwarded to me at Savannah or Macon, or the nearest Medical Officer," one Georgia purveyor advertised.[66]

Even wound bandages were lacking. Hospitals felt this deficiency most keenly. Once again, civilians rose to the challenge. Wives and mothers rummaged through their bedrooms and finery for any suitable material. Cotton was preferable, but the blockade had sorely limited all textiles. So, household shirts, bedsheets, and dresses were torn apart for linear strips to serve as wound dressings. Surgeons were dearly grateful. One wrote: "[I]t was a work of love with the women of the South to make bandages and lint. They often stripped their families and their households of sheets, spreads, and even skirts in order to supply bandages and lint to the hospitals."[67]

Whether military or civilian, professional education suffered as well. There was now a dearth of collegial exchanges with the North. Ordinary lines of communication had been severed. Out of necessity and, perhaps, a touch of innate pride, physicians of the South turned to their own resources for timely updates of medical topics. In 1864 publication began of the *Confederate States Medical and Surgical Journal* (hereafter referred to as the *Journal*), a compendium of clinical information written and published by Southern authors for Southern doctors. It was another brainchild of Surgeon General Moore and served as the official periodical of Confederate medicine. The editors made every effort to provide local practitioners with the latest news in diagnosis and therapeutics, not only from home but also from abroad. It was an effort of the utmost importance, as the publishers emphasized: "Not only as the organ of the Southern medical profession, but as a means of imparting information to those who have, for three years, been debarred from any intercourse with the scientific world, will the publication of a medical periodical be found useful—indeed, an absolute necessity."[68] Fourteen issues of the *Journal* were published between January 1864 and February 1865 on subjects ranging from microscopic pathology of the liver to the efficacy of turpentine as a substitute for quinine in intermittent fevers (malaria). It would attract a larger audience than any southern journal to date. However, after February 1865 the *Journal* abruptly ceased publication. By then, Richmond was under siege, commerce had all but halted—perhaps even paper and ink were lacking—and common morale reached dismal levels.[69]

Other professional groups joined in. The Confederate States Army and Navy Surgeons Association—"for the advancement of science"—organized by faculty of the Medical College in Richmond in 1863, submitted their largely surgical "Transactions" to the *Journal* from the battlegrounds of Chancellorsville, Gettysburg, Manassas, and Richmond.[70] These reports reached a high degree of accuracy and respectability, even drawing attention from foreign journals, such as the prestigious British monthly, *Lancet*: "We cannot but sympathize with the members of the medical profession in the Southern States in their efforts to secure the benefits of professional intercourse . . . In the terrible war, which devastates the South . . . the medical profession play the most beneficent part."[71]

Persistent attrition of Confederate troops, whether from battle, starvation, or disease, depleted the ranks of Lee's Army of Northern Virginia and Joseph Johnston's Army of Tennessee. Union generals Ulysses Grant and William Sherman relentlessly pounded Confederate troops in Virginia, Tennessee, and then Georgia. Sherman's decision in 1864 to drive through the Georgia heartland on a sixty-mile-wide front, wrecking all that stood in the way, demoralized and devitalized southern culture. Moreover, Sherman was able to disrupt and permanently alter not just the physical accouterments of southern businesses but the essence of their society by dismembering the social order and completely demoralizing the spirit of their rebellion. Grant's assault on Richmond and Petersburg, a protracted and bloody affair, eventually broke through Confederate defenses in April 1865. With the Confederate capital in ruins, there was nothing left. Lee surrendered on April 9. Johnston followed suit in May. The war was over. The South collapsed in defeat.

The toll of the war on southern manhood was inconceivable. A generation of young men essentially disappeared. Although exact figures are unknown, it was Jones's belief that, of the six hundred thousand men at arms fielded by the Confederacy during the rebellion, two hundred thousand were lost to disease and battle, two hundred thousand were taken prisoner, and one hundred thousand were discharged for disability or simply deserted.[72] And of those left behind—the families and widows—untold numbers also fell victim to malnutrition, violence, and pestilence. Dixieland was a wasteland, devoid of happiness, wallowing in the curse of ruination and despair.

Abject defeat at war's end toppled all that was sacred in the South. Soil and slavery were the foundations of an agrarian society as if agriculture, to paraphrase historian Drew Faust, was not just a means of support but was the raison d'être for many southerners. The rich earth offered life-sustaining blood—and slavery was its veritable heart. In fact, capitulation of the Confederacy caused such disruption that long-held beliefs in unity of nature, society, and evangelical mission—a Gordian entanglement—now faltered. Class structure as ordained by God made sense in the southern mind, and the necessary labors of servile Blacks toiling the fields had bred a gratifying Christian ministry as so much (contrived) charity bestowed on naïve, laboring pagans. No more. Reunification would now tear traditional southern Christian morality asunder. Victory for the North suddenly liberated Blacks, ill equipped for freedom. Without indentured labor, fertile lands would no longer yield such bountiful profits.[73]

That fragile distinctiveness cherished by the South was melting away, a house of cards tumbling under the steady advance of abolitionist troops and the aimless milling of hundreds of thousands of formerly enslaved people.

And across the bleak landscape of the vanquished wandered Confederate veterans, clothes in tatters, hungry, despondent, harassed by Yankees. Southern women, too, understood the implications of defeat. Georgia resident Eliza Frances Andrews, witnessing the destruction brought on by Sherman's army, wrote in her diary, "The props that held society up are broken. Everything is in a state of disorganization and tumult."[74] Similarly, North Carolina socialite Catherine Devereux Edmondson saw nothing instructive about the war. The "future stands before us dark, forbidding, & stern . . . [full of] all the bitterness of death without the lively hope of Resurrection," she wrote in her diary.[75] There was legitimate worry in all this, aside from disruption of their planter society. Emancipation of Blacks left fields fallow, crops rotting, and famine just around the corner. Confederate bureaucrat Robert Garlick Kean, who traveled through Virginia just after Robert E. Lee's surrender at Appomattox, saw a landscape stripped of all worth and acknowledged that the entire workforce of the country was overthrown, "without preparation or mitigation." That—the abolition of slavery—was the greatest threat to the very survival of the South, in his thinking.[76]

Health care came precariously close to crisis. In his work *Doctoring the South* author Steven Stowe took heed of the chaos of medical practices wrought by the destruction of Dixie. The war had sucked numbers of physicians away from their communities, divesting the countryside of doctors. Indeed, surgeon Joseph Jones estimated 834 surgeons and 1,668 assistant surgeons served in the field, and 22 surgeons plus 51 assistant surgeons served in the Confederate Navy, not counting the doctors who staffed general hospitals and infirmaries throughout the Confederacy.[77] Little medical resources remained for town and country. But, Stowe claimed, at war's end those same doctors eagerly returned. Most had been so disillusioned by the war that, for sanity's sake and out of a sense of agrarian loyalty, they embraced their former practices, now bolstered with newfound knowledge of sanitation, contagions, and surgery. "For the most part," Stowe argued, "the war reconfirmed southern physicians' sense of the primacy of personal experience and the ideal of medicine as a moral endeavor in a local community setting." Despite the horrors of combat, camp illnesses, and overcrowded hospitals, physicians welcomed the relative civility of everyday medicine and the pivotal role they played in hometown communities. In other words, they were only too anxious to return to a lifestyle that, while disrupted by war, was meant to once again honor the centerpieces of southern medicine—patient and family—the so-called orthodoxy of the South.[78] So little of it now remained.

And what about the very people for whom the war was fought? What of the emancipated Africans now freed men and women, released from their human bondage? In fact, their plight had worsened. Surveyor Robert Kean feared that "[o]ne-half of the negroes unable by age, sex, infirmity, or want of character to support and take care of themselves are thrown on their own resources . . . The community is wholly unable . . . to take up the burden of a vast pauper system. The inevitable result will be destitution and suffering on a vast scale."[79] These were truly disheartened people, gathered together out of pity or charity in encampments that would do little but spawn the plagues of the ill-prepared, ill-fed, and health-impoverished congregations. In Charleston, the death rate among Blacks, while a degree greater than whites before the war, climbed dramatically following, almost doubling that of the white population.[80] Historian Jim Downs wrote: "The disease, death, and suffering that plagued freed people during the Civil War years resulted from the simple fact that no one predicted that military engagement and the subsequent emancipation would lead to the largest biological war of the nineteenth century."[81] He contended, and justifiably so, that the mass crowding of injured and sick, coupled with the enormous influx and intermingling of enslaved Blacks into army camps and refugee centers, produced an explosion of contagious ailments. Diseases like pneumonia, typhoid fever, and dysentery could not be treated and killed huge numbers of formerly enslaved people. These were men and women who had been relatively isolated on remote plantations and in small communities prior to their liberation. In those times, sanitation and health care were almost guaranteed by virtue of the enslaver's investment. And doctors were only too willing to comply as long as fat fees flowed from the planters. Africans were a predictable revenue stream.[82] But not now. Hygiene was shocking, and anyway, formerly enslaved people were a liability—no money. Few doctors would touch them.

In Mississippi, garrisoned Union soldiers found a frightful scene, never having traveled through predominately Black communities. "Their condition was appalling. There were men, women, and children in every stage of disease or decrepitude, often nearly naked, with flesh torn by the terrible experiences of their escapes. Sometimes they were intelligent and eager to help themselves; often they were bewildered or stupid or possessed by the wildest notions of what liberty might mean."[83] Vicksburg's caves, formerly home to residents during the siege, now housed nomadic groups of African Americans, victims of nakedness, famine, and disease. It was as if, once again, they were the same ruined people who had exited slave ships after the terrible Middle Passage.

Not that the Union government lacked a plan. The Bureau of Refugees, Freedmen, and Abandoned Lands was formed in March 1865 and would be run by the War Department. Simply known as the Freedmen's Bureau, it was, in theory, designed to oversee the African Americans' transition from slavery to freedom. To that end the bureau hoped to encourage education and self-sufficiency among newly freed people—including tending the sick. But the burden of care proved unmanageable. Waves of epidemic disease, smallpox among them, carried home by returning soldiers, swept over the Black populations—men, women, and children. And in 1866 Asiatic cholera, brought upstream by steamships from New Orleans, annihilated even more. For those destitute Africans who already lived in unsanitary conditions, it was a veritable death sentence. And when cholera abated that summer, yellow fever took its place. Government resources foundered, and the burden of care fell to physicians strapped financially themselves, hardly able to curb the socioeconomic conditions that fueled these plagues.[84]

Now, would their misery finally register? Not a chance. Penniless and destitute, African Americans drifted like refugees from a holocaust, welcomed by neither victor nor vanquished. Those Yankee opportunists who claimed the war had unleashed a moral enlightenment still failed to understand the inequality of it all. And few southerners cared. Sociologist John Franklin wrote that southern educators like the fiery Rev. C. K. Marshall of Mississippi predicted an end to the "Negro" race by 1920—simply because they would all be dead. Newspapers such as the Natchez *Democrat* proclaimed that "the child is already born who will behold the last Negro in the state of Mississippi." Those were not isolated comments. In South Carolina, white supremacists felt if they could not retain Africans in slavery, they were of the mind to get rid of them entirely.[85] Equality, in the postwar South, was a transient notion among a minority of idealistic whites.

As for the medical arts, advances in understanding of sanitation and contagions on both sides would provide for a healthier, safer public—but not for a while and not for everyone. "Public health" was still a foreign term. As any war does, the Civil War "created the setting for the most significant medical experience of the nineteenth-century United States." And importantly, over time, the distinctiveness of southern disease would melt away so that a true blending of southern and northern medicine could allow for a unified effort to decipher and eradicate epidemic maladies of the entire nation.

In the hearts of southerners, even men of science and learning, perhaps much had changed indeed, but much would never change. In fact, for southerners, the destructiveness of war brought about a bewilderment of uncompensated ravages, destroying towns, homes, hospitals, and practices. An upsetting of the social order and the southern way produced medical communities bereft of direction and purpose. Distinctiveness—that hallmark of southern ethos—too, had been shattered by a rejection of all customs southern and, shortly, by the imposition of northern-borne "reconstruction." As if the long heritage of the earth and its sanctity—that agricultural soul of the South—was another stiffening corpse on the battlefield. Would they all soon relinquish the values, prejudices, and convictions of antiquity? Not likely. Enlightenment, that expected awakening to the righteous beliefs imposed by countrymen to the North, might sound forth in idle conversation, but bitterness over the war and the rejection of their coveted liberties—even manhood itself—would fester like latent cancers deep in emotional recesses. And in small ways, so innocent and professional it would seem, a pride in Dixie would come out—that distinctiveness, that honor, that noble mannerism so peculiar to the South.

Confederate icon Samuel Preston Moore took an oath of amnesty on June 22, 1865, and returned to his destroyed Richmond. There he entered a quiet civilian life and involved himself in civic affairs. Only rarely did the brilliant humanitarian ever practice medicine again.

As journalist James Shepherd Pike wrote almost a century and a half ago: "There is in the South today an enormous mass of inherited worth, and virtue, and capacity, and wisdom, and every solid element of citizenship, that has an indefeasible right to demand recognition, and justice, and fraternal consideration. The commonest sentiments of humanity require it."[86] Indeed, in the stubbornness of these former Confederates, the bitterness of defeat may have even more boldly cemented a pride in southern distinctiveness.

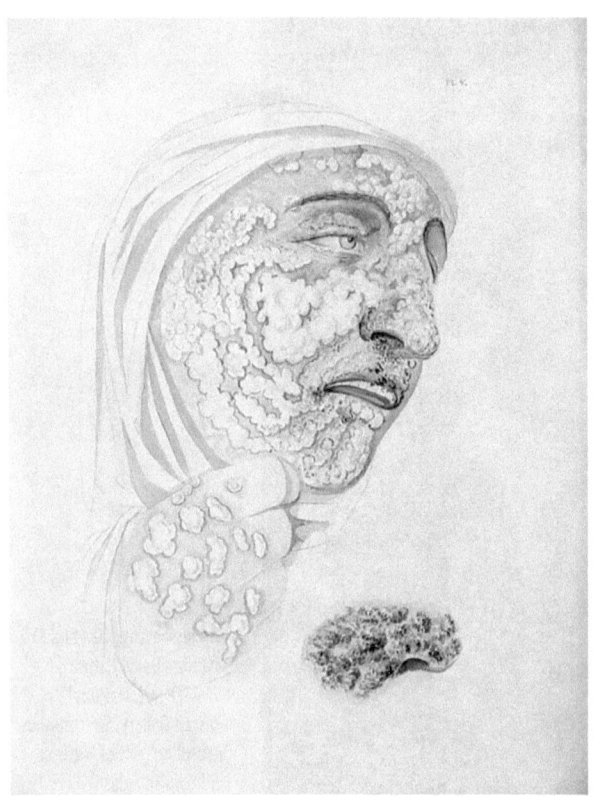

Confluent smallpox eruptions; John D. Fisher, *Description of the Distinct, Confluent, and Inoculated Small Pox Varioloid Disease Cow Pox and Chicken Pox* (Boston: Lilly, Wait & Co., 1834)

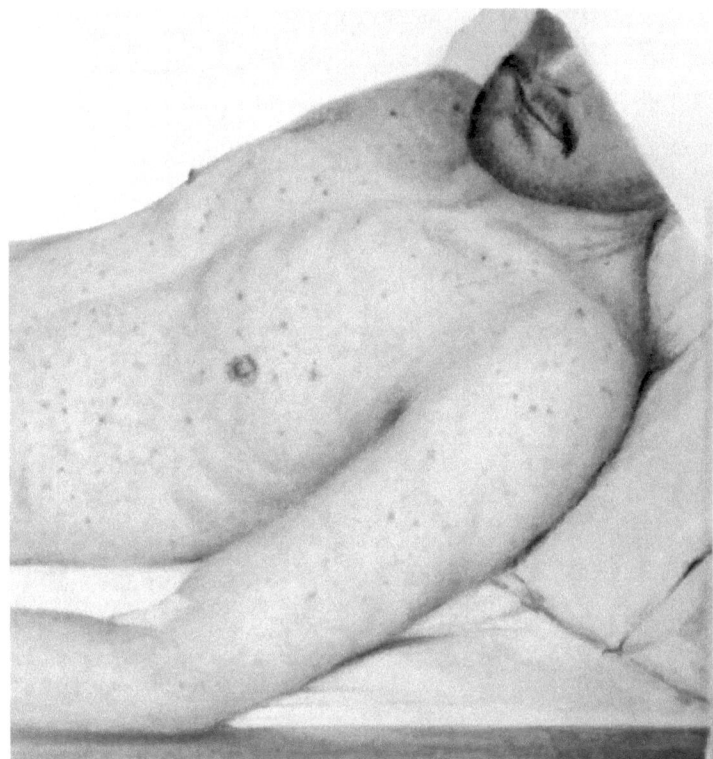

The macular rash of typhus, or so-called jail fever; Georg Jochman, *Lehrbuch der Infektionskrankheiten fur Arzte und Studierende* (Berlin: Von Julius Springer, 1914)

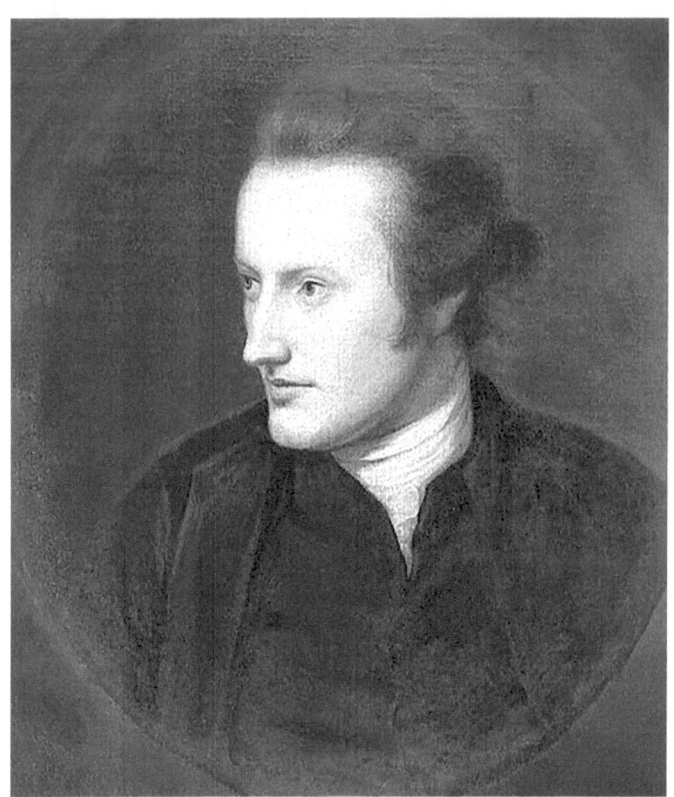

Charleston physician and historian David Ramsay; Wilson Peale, National Portrait Gallery, Smithsonian Institution (Gift of Pattison and Carolyn Fulton)

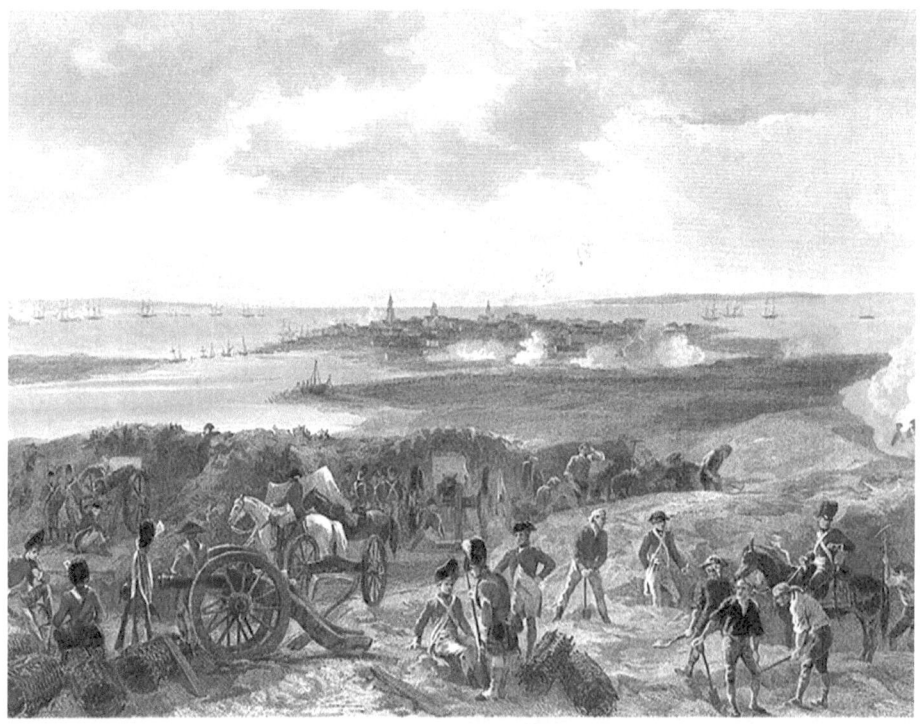

Siege of Charleston, 1780; Alonzo Chappel (1828–1887)

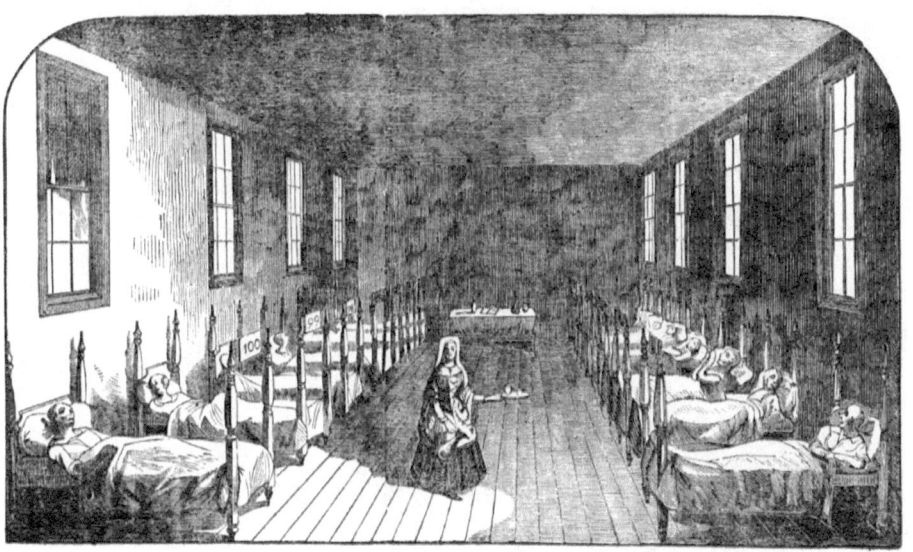

Sick Wards of Charity Hospital, New Orleans, 1853; Anonymous, *History of the Yellow Fever in New Orleans* (Philadelphia: C.W. Kenworthy, 1854)

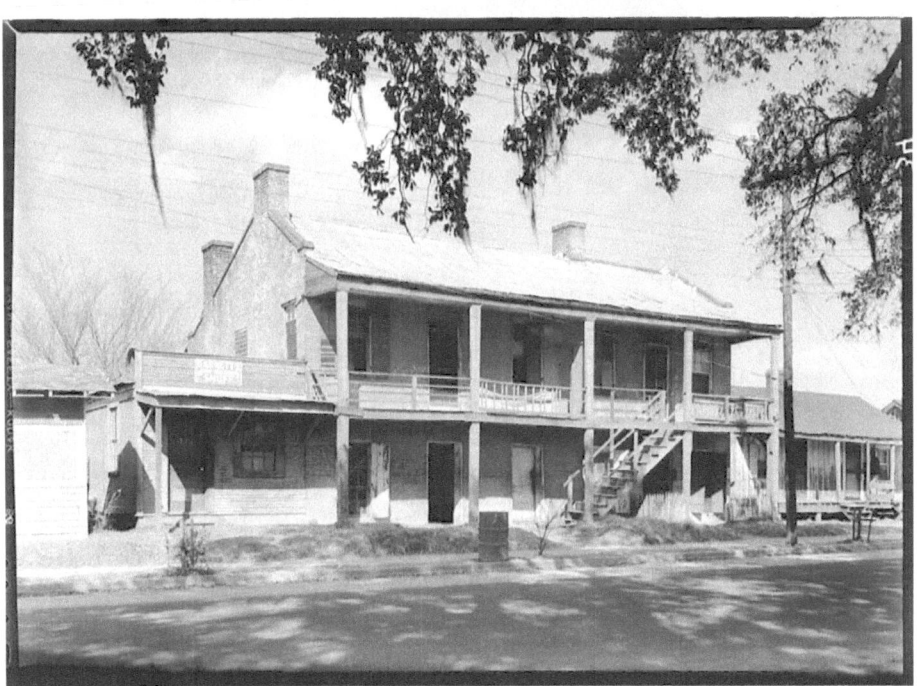

Former hospital for the enslaved (sick house), Natchez, Adams County, Mississippi
(Library of Congress, Prints and Photographs Division, Washington, DC)

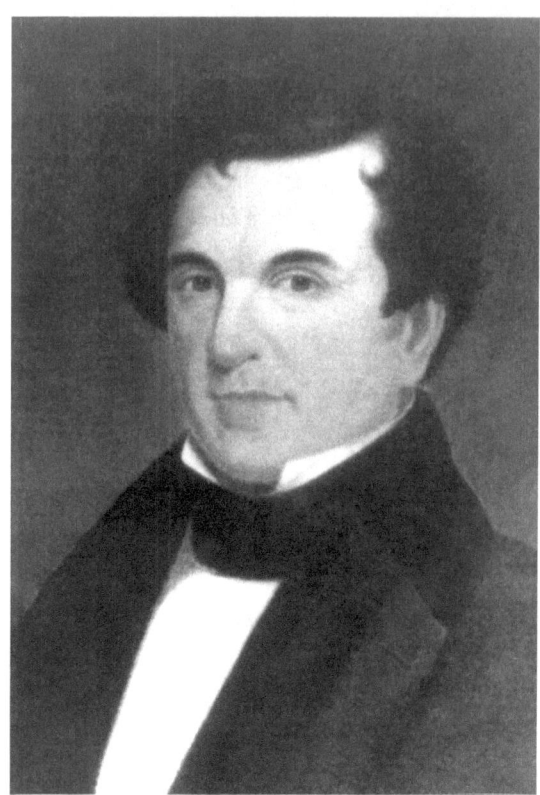

Milton Antony of Augusta, Georgia; unknown artist (Courtesy of Historical Collections and Archives, Robert S. Greenblatt, MD Library, Georgia Health Sciences University)

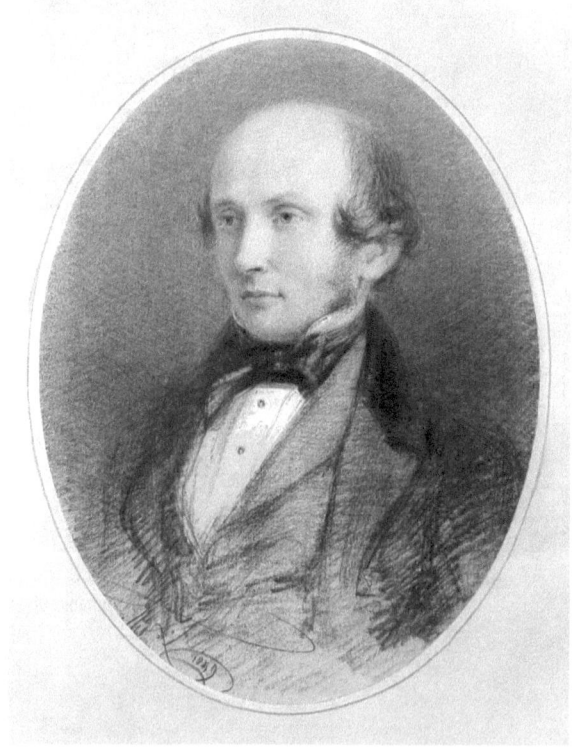

Samuel A. Cartwright; Thomas Landseer (Wellcome Collection)

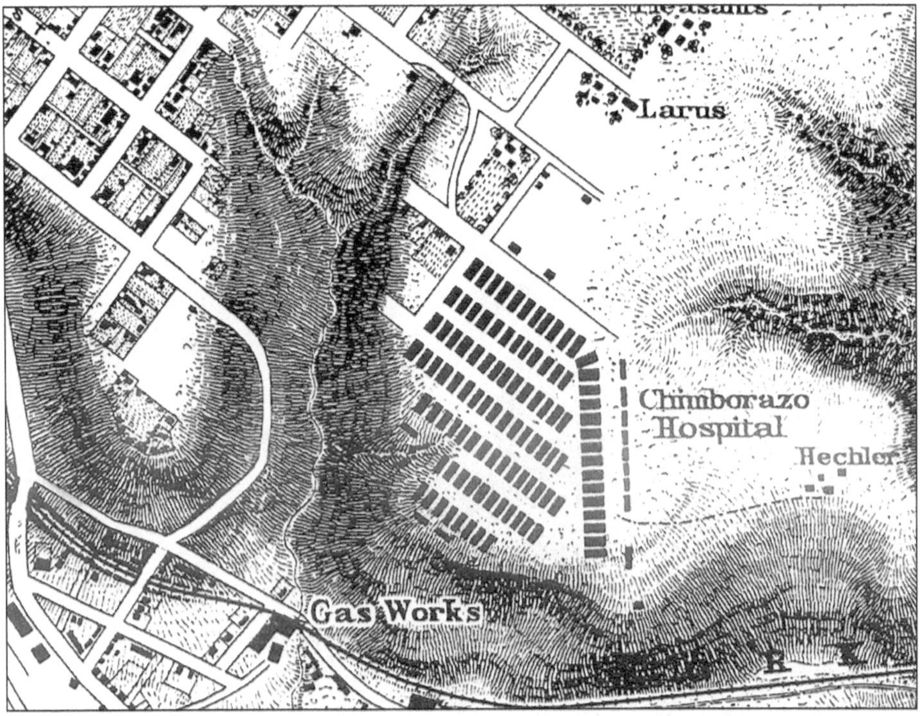

Chimborazo Hospital Map (National Archives and Records Administration, Record Group 77, Map G, 204, 55)

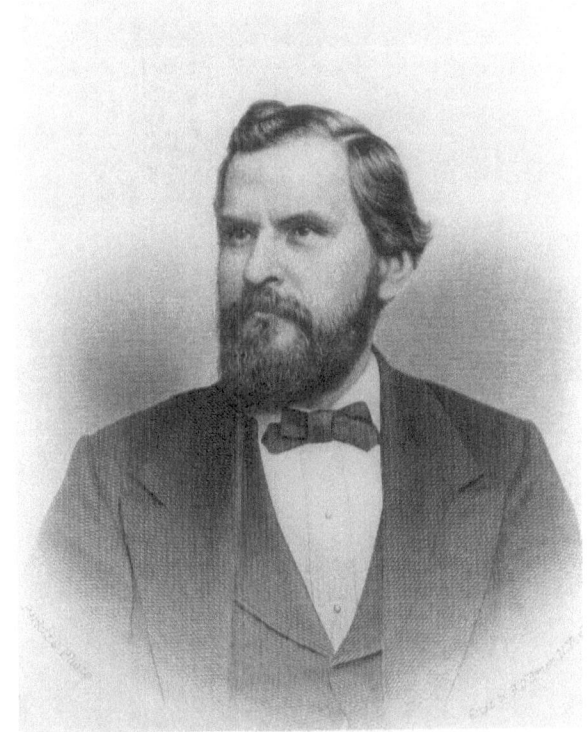

John Julian Chisolm (Courtesy of the Waring Historical Library, MUSC, Charleston, South Carolina)

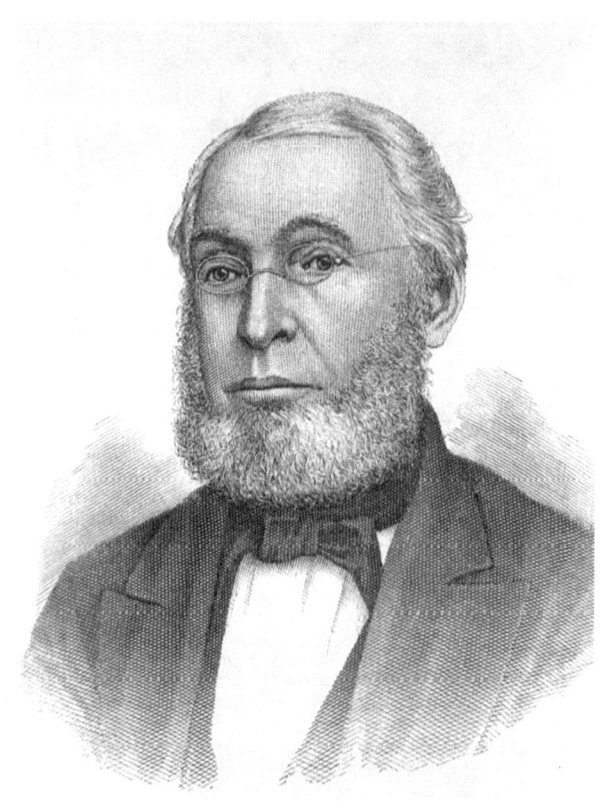

Paul F. Eve (National Library of Medicine)

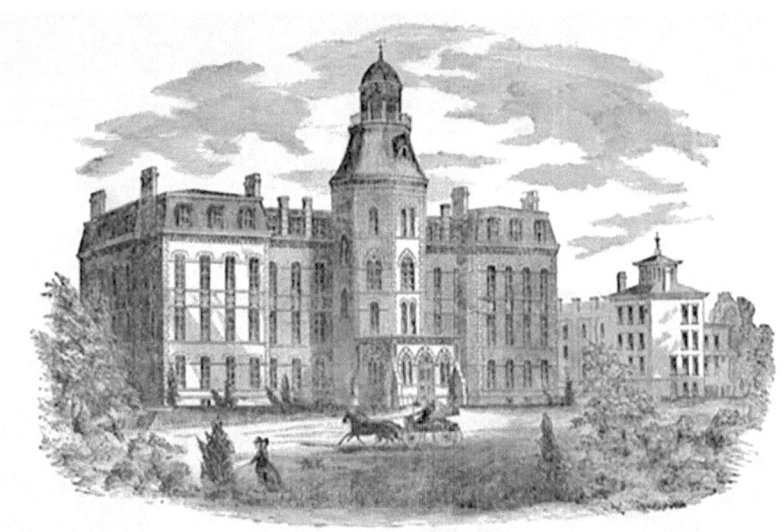

Howard University, 1868–1869
(Miriam and Ira D. Wallach Division of Art, Prints and Photographs: Print Collection, New York Public Library)

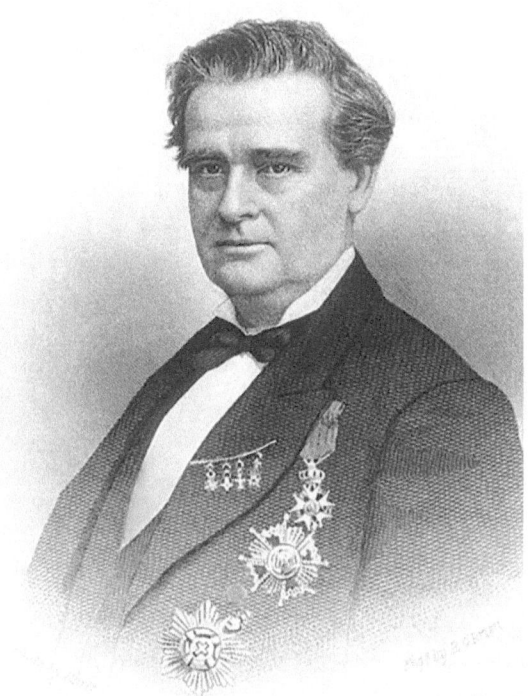

James Marion Sims; Lucius R. O'Brien, engraver
(National Library of Medicine)

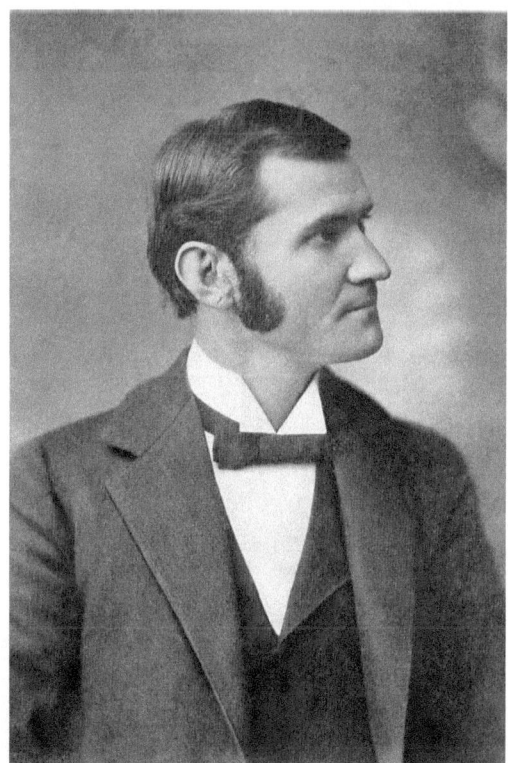

William Elias Brownlee Davis, cofounder of the
Southern Surgical and Gynecological Association
(Reynolds-Finley Historical Library, University of
Alabama, Birmingham)

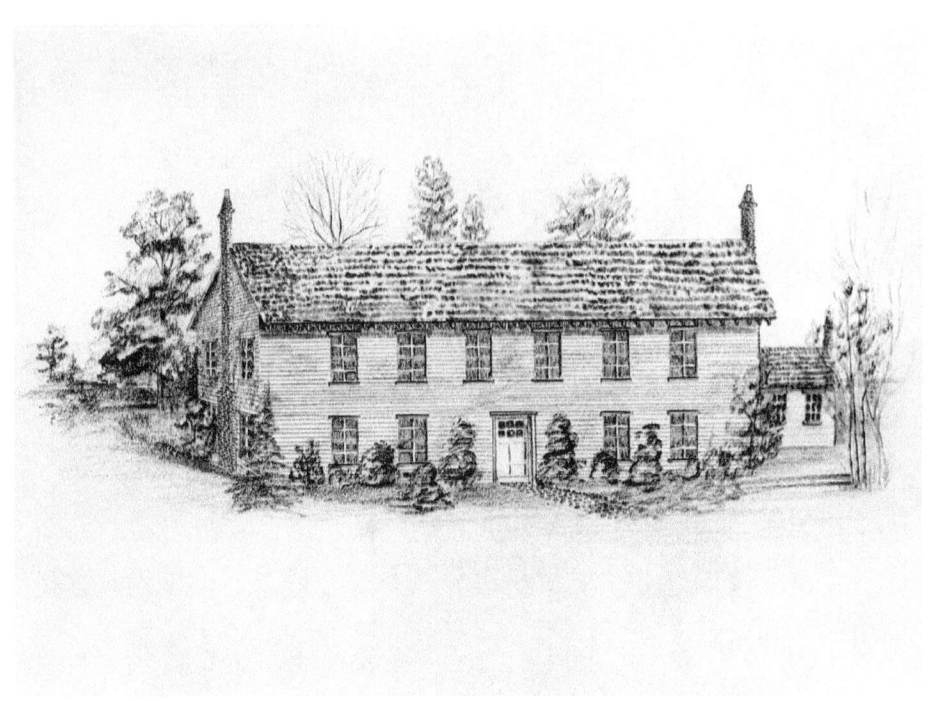

Augusta City Hospital around 1818
(Courtesy of Historical Collections and Archives, Robert B. Greenblatt, MD Library, Augusta University)

CHAPTER ELEVEN

AN ABOMINATION OF HEALTH

Reconstruction of the South

*As the carcass invites the vulture, this prostrate land
drew adventurers from all points of the compass.*
—JOURNALIST AMBROSE BIERCE, 1865

"The evils of the South are of her own procuring. They are not Northern inflictions," so wrote clergyman Henry Ward Beecher in 1887.[1] The victorious North, resplendent in its effort to unite the Union once again, descended on the South with the will of conquerors intent on sweeping away an immoral and repugnant culture. Even so, federal agents, in all their pomposity, found a scene of stark annihilation. The report of General Carl Shurz, sent by President Andrew Johnson in 1865 to investigate conditions in the South, gave an alarming warning: "It is, indeed, difficult to imagine circumstances more unfavorable for the development of a calm and unprejudiced public opinion than those under which the southern people are at present laboring. The war has not only defeated their political aspirations, but it has broken up their whole social organization."[2] In so many ways, the South was broke. Millions of dollars had disappeared through devaluation of former human property, destroyed real estate, or accumulated Confederate debt. "With this went the moral effect of an unsuccessful war with all its letting down of social standards and quickening hatred and discouragement," sociologist W. E. B. Du Bois wrote in 1910.[3] Of course, the plight of millions of formerly enslaved

Africans was unimaginable, many turned loose without means of any kind: financial, intellectual, or skillful. The most apparent need, Congress knew, was to integrate these people as useful—and free—members of a new southern economy. Yet even though conditions were abominable for Blacks, top priority went to the white communities. In Alabama, representatives from the Freedmen's Bureau gave a startling portrayal in 1865 of the suffering of whites, temporarily at least, side-stepping the more tenuous predicament of the people they formerly enslaved.

> By far the greater suffering exists among the whites. Their scanty supplies have been exhausted, and now they look to government alone for support. Some are without homes of any description . . . The general destitution has rendered many kindly disposed people unable to do anything for the negroes who were formerly their slaves . . . there is much suffering among the aged and infirm, the sick and the helpless.[4]

Women, now widowed, and their children, this same reporter continued, were seen begging for food door to door. Drought and a piddling harvest added to their misery. It would be hard to imagine a more volatile situation for hatred of the opportunists who ventured south to join, lawfully or unlawfully, in reconstruction. While a politeness so typical of southern customs exuded acceptance, there was deep loathing for the Yankees with whom they were forced to interact. And even more, this "unfriendly spirit," as Carl Schurz related, "is all mildness and affection compared with the popular temper which in the south vents itself in a variety of ways and on all possible occasions." Even though he may be shown common respect, the term "Yankee" still implied "those traits of character which the southern press has been so long in the habit of attributing to northern people." "Yankee wickedness" it was called.[5] Men folk and women concealed their distaste for the northern "carpetbaggers," as they came to be known.[6] Rarely openly hostile, many southerners simply abided by imposed dictates and submitted to concessions in hopes of having themselves restored soon to power. Only then could they arrange a social order of their own preference—much akin to the Confederacy that had so recently slipped from their grasp.

The mismanagement of rebuilding under Lincoln's successor, President Andrew Johnson, added immeasurably to the gloom of southern whites. Was it intentional that Johnson now punished the South? Many clergy felt so. One New York minister announced from the pulpit that the new president (Johnson) had been called to "hew the rebels in pieces before the Lord." Johnson's ineptitude to address southern ills was not so much incompetence, then, as divine retribution. It was as if a furious God had joined ranks with the North to purge wickedness from the South.[7]

There was no escaping the utter wreckage. It was "disorder worse than war, and oppression unequaled in American annals."[8] Poverty and more poverty were the plight of Dixie. Emancipation had dismantled a vast free enterprise market and loosed enormous sums of capital investments. Journalist and author Ambrose Bierce observed in his visits through occupied Alabama after the war, "As the carcass invites the vulture, this prostrate land drew adventurers from all points of the compass." Many of these vultures, he sadly found, were in the employment of the United States government.[9] Some were scoundrels, pure and simple. Others had a more beneficent motive, albeit badly strategized. In a hurried effort to integrate a fractured society, northern officials handed choice state government positions to poorly prepared African Americans only recently freed from slavery. As such, Blacks often were merely puppets, acting at the behest of northern scoundrels who calculated their own nefarious ends.

Meanwhile, the conduct of true southerners "never yielded moral support to the corrupt legislation surrounding them, and exhibited extraordinary wisdom, endurance, patience, and subordination to law.[10] It was manifest resilience in the face of demolished infrastructure. Major southern cities—those magnets for innovation and education—were in shambles. Affluence disappeared; dignity was a distant remembrance. The South's agricultural and manufacturing infrastructure almost ceased to exist. Mainstay crops of the Deep South, cotton and corn, fell precipitously between 1860 and 1880 in Alabama, Mississippi, and Louisiana—up to 40 percent of pre-war levels.[11] In many areas, little remained but a scorched countryside and homeless inhabitants. Colleges across the region had been sacked, looted, burned, and vacated. Financial support ebbed because southern finances had disintegrated. Historian Joseph Stetar wrote that "both Southern culture and higher education were, in the latter third of the nineteenth century, distinct from those in other sections of the nation." Experimentalism and rationalism did not rise to the forefront as they had in the Northeast. Instead, southern learning focused on mental discipline, piety—that time-honored southern virtue—and Christian education. Innovation fell by the wayside.[12]

It was not until the congressional elections of 1866 that the new Republican majority was able to effect legislation, including the Fourteenth Amendment, which constitutionally confirmed civil and equal rights to all Americans. It was praised as a vital step to reform and reconstitution of a free-labor economy. That same Congress, a year earlier, established the Freedmen's Bureau as a gateway vehicle for newly freed Blacks. With southern state governments in disarray, it was the only practical means of carrying out federal policies and federal assistance. Among a number of humanitarian functions, health was a major interest of the bureau. It at least offered a temporary substitute: medical aid to the impoverished—both Black and white. Yet programs provided by the bureau were not free. States needed to contribute—and some states simply would not or could not. For example, North Carolina appropriated a mere $0.80 per capita in 1866 compared to $3.59 for Arkansas.[13]

Physicians, so eager to rejoin their hometowns, could not subsist on meager payments. So depleted were the towns and so destitute the residents that no one sought or could pay for medical services. One surgeon, finding his community of Columbia, South Carolina, in ashes, relocated his entire family to Charleston: "I wagoned [sic] my way to Charleston with all my dependents, where living in two rooms I made my own fires, helped cook, and trudged around on foot for a year to get a bone at market, or the scant loaf of bread that served our frugal meal."[14] He was not alone. Some absconded to parts North and West, in search of opportunity. With licensing laws defunct, practitioners of all types filled the void, rogues so perverse as to be frankly criminals. The South had become a wasteland for medicine: communities stripped of doctors, professional schools shuttered, and collegiality stifled. From 1861 to 1865 medical initiatives had all but stopped. Educationally, medical colleges were closed, faculties had been disbanded, most medical journals ceased, and much of community care diverted to the all-important war effort, sucking many able-bodied physicians into the ranks of the Confederate military. A vacuum of medical knowledge and initiative resulted.

For those wanting to ignite a sputtering academia, it was a bleak picture indeed. Yet only there could the future of the South be rescued. All eyes were on urban centers of education that existed before the war. But they were in disarray. The ravaged state of Georgia was a prime example.

During the four years of war, Atlanta, Georgia, had become a Confederate boomtown, the population doubling from 1860 to 1864. As a manufacturing center, Atlanta was a giant Confederate industrial mill, producing such essential war items as shot and shell, rails, carriages, and tents. Extensive warehousing provided a ready source of war material for Confederate forces. General William Sherman knew it and made the destruction of Atlanta his priority. Shrewdly, though, Sherman may have laid waste to much of the town, but he retained intact those foundries to maintain production for Union troops.

The Atlanta Medical College, founded in 1854, emptied its lecture halls and laboratories in 1861 to fill, instead, with hospital beds. All educational activities of the college ceased. The city, which boasted twenty-six hospitals to house Confederate troops during the war, could count none remaining afterward. Regardless of race, wealth, or social status, no health facility stood to treat anyone. At the college, buildings were used by Confederate forces to house both Confederate and Union casualties. But "burglarious and thieving achievements" abounded as Union armies marched in so that, at war's end, there was "practically complete destruction" of physical equipment as well as financial resources.[15]

Yet the structure itself remained standing and survived Sherman's devastation. It all happened by ruse. Professor Pierre D'Alvigny of the medical faculty enlisted some quite healthy attendants to play the role of bed-ridden patients so that when the Union officer in charge of the burning arrived, he was faced with the inconceivable notion of burning men alive (the truly sick patients had already been moved). Told to evacuate the "patients" by morning, D'Alvigny complied, but by that time, federal troops had departed, and the college was saved. In August 1865 the faculty reassembled, and by the following February courses were again offered.[16] By March 1866, the Atlanta Medical College was fully operational. The *Atlanta Medical and Surgical Journal* that month boasted: "Medical teaching has been re-established, and the prospects of Atlanta Medical College are far better for the ensuing Regular Summer Session, than the most sanguine could reasonably have anticipated, with the ruined condition of the country, and with the dilapidated condition of the college buildings."[17] The fact that the formerly prestigious journal had even reemerged furnished a spark of optimism for the medical community. "After over four years of absence, the editors went on, "we, under embarrassing circumstances . . . hope to be able . . . to furnish the medical reader with a periodical . . . useful to him as a practitioner."[18] Readers once again eagerly digested the discoveries in anatomy and physiology that could now filter into the South from such exotic places as Paris, Berlin, and Vienna.

Still, the surrounding devastation could not be ignored. Resentment had roosted in the hearts of many of Atlanta's citizens, including academicians. Newly recruited surgery professor Samuel Hollingsworth Stout, former enslaver and Confederate physician, told his graduating students that year (1866): "That pile of ruins, those blackened walls, that line of rifle-pits, those redoubts, those fields, beneath which lie the Federal and Confederate dead, every living man and woman, and almost every child . . . have a tale to tell of devastation and desolation."[19]

Although Sherman had spared his wrath on Augusta, Georgia, after the war, the town was beset with abolitionists and, if not bad enough, the plague of typhoid fever. Sicknesses of mind and body, the populace reckoned. As for the Medical College of Georgia, so illustrious in former days, author Phinizy Spalding wrote: "[I]ts spirit, if not broken, was stilled. The numbers, the money, the influence, the enthusiasm, the drive, the determination to try something new—all were misplaced in defeat."[20] And with the economy flattened by war and disappearance of its bonded labor force, little remained to endow the college. As a result, enrollment there, too, lapsed. Desperate for financial security, trustees approached the University of Georgia in Athens. State support might salvage the medical college. Trustees of both institutions reached a favorable agreement in 1873, merging the two institutions, the Medical College now serving as the university's Medical Department.

But troubles for the college were not over. The overarching issue remained the bankrupt condition of state (and southern) economics. Such upheaval wrought by the war caused a total disruption of agrarian commerce—the engine that drove higher education. The end result was a precipitous drop in enrollment. Only fourteen students would graduate in 1873 and 1874. Like the *Atlanta Medical and Surgical Journal*, in the summer of 1866 the prominent *Southern Medical and Surgical Journal*, on hiatus during the war, revived under new editorship at the Medical College of Georgia to educate readers on recent medical breakthroughs both at home and abroad. In all their scholarship, though, the journal's editors could not refrain from prefacing their scientific publications with diatribes on the injustice of the war and the inhumanity of perceived Yankee vengeance: "We cannot close our eyes to the facts that our armies were vanquished . . . by superior numbers and by starvation, and our records of honor as a people, captured and burned; and that our houses and lands are desolate, our cities burned, and our people distressed and afflicted."[21] The wrecked southern economy, however, would handicap this periodical. Production and distribution were expensive, and before long, for some, money ran out. The *Southern Medical and Surgical Journal*, so respected in antebellum times, folded in 1867 from lack of funds. It had functioned for barely a year, and its failure struck another major blow to Augusta's Medical College.

In the former Confederate capital of Richmond, the Medical College of Virginia had remained open and, in fact, graduated students each year of the war. However, workers at the Richmond Almshouse and City Hospital shortly became strapped for bare necessities such as salt, bacon, meat, chloroform, morphine, and Epsom salts. In 1865, the City Hospital's sole ambulance horse was sold at auction (and probably eaten), patients were moved back to the original Egyptian building, and rooms were rented for profit. By July 1865 Virginia was close to financial ruin and the college was broke. Still, classes continued, albeit in the most spartan of fashion. Teachers were paid a pittance and, in fact, were tapped for donations. Enrollment, of necessity, declined in the postwar years, from more than fifty to fewer than twenty. In 1866 the reconstituted Virginia General Assembly provided financial relief by the appropriation of funds to compensate faculty for their aid to the college. Then the slow ascendancy to solvency. In 1867 the college opened its first outpatient clinic, supported in part by the Freedmen's Bureau. The facility made no distinction of color or status. Black and white, sick and poor were all admitted.

Jefferson's proud university in Charlottesville also had not wavered in its mission. Following Lee's surrender, the teaching staff promptly resumed their educational activities. There had been rumors leaked to the public of sacking and burning by Union troops, but these were quickly dispelled. Yes, the dormitories had been converted to hospitals but not destroyed. And yes, Virginia's agricultural commerce had been polluted "following the triumph of the destructive measures of Black Republicans," but the public ignored naysayers and professed undiminished confidence in their institution of higher learning. In fact, the war and all its horrible inflictions, both from wounds and disease, had provided unsurpassed clinical material for instruction for the Department of Medicine. So, unimpeded by the direct ravages of wartime, the university's unique mixture of didactic teaching and bedside training carried forward. In fact, the medical curriculum now extended almost a full year. Its professors bragged that despite the bloody ramifications of a "sectional war" inflicted chiefly on Virginia, by the following year (1866) an amazing 258 students completed studies and graduated.[22]

Unlike Virginia, nearly on the front lines of the war, South Carolina avoided terrible battlefield slaughters. Yet it still suffered a share of war's devastation. Sherman's army crisscrossed the state in rampages of violence and pillage. The *Columbia Phoenix* paper reported: "The march of the Federals into our State was characterized by such scenes of license, plunder, and conflagration as very soon showed that the threats of the Northern press, and of their soldiery, were not to be regarded as a mere *brutum fulmen* [empty threat] . . . fugitives lined the roads, with wives and children, and horses and stock and cattle, seeking refuge from the pursuers."[23] Union artillery had not only pummeled Columbia but also shelled Charleston, the citadel of secession. The Medical College of the State of South Carolina had suffered dearly. Shells damaged buildings, and looters robbed the museum of furniture and anatomic preparations. A near bankrupt South Carolina could offer almost nothing to rebuild, and the destitute citizenry could provide little more. Only through painful auctioning of priceless commodities such as furniture, drapes, and wax models could enough money be raised to nervously open for the autumn session of 1865. Even the Roper Hospital, again in civilian hands, began admitting patients into a grimy but functional interior.

Yet the Charleston school's coffers barely met expenses, and many Carolinians were wary of its future. In a bizarre turn of events, trustees of the University of South Carolina in Columbia proposed a new medical school. On an undergraduate campus stretched thin by finances (only forty-five students entered the fall of 1866), assembly of a medical faculty was especially daunting. Money was scarce (as of May 1868 the total expenditure on the medical department amounted to a mere $299) and equipment meager. None of this set well in Charleston. The faculty there sent a searing objection to the state legislature in 1869:

> The proposed plan [Columbia's medical college] is unnecessary and uncalled for, because the State already possesses one Medical College advantageously located in a large and prosperous city, easy of access from every point . . . commodious buildings and lecture rooms . . . abundant supply of anatomical material, and several hospitals of extensive accommodation . . . Where, then is the necessity for a second Medical College in the State?[24]

Of course, the Columbia faculty countered with arguments that their new school was more centrally located, a part of the state-supported university, and was already housed in available university buildings. They proposed an aggressive curriculum of two full years encompassing literary, scientific, and professional courses, with bedside instruction in practical items such as "application of the bandage, the splint and the scalpel." Magnanimously, they advertised free schooling and admission to students both Black and white. The legislature sided with Columbia. Eight students entered in the first class, without scholastic requirements. Four students graduated in 1868, three in 1869, four in 1870, one in 1871, seven in 1872, and three in 1873. Integration proved a dismal failure, though. Following admittance of Henry E. Hayne, an African American, faculty resigned en masse, an event from which the school never recovered. From there on, there were no graduates. The school ceased to function entirely in 1876.[25]

In New Orleans, a city awoke from the nightmare of occupation and federal tyranny. At the start of the Civil War, New Orleans had become the largest city in the South. It was a major port of trade and a funnel for literally all the exports flowing from the Mississippi Valley. Yet it had become an atypical southern town, populated with as many "foreigners" as locals. "New Orleans was geographically southern but culturally sui generis," wrote Howard Hunter. Historian Ted Tunnell characterized it this way: "[T]he Southern people as a whole were notable for their homogeneity; the people of New Orleans were notable for their diversity."[26] It added an aura of sophistication to the community, as if a northern town with all its immigrants had been lifted and planted in the Louisiana swamps. Medically speaking, the city was awash with disease and pestilence, just as it had been before the war. Stone's Medical College of Louisiana had prospered and filled annually with students eager to encounter the mysterious diseases of Charity Hospital.

Nearby, Fenner's New Orleans School of Medicine had been equally successful. Yet educational prosperity ceased in 1862. With Union troops bivouacked in the city itself and Benjamin Butler's iron rule, all sessions at both schools stopped. Refusing to take any oath of loyalty, Fenner left New Orleans for Mobile, Alabama, to serve as a volunteer surgeon. Upon his return in 1865, his finances were in ruin, and he was almost destitute. Through herculean efforts, Fenner was able to gather a faculty, fill the dissecting room with cadavers, dust off the museum specimens, and restore the grandeur of his beloved medical school. At the same time, he revived his *New Orleans Medical and Surgical Journal*, publishing again by 1866. For this, Fenner felt a special imperative. Like other southern scholars, he knew journals were the lifeblood of knowledge for his southern colleagues, strapped as they were with years of isolation and academic inattention.[27]

Yet the inveterate clinician, teacher, and organizer, exhausted by the stresses of Civil War, relocation, financial ruin, and the strain of rebuilding, finally wore out. He died in May 1866. His terminal illness was a short one, characterized by paroxysms of fever and delirium, as if the long, arduous stress of reforming medicine in his adopted city finally triumphed. His legacy was an honorable one. He was thought of as a kind, charitable man, devoted to the service of others. In a sense, he, too, was a casualty of the war. His New Orleans School of Medicine, almost completely reliant on private tuition, struggled with sagging admissions and finally closed its doors in 1870. Yet his *New Orleans Medical and Surgical Journal* flourished once again as a major medium of southern medical information.[28]

⸺

And what of those formerly enslaved people, freed by emancipation but so poorly equipped to integrate into "white" society. They were little more than shabby mobs, huddled in stark encampments astride shattered cities. Some estimated four million Blacks had been freed. They became a population particularly vulnerable yet particularly unprotected. Hundreds of thousands of freed Blacks were at the mercy of a health care system—or lack thereof—that, for them, was nonexistent. Newly designated African *Americans* sought care at traditional almshouses and charity hospitals built explicitly for that purpose. Yet southerners refused to take them in—too many whites filled the beds. Some charitable doctors, though willing to treat Blacks, went uncompensated for their care and soon quit. Bereft of physicians, shunned by hospitals, and deprived of medicines, Blacks languished in refugee camps or shifted through cities to become the new urban poor. The Black population of Charleston rose sharply after the war, formerly enslaved men and women flocking to the city from outlying low country in search of jobs, shelter, or public aid. But they came to a community destitute and thinned in numbers, hardly able to employ its white residents, let alone Black newcomers.

While health of whites actually improved following the war, that of emancipated Africans had decidedly worsened.[29] Crowded, unsanitary conditions almost certainly contributed. Diseases like tuberculosis soared. Malaria and syphilis raged in tent cities and hovels. Who now to care? Incompetent healers and ineffectual nostrums peddled by scallywags slithered in. It was "a crying shame," not a few declared.[30] Was this bedlam preferable to slavery? Some thought not: "[W]hen one considers the strict; almost domestic control under which the slaves were kept in Charleston, how they were cared for when young and provided for when old, and how their number in the city was kept down to the actual demand for their services, one finds natural reasons enough for an increased liability to death in the severe ordeal they have passed through since their emancipation."[31] Such scenes fostered deeper racism. Conjured inborne deficiencies were to blame: less intelligence, less education, improper diets, inadequate clothing, poor ventilation, and, in general, unhealthy habits. "[A]s a slave he seemed hardy enough, his health being guarded by his master... His physical condition today does not appear very stable or encouraging, for he [the Black man] is showing a striking susceptibility to disease in general," one Texas epidemiologist opined.[32] Rue the days of freedom, he implied; slavery was a fitter option.

There were but few champions for the Black cause. In General Oliver Howard, commissioner for the Freedmen's Bureau from 1865 to 1874, Black America found one. During the war, Howard witnessed the horrid conditions of camps for those formerly enslaved, usually adjacent to army bivouacs and laden with substandard sanitation. Under such conditions many army physicians loathed caring for these wretched people and considered them not even the worth of cattle.[33] In cities, such Black slums could be found on the fringes, and Howard had seen there, too, a refusal of municipal governments to address them. There was no denying that the white South seemed to care less. African Americans languished in dens of filth and depravity at the mercy of common diseases. For any man of compassion, these were appalling sights. Despite the bureaucracy of his position, Howard hounded Washington to mobilize available resources for the sake of his entrusted Black subjects. He created a medical department within the bureau, then directed his staff to set up hospitals, dispensaries, and home visitation programs for the destitute. So successful were his efforts that near its peak operation, from September 1, 1866, to September 1 1867, his medical program ran forty-six hospitals and forty-eight asylums and dispensaries manned by 105 commissioned and private surgeons who cared for 135,296 freed men and women. He saw to it that his hired doctors, nurses, and administrators did not shirk their duties. Overall hospital mortality was said to be a respectable 3.4 percent.[34]

What the Freedmen's Bureau could not directly address, though, was, in Howard's mind, a glaringly obvious problem. There were hardly any Black physicians. In fact, there were precious few Blacks around with any higher schooling. For Howard, the solution was obvious. Education was the key to Black relief. Relief from what, War Secretary Edward Stanton asked in 1865. "Relief from beggary and dependence," was Howard's response.[35] With Stanton's tacit approval, Howard, as bureau commissioner, made it happen. Schools of higher education appeared throughout the South in 1866 and 1867: Charleston, Atlanta, Macon, Savannah, Memphis, Mobile, Nashville, and New Orleans. Locally, in Washington, Howard met with members of the First Congregational Church. At first, talk centered on educating Black preachers and founding a theological school. It would be named, the group insisted, the "Howard Theological Institute." No, Howard urged, far more was needed. Education for all, clerical and lay—Black and white. The name and scope changed to the "Howard Theological and Normal Institute" and, finally, in January 1867 "Howard University." According to archivist Walter Dyson, "[I]t was impossible to decide which the freedmen needed more—doctors for their souls or doctors for their bodies."[36] They needed both. Liberal arts, theology, and medicine courses all appeared on the solicitations.

President Andrew Johnson approved the Howard University charter in 1867, and classes began for the Medical Department in November the following year. Five professors met eight students that first day of class. Dr. Alexander Augusta was the lone Black faculty member—the demonstrator in anatomy (another Black physician, Anderson Abbott, donated his time to the school as an instructor).[37] The infirmed patients of the Washington Freedmen's Hospital, which occupied the grounds of a former Black refugee camp, provided subjects for bedside teaching. Supported by the Freedmen's Bureau until 1879, Congress maintained the school with special appropriations thereafter. While there is little doubt Howard, who was elected the university's first president, focused on Black education, the colleges within were open to applicants of all backgrounds and ethnicities. By 1880 Howard University had graduated a total of seventy-seven medical students, six of whom were women.[38] Yet bigotry was rife. The new Medical Society of the District of Columbia refused membership to Black physicians and expelled members who taught at Howard. Such disputes did not end there but extended to the staid American Medical Association and even to the floor of the United States Senate. In white public opinion, emancipation did not mean equality; it only meant that the Black, the "Negro" of whatever intelligence, motivation, and education, was no longer a bonded slave.[39]

Impressive as his accomplishments were, Howard's manners and determination irritated not a few of his fellow bureaucrats. In 1872 President Grant abruptly sent Howard to the Southwest as "Peace Commissioner" to the Native Americans. It was a thinly veiled attempt to remove him from the Freedmen's Bureau so that Congress could shut it down, which they promptly did. Only one hospital and one infirmary remained, treating a mere 1,500 patients.[40] As the Freedmen's Bureau faded, a two-tiered system developed whereby Black health care became progressively segregated, isolated, and disparate from whites. The freedmen's hospitals fell into disrepair, often dirty and run-down. Without Howard's oversight, their administration too easily turned corrupt. The corresponding white systems, resplendent in private funding, more and more ignored the plight of the sicker and needier African Americans. It was all sublimely justified by the hint of social Darwinism wafting in the political breeze, that Black Americans—unfit as they were perceived to be—might slowly die off.

Howard was not alone. Nashville, Tennessee, resident George Whipple Hubbard (1841–1921), a former Union corpsman during the war and eventual graduate of Vanderbilt University Medical School in 1875, was another dismayed at the sorry plight of freed Blacks. He had lingered in wartime Nashville and then accompanied Sherman on his march into Georgia. Looming large in all that, he saw, was a developing crisis in health care.

Nashville itself was spared the ravages of some southern cities. Still, following the collapse of the Confederacy, the community, at heart a richly southern city, abounded in human misery. While affluent whites who had fought for the South or North warmed in their spacious salons, the dregs of their community, freed people with nowhere to go and with no money and few jobs, were homeless. Back streets and alleys filled with vagrants in search of federal troops who might furnish sustenance or shelter. They settled in shantytowns within the city, shacks of filth, disease, and violence. But even the more livable sections of town were not much better. Sanitation was primitive. Aside from the homes of the wealthy, municipal waste, rotting food, and excrement were tossed out of windows or piled on sidewalks and left to fester in the streets. The odor was stifling, reminding visitors of the stench of slaughterhouses.

Weak public initiatives could do little to change that. For Blacks, they remained where they had first camped, in their hovels of wood, paper, or less. Illness was rampant; distempers of the South rose with a vengeance to squelch any semblance of vitality. So densely packed were the living quarters of some that disease took each family member in short succession. Formerly enslaved people knew little about hygiene and practiced less. As elsewhere, physicians were inaccessible; there was no money to pay them. Only two in the whole community were Black physicians.[41] The alternative, then, was voodoo, sorcery, midwifery, bleeders, and herb practitioners. As a result, Black people died at an appalling rate, far in excess of their proportion in the general population. Would white America allow that to continue?

Hubbard thought not. Like Howard, he knew that education held the key to Black self-sufficiency. A northerner by birth (New Hampshire), Hubbard was no fan of slavery and loathed the wretched condition of a people mishandled and mistreated and now literally forced into another form of economic bondage. There had to be a practical solution. No better place than his chosen home of Nashville to start his work, he supposed. A passionate man, he was said to have "the vision of a seer, the courage of a warrior and the faith of a saint."[42] His unlikely collaborator was a former Confederate surgeon, Tennessean William Sneed. After the Confederate surrender, Sneed had joined the faculty of the old University of Nashville medical college. At the merger of the medical college with Vanderbilt University in 1873, Sneed was swayed by Hubbard's humanitarian activities and, instead of the heavily endowed Vanderbilt, staked his fortunes with the former Yankee. In fact, he and Hubbard became such close friends that it was Sneed who urged Hubbard to complete his doctorate in medicine at Vanderbilt. As their home for Black medical education, Hubbard and Sneed set their sights on the small local Central Tennessee College for freedmen, at the time run by the Methodist minister John Braden.[43] Braden quickly agreed to the merger but persuaded Hubbard and Sneed to expand their vision by providing bona fide medical schooling for Blacks. Benefactors such as the wealthy Samuel Meharry, the John F. Slater Fund, and the Methodist community provided the funds for their new freedmen's medical school, which began operations in 1876. Hubbard and Sneed were the only two faculty.[44]

For Blacks this was to be no easy path. To begin medical studies at Central Tennessee College, students were to have an impeccable Christian character and be proficient in "common English branches." The medical curriculum consisted of two five-month terms studying, in the first year, anatomy, physiology, chemistry, and pharmacology. The second year of coursework was largely clinical: surgery, obstetrics, diseases of children, and theory and practice of medicine.[45] To graduate, a student must have completed all coursework, passed an examination, and submitted a thesis.

The first class of five Black students attended lectures in a building previously used as a barn (Samuel Meharry and his brothers would shortly fund a new four-story structure). Since most were formerly enslaved and lacking even rudimentary education, simple instruction in spelling, reading, and writing consumed much of their time. The major impediment for the first few classes were poor health, poverty, and other familial distractions that simply made it impossible to keep up with the coursework. For the class of 1877, only one of the students, James Jamison, was able to successfully graduate, and only 3 more the following year. Yet by 1890, Central Tennessee Medical College (it would not be named Meharry Medical College until 1915) had graduated 116 Black physicians, all men.[46]

Meharry would stand alone (to this day) as the only medical school—and southern at that—devoted entirely to the education of Black physicians.

The Union policy of Reconstruction was a dismal failure for the South. Ingrained hatred of all things northern, a ruined lucrative agricultural economy, and unabated disgust for freed Black people did little in southern minds to ingratiate them to opportunists who professed a resurrection of southern dignity. Most profound of all was the desperation of millions of emancipated Blacks who were sick, ignorant, and still beholden to white approval and acceptance. For a time after the war, southern distinctiveness still reigned in the hearts of defeated rebel patriots, despite their token effort to comply with the burdensome oppression of reparation. All the while the masses of displaced Black refugees clogged cities and towns and bred sickness and virulent contagions now so characteristic of a beaten, destroyed landscape. Bondage would continue in the minds of African Americans, slavery now no longer geographical but intellectual and cultural. While perhaps for all the best intentions initially, in the words of essayist Richard Hume, "[Reconstruction policies] fell victim to racial prejudice, the heritage of slavery, postwar bitterness, governmental corruption, southern violence, and waning northern idealism."[47]

CHAPTER TWELVE

SURGERY AS SOUTHERN MEDICAL REDEMPTION

> Does all history, does even the field of romance, furnish heroes superior or patriots more noble?
> —FORMER CONFEDERATE SURGEON HUNTER MCGUIRE, 1890

The nineteenth century became the century of scientific revolution. Concepts of disease and manners of therapeutics would change drastically over those one hundred years. Gradually displaced were ideas of sickness stemming from Hippocratic beliefs held for millennia. Traditionally, physicians insisted that disease manifested by systemic imbalance, either excessive excitement or debilitating enfeeblement—calling for the so-called "heroic" therapy described by historian John Harley Warner.[1] "[T]he term *heroic therapy* has conjured up images of earnest physicians engaged in violent purging and puking, copious bloodletting, sweating, and blistering—all in the name of healing," and all so very American. The thoughtful doctor sat at the bedside, querying, listening, auscultating, percussing, and probing. It was the ancient art of physic. The history and physical examination told all. Based on his interpretation, remedies were prescribed, aimed at restoring imbalance; and response to therapeutics—the more violent the better—was meant to promote internal restoration of equilibrium—and verification of the doctor's diagnosis. Of course, mitigating factors were considered paramount: gender, race, even moral status. Superimposed, particularly in the South, were those climatic influences such as heat, humidity, stagnant waters, and the invisible toxins of decaying matter.

Disease was then a consequence not of pathologic interior genesis but of the disturbances of temperament and constitution aided by the effects of weather and soil. Such mystical happenings, barely understood by men of learning, fit nicely into a paradigm of health care readily comprehended by the lay community and transformed into a workable style of folk medicine, that is, the desired effect of nostrums correlated with a likely correction of core disorders. Warner added that "[b]y the 1830s the South had developed a minority consciousness through its colonial agrarian economy, dependence upon slavery, and loss of political power." No less was the rising sentiment of disparities in health. There also seemed, in Warner's thinking, that "the low standing of intellectual inquiry in the South further exacerbated the sense of marginality that thinking Southern physicians experienced."[2] In more enlightened places—basically the North and its pipelines to Europe—revolutionary work in experimental medicine realigned medical thinking away from Hippocratic supposition and into the realm of empiricism: measurable and definable alterations of anatomy and physiology. Less certain became the brutal heroic treatments of the past—the profuse bloodletting and purging—and less enthusiastic were clinicians to use standard pharmaceuticals—botanical and mercurial.

The impact of the experimental age was slow to penetrate the antebellum South and even slower following the Civil War, with its near total dismantling of southern colleges and universities. Wartime reliance on backyard botanicals and their anecdotal benefits cemented, for a time, their place in the southern pharmacopoeia. In the South, sicknesses continued to swirl in the miasmas of a bygone age. As only southerners could, physicians stubbornly held to their outmoded beliefs. The South was a sacred fountain of honor, grace, and religion. Such independence, refinement, and distinctiveness must not pass, even as its bid for secession failed so horribly. Men of the South—doctors included—were proud of their historical importance in forging the United States during the American Revolution and felt their talents equaled or exceeded those of their northern counterparts. There remained still the southern physician's conviction that a vital dynamism permeated the land and its people, that a separate identity was irrevocable. There innately remained a regional character in medicine as well as politics, culture, and custom. As before the Civil War, southern doctors were still committed to cultivate, educate, and disseminate their brand of medical and surgical science. That raucous spokesperson for southern medicine Samuel Cartwright had called southern climates and illnesses more akin to those of the Mediterranean, Greece and Italy, and summoned the teachings of Hippocrates as more relevant for southern clinicians. Southern physicians have an advantage over their northern counterparts, Cartwright argued. They had studied medicine twice: first in northern cities to get a diploma, then in studying diseases "of their own country" to become successful practitioners. So, in a sense, they were twice as good.³ Of course, the core principle of southern medical training was exactly that: keep southern students close to where they will practice. Teach them the peculiarities of southern health and southern disease. "Medicine is only successfully learned by practical and personal experience ... It is the greatest folly imaginable for Southern students to be going to Paris and Philadelphia to learn Southern medicine," so wrote the editors of the *Georgia Blister and Critic* in 1854 in that "blistering" avocation of southern medical education.⁴

Nevertheless, the war changed much. Crowded military camps and prisons brought home the worth of sanitary measures. Confederate doctors soon realized the centrality of hygienic practices in diminishing camp diseases, staving off gangrene, and reducing wound infections. Bedside measurements of pulse and temperature provided tempting clues that physiologic parameters reflected efficacy of treatment. Hippocratic humoral theories gave way to physiologic diagnostics and experimental therapeutics. War had awakened a new era in medicine, even in recalcitrant Dixie.

Most obvious, it had awakened the powers of a new surgical craft. Prior to the war, few practitioners anywhere had the stomach for it. In colonial times, such skills were rarely emphasized and seldom practiced. In America as a whole, surgery, as a calling, hardly existed.⁵ For the most part, there was little distinction made between physicians and surgeons anyway—practitioners were expected to do both. Revolutionary War doctor James Tilton commented that, while the British could divide the practice of "physic" and surgery due to their "high degree of civilization and luxury," it was not the same in the North American colonies. "It is, however, very different in our country, where every medical character, practices both professions; and it is found, by experience ... to be impracticable to separate these duties."⁶ As a result, surgery was far from the scholarly profession that "physic" as a whole claimed. "Surgical ailments in the United States are almost unknown," declared Samuel Cartwright.⁷ No doubt, much of this was due to the brutal nature of pre-anesthetic procedures where speed was paramount and the wails of patients almost intolerable. And even if possible to complete, flagrant infections carried off not a few survivors of the brutal business. Seldom were clinicians tempted to embark on such barbarism.

This was especially true in the South, where conditions for surgery were often primitive and confined to home or hovel. Few doctors risked their precarious reputations by trying such deeds. General practitioners were prepared, where necessary, to set fractures, sew lacerations, or carve out ugly tumors, but only in the direst of circumstances. More tolerable were the examinations, the bleedings, the pharmaceuticals, and the birthings, where at least short-term survival was more likely. In fact, reports of surgical cases by individual physicians rarely topped a handful. A few submitted their individual cases more as testimony to bravado than rational thinking. Even fewer reported more. Surgeon T. P. Bailey of South Carolina, for example, presented a grand total of four operations in the *Charleston Medical Journal and Review* of 1859—an almost unthinkable collection.[8] Cartwright made the sarcastic but, for once, accurate remark that may have typified all of antebellum southern surgery: "The medical world are [*sic*] not looking to the far distant Mississippi for any discovery in surgery."[9] In fact, later on, when reviewing all the surgical progress of the century since the Declaration of Independence, Philadelphia surgeon Samuel Gross rarely mentioned southern surgeons and certainly withheld the label of pioneer. Most of the notable milestones achieved by surgeons happened in the North.[10]

It was not so in Europe. Specialization in the surgical arts had already gathered momentum even before the mid-nineteenth century, encouraged by the likes of Frenchman Antoine-François Fourcroy, who had espoused such practices to the National Assembly in Paris in 1794: "Medicine and surgery are two branches of the same science; to study them separately is to abandon theory to stretches of imagination and practice to blind pursuits. To bring them together and consolidate them is to enlighten them mutually and to accelerate their progress. Those pupils who prefer the routine of operating will indulge more particularly in this aspect of the art of healing."[11]

In point of fact, according to historian Toby Gelfand, in France at the close of the eighteenth century, the surgical arts—even preceding anesthesia—had risen to such distinction that the ablest practitioners were, in fact, surgeons. These egotistical masters erected huge clinics in Paris and by the power of their craft shifted centers of learning from the lecture halls of elite colleges to the wards of the great Parisian hospitals.[12] From Germany came reports of laboratories intent on unraveling the mysteries of human pathology and expertly versed in the nuances of anatomy. Richard Shryock claimed the transformation of surgery toward specialization was not even so much the advent of anesthesia or antisepsis but more emphatically a response to newer concepts of disease, not as humoral disorders, but focusing on anatomic regions producing characteristic and reproducible symptoms and signs.[13] The clinics of Theodor Billroth in Vienna, Austria, and Emil Kocher in Bern, Switzerland, were alive with direct surgical attacks on the seats of disease—tumors, cysts, congenital deformities now the target of the surgeon's knife. A few visionaries in America took up the cause, mimicking their European colleagues. Physician John Jones urged practitioners of the art to be complete physicians, as much physic as surgeon. "It can no longer remain a doubt," Jones wrote in 1775 (and could have written today), "with any unprejudiced person, that an enlightened mind, united to the person of an operator, must and will constitute the most accomplished and successful Surgeon."[14] One must not separate surgery and the ancient art of physic, he insisted.

Little of that attitude permeated southern physicians, encased as they were in the sanctity of general practice. However, while few practiced the surgical arts—and fewer, still, exclusively—there were exceptions notable by their daring. The Kentuckian Ephraim McDowell (1771–1830) had boldly removed a fifteen-pound ovarian tumor from a long-suffering woman in 1809 without the benefit of sterility or anesthesia, and then operated on two more women for similar problems over the next seven years. All three survived his operation. It was an audacious and remarkable feat in an age where such interventions were considered almost madness and bordered on barbarism.[15] Another South Carolinian, J. Marion Sims (1813–1883), startled the academic world with his remarkable ability to repair the troublesome vesico-vaginal fistula—an abnormal communication between urinary bladder and vagina. Sims was typical of southern country practitioners. Educated in Philadelphia, there was no doubt he would return to the South, soon settling into a small-town practice in Montgomery, Alabama. He began as caregiver to the well-heeled, but slowly his surgical dexterity earned him an additional reputation as "a judicious practitioner and as a skillful surgeon." He had an ambition for surgery, he admitted, and, not lacking self-confidence (or humility), performed "all sorts of beautiful and brilliant operations." Foremost among these, of course, was his work on the vexing bladder fistulas. These consequences of childbirth had perplexed some of the outstanding minds of the day, even the likes of the French master Guillaume Dupuytren. Sims trumped them all. He used a specially made speculum and fine silver wire suture to close the fistulas in three despondent enslaved women ("servants" he called them), all kept in a small hospital behind his house and done free of charge. That he called these early efforts "experiments" had given rise to the notion that Sims was abusing enslaved women, an accusation, which on closer inspection was largely groundless. In fact, Sims, who was summoned in desperation by each of these women's enslavers, volunteered to try to relieve their suffering at his own time and expense. The triumphs he enjoyed from these early cases shortly drew patrons everywhere. For his success, he was awarded international recognition, a singular bright spot in antebellum southern surgery.[16]

A classic of Confederate surgeons was Paul Fitzsimmons Eve (1806–1877). Eve was a Georgian by birth, born just south of Augusta. Before moving to Georgia, his father had served in the Revolutionary War and had been Pennsylvania classmates with Benjamin Rush and Continental surgeon William Shippen Jr. No doubt at his father's prompting (and likely connections), the son also headed north to the University of Pennsylvania for his medical schooling. It was in Europe, however, that his love of surgery ripened with instructions by the legendary Astley Cooper, Dominique Larrey, and Philibert Roux. He had not seen anatomy exposed in such detail nor the meticulous techniques of these men who had devoted their lives to the surgical arts. Even more, for such a man of fortune, Eve found himself at the Paris barricades July 26, 1830, for the so-called "July Revolution." He was quickly pressed into service and treated a number of battle casualties. An inveterate opportunist, he then traveled to Poland, serving as surgeon at the front in the short Polish-Russian War of 1830–1831. For that he would receive the Polish Golden Cross of Honor (and endure a hefty dose of cholera).[17] He then returned to Augusta, Georgia, where he had been appointed to the faculty of the Medical College of Georgia and practiced there until 1851. Eve was convinced of southern medical distinctiveness, fueled by its peculiar institution—slavery. In his inaugural address to new students at the Medical College in October 1837 he pointed out: "[W]ould you not expect a marked difference between the information given here at the South and that at the north, on the diseases to which the *negro* is most subject ... Where would you go to study ... his peculiar habits, the causes, progress, and more especially the proper *treatment* of his *particular affections!*" [italics his].[18] Indeed, half or more of a southern physician's practice were bound to be enslaved men, women, and children. Eve simply confronted reality. Conditions for enslaved Africans were harsh—unhealthy housing, sanitation, and diets. It was in that environment his students were to practice. The moral commitment of physicians to serve demanded full instruction on their prospective clientele.[19]

But Eve could not resist the seduction of military matters. He participated as a physician volunteer in the Mexican-American War in 1846 and treated wounded from the Battle of Monterey that May. He even traveled again to Europe and visited the battlefields of the Second War of Italian Independence in 1859.

Along with his propensity for danger, Eve was also a gifted technician. While in Augusta, he astounded the medical community by performing the first removal of an entire uterus—the first total hysterectomy in the United States. Unbelievably, the woman survived her operation and recovered, only to die some months later, likely from recurrent cancer.[20] In 1851 Eve left Augusta to take a faculty position at the University of Nashville. His surgical practice was prodigious and, in fact, so expansive that he published his work in 1857 as *A Collection of Remarkable Cases in Surgery* ("uncommon events and strange circumstances," he prefaced).[21] His operations spanned cranium, chest, abdomen, pelvis, and extremities. Most notable were his presentation of abdominal cases, a number of wounds among them from penetrating trauma, including his encounter with a young man whose abdomen had been sliced open. Protruding through was a large, dilated stomach, full of gas and food. Eve had to open the stomach and empty its contents, shoveling out food, until he could sew it up and push it back into the abdominal cavity. Such a feat was almost unheard of for the day; even more remarkable for the times: the patient survived. With Tennessee's secession in June 1861, Eve was assigned as surgeon in the Confederate States Army. Fleeing Nashville with the approach of Grant's forces in February 1862, Eve was chosen to head the four-hundred-bed Gate City Hospital in Atlanta, a second-rate hotel turned into an infirmary and packed with too many mangy war wounded.[22] Following his service in the Confederate Army in the Civil War, Eve returned to Nashville and eventually took a professorship at the newly opened Vanderbilt University. He died in 1877 at the age of seventy-one while returning home from a house call.

Georgian Robert Battey (1828–1895) would become a controversial figure in southern surgery. Battey had received his medical education in Philadelphia at Thomas Jefferson Medical College. He studied under the accomplished obstetrician Charles Meigs there and developed a special interest in female disorders. Battey soon returned to Rome, Georgia, to practice. Miegs had given him a curiosity about gynecological problems, particularly troublesome fistulas between urinary bladder and vagina, so-called vesico-vaginal fistulas. In Rome, Battey, fascinated by such scourges, successfully repaired his first such fistula in 1858. But it was not there that Battey would make his mark. Of capable means, Battey, as many affluent physicians did, traveled to Europe to bolster his medical expertise. In England, he met Thomas Spencer Wells, who had by that time performed numerous ovarian operations. Wells's results were revolutionary, almost 150 operations without a single death, whereas in America the death toll approached one in four. Wells's passion for the procedure was infectious, and Battey returned to America anxious to imitate his English mentor. The Civil War intervened, though, and Battey found himself a Confederate Army surgeon, placed in charge of Atlanta's four-hundred-bed Fair Ground Hospital No. 2. There, he spent more time battling diarrheas and pneumonias than the nuances of pelvic surgery. Following the war, he returned to Rome, where, in 1869, he finally was able to copy Wells's methods and removed a thirty-pound ovarian tumor from the wife of a physician. In 1872 he completed his first bilateral oophorectomy on a young woman suffering various nervous complaints and pelvic inflammatory disorders. Contemporaries assumed that women's behavior—hysteria it was often labeled—must come from some derangement of her ovaries. It was only logical in such distressed states that the ovaries should be removed. Over the next two decades, Battey complied and did a number of oophorectomies for admittedly ill-defined symptoms. His results, like Wells's, were astonishing; his explanation simple: "clean hands and appliances," a clean operating room (oftentimes the patient's house), "pure atmosphere and free ventilation," skilled nursing, antiseptic solutions and spray, and careful technique.[23]

Battey's dazzling bravado earned him the chair of Obstetrics at the Atlanta Medical College. The popularity of his operation spread as a potential cure for all types of female maladies, including "insanity." Battey himself claimed that oophorectomy might benefit a number of mental disorders. Soon, he had proposed his own terminology: "oophoro-mania," "oophoro-epilepsy," and "ooporalgia." Not a few of his patients had the operation in their twenties—amounting to a surgical menopause—for various "nervous" disorders. "In my experience," he would write, "the time required for the disappearance of nervous disorders [after oophorectomy] has been quite variable." He claimed one-third were "cured," and, he added, the indications in his mind were solid. Nervous problems—mania, hysteria, neuralgia—are best treated by castration. A number of colleagues who followed his example and liberally castrated young women loudly agreed. The matter of premature menopause, however, was conveniently ignored.[24]

Oophorectomies skyrocketed. One estimate put the figure at 150,000 women sterilized.[25] Battey tried to temper enthusiasm of his colleagues, but he remained convinced oophorectomy could be beneficial.[26] The female public felt differently. Battey was caught at the center of a feminine maelstrom. This was needless castration of women, critics protested. Southern surgeons were quick to run to his defense. "[W]e must protest against the wholesale condemnation of a great life-saving procedure and a large and respectable body of earnest practitioners on account of the recklessness of a few," declared the respected surgeon Lewis McMurtry of Louisville.[27]

For surgeons of Battey's ilk, it was a heady time, one not necessarily in tune with proper scientific scrutiny. Historian Lawrence Longo claimed, "The Achilles' heel of medicine [and, particularly, surgery] is it's too frequent and ready espousal of untested procedures or unproven theories."[28] Fortunately, by the turn of the century the numbers of oophorectomies had dropped precipitously. The general feeling pervaded that ovaries did not "have the paramount reflex power generally attributed to them." "Reforms in medicine," Longo said, "have always come from without the profession." Unfortunately, such changes can occur at a glacial pace.

Yet without question, the Civil War contributed to a rising enthusiasm for the surgical arts. Joseph Lister's antisepsis, William T. G. Morton's ether, and James Young Simpson's use of chloroform added to the optimism that, now, surgeons could venture into the human body in ways totally unthinkable decades before. Military doctors had witnessed firsthand the blissful effects of anesthesia in field hospitals and would soon appreciate the sterilizing outcomes of Lister's carbolic acid.[29] Men with the boldness of Battey and the finesse of Eve dispelled notions of surgical barbarity and acquainted the public with a valuable arm of therapeutics.

But in the South, these same surgeons also returned home beaten. Apart from the thrill, the gore, and the piles of limbs, for ex-Confederate medical officers war had chilled enthusiasm. Widespread destruction and so many ugly deaths wiped out any semblance of progressive thinking, even in the face of occasional dazzling successes. Doctors were spent, their minds numb to the sorrows. Their South was an intellectual wasteland as well as an economic one.

Immediate concerns of family and community took precedence. Basic human needs now unanswered, doctors, for all their worth, tended to the essentials.

How to recover? It would take decades. North Carolinian John Wesley Long reflected in 1914, "Those of you who live in the large cities of the North and West cannot appreciate the disadvantages under which the southern surgeons labored. If this was true in antebellum days, it was a hundredfold more so following the war."[30] Ill health and epidemics in their war-torn country consumed the energy of practitioners. In those first postbellum years, there was little space for inventiveness.

A New South, progressives believed, must break with traditions of the past: leave behind the old, purely countrified values. Animosity to and rejection of northern intrusion and industrialism gradually gave way to resignation, acceptance, and even imitation of manufacturing incentives and economic diversity—perhaps the mourning process of a culture come full circle. This, of necessity, led to a certain abdication of southern autonomy and a willingness to consider integration with northern ideology not as a total divestment of southern conventions but as an embrace of the republic as a whole. Yet this did not apply to attitudes. "[T]here was no revolution in basic ideology [in this "new" South] and no intention of relinquishing the central Southern position and surrendering bodily to Yankee civilization . . . the turn to Progress clearly flowed straight out of [the] past and constituted . . . an emanation from the will to maintain the South in its essential integrity," so spoke author W. J. Cash of the New South of the 1880s.[31]

Still, resignation did not oust a seething racism brewing beneath. For one, ex-Confederate doctor Hunter McGuire stood in defense of southern ethos. McGuire had served with distinction under Stonewall Jackson's command. In fact, he had amputated Jackson's left arm at the Battle of Chancellorsville. A tireless devotee of the art, he was not one to settle with mediocrity. McGuire would later say, "Does all history, does even the field of romance, furnish heroes superior or patriots more noble?"[32] It was certainly foremost for Samuel Stout in 1866 when he said a "high and holy task" was "to preserve the civilization of the Southern people."[33] More worrisome even were the remarks made in the *Atlanta Medical and Surgical Journal* in 1868 depicting "the Negro" as of immovable character that "stamps him a barbarian of barbarians." Science must settle this issue, the editors argued, "the beginning and the end of the negro will be indisputably revealed," alluding to his "subordinate position" and curious habits and behavior.[34] Even the legendary New Orleans surgeon Rudolph Matas, in his extensive 1896 treatise entitled "The Surgical Peculiarities of the American Negro," wise and discerning as he was, could not refrain to declare that the African American was "ethnologically inferior and passive," struggling for existence with a "superior, aggressive, and dominant population."[35]

Yet technology was on the advance. In more urbanized areas, surgery was viewed as a new, expanded arm of medicine and product of technology. Drawn to the modern clinics of Europe, Americans flocked to France and across the Rhine for training. Gawking students, their excitement almost palpable, packed the amphitheaters of Theodor Billroth, Emil Kocher, and Anton Eiselsberg. It was estimated that between 1870 and 1914 173 clinical institutes, many specialty oriented, were erected alongside German universities in which fifteen thousand Americans took some sort of graduate training. The German system of education had broad appeal to visitors, impressed by the intensity of training and breadth of clinical material. Back home, armed with a wealth of Germanic know-how, returning academicians sought to mimic the German model. American universities strengthened their links with hospitals, organized pavilions according to surgical disciplines, and fostered specialty-centered patient care.[36] Even in the war-ravaged South, the newly conceived hospital and medical school of Vanderbilt University in Nashville, richly endowed by its founder, sought the best clinicians in the country.

Not all subscribed to specialization. Organized medicine in the United States took a dim view. As a political and bureaucratic force, the American Medical Association (AMA) was the guardian of the generalist. Outspoken in its criticism of specialism, the AMA felt that traditional Hippocratic methods were being exchanged for purely technical abilities and that technology would replace the bedside manners of clinicians—up to that time the mainstay of physician therapeutics. Even some surgical practitioners argued against specialization as not the American brand of medicine. The editor of the influential journal *Medical Record*, George Shrady, wrote a scathing editorial in 1875 condemning the trend. No doubt specialism has been an "incalculable benefit" to scientific medicine, he commented, but "not only is talent, in many cases, misdirected, but the legitimate claims of general practice are ignored." Even though an accomplished war surgeon himself, Shrady feared overenthusiastic specialists descending on the unsuspecting patients—as if specialists were creating a demand rather than addressing one. Specialists, he warned, were increasing far beyond a reasonable demand for their services.[37]

But American surgeons paid little heed. They were now the darlings of medicine, congregating to solidify training and share experiences. Progress seemed exponential. To disseminate the surge of information and practices, specialty societies appeared. As the premier effort, the American Surgical Association came together in 1880. At his presidential address before that organization, Philadelphian Samuel D. Gross endeavored to "unite these men [surgeons] into one harmonious whole, for the benefit of all," not by striking a blow to the AMA, but by "rousing it from its Rip Van Winkle slumbers, and infusing new life into it." Gross went on to say that "we hope to make the American Surgical Association an altar upon which we may annually lay our contributions to Surgical Science."[38] The effort attracted the brightest and most talented surgeons from cities across the country—except, that is, from the South. Even by 1884, of the ninety-three active members, only thirteen (14 percent) were from the former Confederate states (although William Briggs of Nashville was its second president).[39]

In the South, as only southerners could, physicians stubbornly held to their traditional beliefs. Theirs was a sacred repository of honor, grace, and religion. Such independence, refinement, and distinctiveness must not pass, even as its bid for secession failed so horribly. Men of the South—doctors included—were proud of their historical importance in forging the United States during the American Revolution and felt their talents equaled or exceeded those of their northern counterparts. There remained still the southern physician's conviction that a vital energy permeated the land and its people, that a separate identity was irrevocable. In their minds, a regional character in medicine had been firmly established. Southern doctors remained committed to cultivate, educate, and disseminate their kind of medical and surgical science. At the same time, they were keenly aware that a surgical phoenix should arise from southern ashes.

Resurrection began in Birmingham, Alabama, in 1887. Two brothers, William and John Davis, jointly in practice there, managed to bring together enough surgeons and gynecologists to form a local scientific society. The Davis brothers themselves were fifth-generation physicians. Their grandfather was an early settler in the Alabama territory; their father, Elias Davis, had been an officer in the Army of the Confederacy and was killed while commanding sharpshooters at Petersburg. John Daniel Sinkler Davis, the older brother, had graduated from the Medical College of Georgia at age twenty. His younger brother, William Elias Brownlee Davis, attended Vanderbilt University and the University of Louisville as well as Bellevue Medical College in New York. He had graduated in 1884 and returned home to Birmingham to join John in practice. They were convinced that surgery was now a legitimate specialty and that fellow practitioners were obliged to share experiences, particularly in the war-ruined South. First, they authored a local scientific journal called the *Alabama Medical and Surgical Journal*. Using it as a forum, they promoted their new surgical society in the first edition in December 1886:

> The [Alabama Surgical and Gynecological] Association will be organized in Birmingham on the 15th of December, and will have purely for its object the advancement of surgery and gynecology in the State . . . It will be organized for scientific purposes and will conflict with no association now in existence . . . It will afford a field for active workers in the departments of surgery and gynecology never before enjoyed by Alabama physicians.[40]

Their long-term plans were for this local group to be a launching pad for a state society of surgeons and gynecologists and even expand to include all of the South in an association of like-minded individuals. Surgeons were becoming a cliquish group. Armored with a bravado that bordered at times on callousness, they could still harbor deep emotional ties with their patients for the pain they might cause and looked to each other for empathetic support and advice. For this, congregations of surgical specialists could provide comfort and confidence in numbers.

Yet the Davis brothers, as editors of the *Alabama Medical and Surgical Journal*, had already run afoul of an influential physician in the state, Jerome Cochran, on a separate issue of licensure. The Davises felt licensure should be a state rather than county mandate. Miffed at their insolence, Cochran, an inveterate generalist, retaliated by throwing his considerable political weight against the new surgical association, feeling it would weaken the established Alabama Medical Association, *and* he managed to keep licensure a county, rather than state, matter. This was a slap in the face to the Davis brothers, who felt their now precarious political standing would jeopardize success of their surgical group. Broader support was needed, far beyond the parochialism of Alabama. The Davises appealed to the entire Southeast, inviting both surgeons and gynecologists to attend their inaugural 1887 meeting in Birmingham.

Almost eighty favorable responses were returned, including such scholars as William David Haggard, professor of obstetrics at Vanderbilt University. Dr. Haggard attended the first session on October 11, 1887, and quickly became an advocate, confident, like the Davises, of its importance in uniting southern surgeons. Other attendees agreed, and on the second day of the meeting, there was such enthusiasm that a motion unanimously carried to rename the Alabama Surgical and Gynecological Association the Southern Surgical and Gynecological Association. Haggard was nominated the first president.

Despite the excitement, it proved an inauspicious start. The impoverished, agrarian South simply could not generate a sufficient membership. Even by widening the net to include part-time surgical practitioners, there were still meager numbers. William Davis suspected that many southern surgeons had fled north, fearful that the depressed postwar economy would not support a surgical practice. Yankees agreed. One cynical northern editor even commented that "one hundred men could not be found in the South who would pay ten dollars annual due." It was then that the association decided to open membership to the entire country. Despite unease about historical peculiarities of southern medicine, surgeons north and west saw value. The Davises watched their Southern Surgical and Gynecological Association flourish by the end of the century. Thanks to them, the South would have its redemption. "[T]he history of surgery would be incomplete and gynecology unwritten but for these bright stars of the South," a reference not only to pioneers like Eve, Sims, and Battey but also the youthful conviction of the Davis brothers.[41]

So it was, on November 13, 1889, that most illustrious of Confederate surgeons, Hunter McGuire, stood before the newly formed Southern Surgical and Gynecological Association in Nashville, Tennessee, to deliver his presidential address at their second convention. McGuire did not mince words. "The South has not kept pace with the North in medical progress and development," he said. McGuire went on to say that "social conditions of the South ... denied to the medical men ... the opportunities which were conducive to the progress and development of medicine." Yet he did not apologize for the recent troubles. In the late "'civil contest," a conflict, he erroneously insisted, that was more about sovereignty than slavery, "the men of the South once more displayed the same great qualities that had characterized their ancestors in the American Revolution." As for the Reconstruction South, McGuire refused to admit anything had changed. "For there is no New South," he insisted, "the blood of her patriots of the past flows in the veins of her people to-day, *unmixed by any other strain* [italics added]." He was unashamed of his Dixie pride. "As Southern men, let us show to the world ... we have still the stamina of our forefathers ... let us strive to be first in scientific attainment, first in integrity, first in high purpose for the good of mankind." His intent was not parochial. Instead, he urged a willingness of southern surgeons to embrace and foster scientific advances countrywide, and in fact, he seemed to rally them to take the lead.[42]

McGuire's oratory had an impact. Just four years following the inaugural meeting, President Bedford Brown of Virginia proudly announced that the young Southern Surgical and Gynecological Association had enabled "our Southern country ... to reap fully the benefits of its talents, learning, and labors" for which "the organization of a home association for the development of surgery and gynecology was imperatively demanded." Surgeons of the association, he added, were bearing their part in the grand cause of civilization and enlightenment in the resurrecting South. Reflecting on the sprouting age of technology, he emphasized that "[w]e need in our Southern country, practical men, practical ideas, practical methods and knowledge." Clearly, visionaries such as he recognized the role science was to play in the reinvention of a New South.[43] No civilized nation had been reduced to such desolation and impoverishment, Brown pointed out. "It is an evidence of Southern spirit, energy, enterprise, recuperative power, and courageous determination to rise above its desolated condition and conquer success and prosperity," he concluded. Despite the pessimistic outlook for the ruined South, the medical profession was one rare beacon of recuperation, a "pillar of civilization and national refinement." However, in all the enlightened remarks of his discourse, there might have still been a reluctance to fully incorporate his African American brethren as one race, the human race.

He concluded his remarks by pointing out: "[W]e stand here also the blood, the bone, and the sinew of the greatest and grandest race on this earth, and I feel that in the hands of this noble race, which has done so much for the glory and civilization of this world, and whose history has been so wonderful in the past, our Southern history, or interests, our institutions, our civilization are safe."[44]

And what of the Davis brothers? William Davis, in the meantime, had become a student of liver and biliary surgery, performing a number of experiments on animals to determine the best way of repairing the common bile duct in gallstone disease. He was nominated as president of his own Southern Surgical and Gynecological Association in 1903. Despite the initial opposition of the influential Jerome Cochran (who indeed had come quite close to wrecking their efforts to organize a surgical society), Davis, in his presidential address, was quick to forgive: "[W]hen he [Jerome Cochran] saw that the Association had succeeded and realized that I had been loyal to the State Association, he became not only my friend, but a supporter of the Southern Association."[45]

Three months later, William was dead, killed in a freak accident at a railroad crossing in Birmingham. He had stopped his horse and buggy to let a train pass but, in calming his horse, his foot caught in the tracks. He stumbled and fell into the wheels of passing cars. His eulogy was effusive. "As a lightning bolt from out the clear sky came the terrible accident which ushered into eternity the noble spirit of Dr. Davis," Richard Douglas of Nashville elegantly wrote. "For him our profession knew no sectional limitations." And in final tribute to William's efforts to resurrect pride in southern surgery, Douglas finished, "[A]s a master mason is chosen to square the corners and bridge the arches in our architectural piles, so he, the master workman in our profession, was appointed to construct the Southern corner of the magnificent edifice of national medical science." It was a bid for unity, for progress, for a new South, and as a profession, surgeons were at the forefront. A specialty spurred by scientific achievement, it represented the new medicine, and the South seemed fertile ground for inoculation.[46]

John also was an avid student of surgery. During the years of the Southern Surgical and Gynecological Association, he presented his work on general and abdominal surgery, demonstrating as early as 1889 his catgut sutures, which he had used to fix intestinal perforations and sewing intestinal anastomoses. His crusade for southern surgical excellence did not diminish. Together with his brother, he was instrumental in organizing a medical college in Birmingham in 1894 that would eventually become the University of Alabama.

Thanks in part to the Davis brothers, the South did rise again, if only in the form of professional distinction. Still, could the antebellum days of the beloved Southland be so easily dismissed? Hardly not. Even southerners generations far removed from those times still commemorate some of their parochial ideals. A landed aristocracy, affluence, decorous lifestyles, and anachronistic customs captivated those nostalgic for the feudal underpinnings of bygone eras. That the South harbored sentiments and behavior so different from more enlightened regions was not considered abhorrent but honorable, even though implicit in such attitudes was a basic inequality of human existence. That physicians shared those feelings is arguable, but there is no doubt they valued a southern pride in their quest for intellectual and professional merit. It is commendable that they were among the first to embrace a true unification with the North as one United States and as one profession. It is also notable that their nostalgia—if indeed that is the proper word—be a melancholy born not of brutal subjugation and abuse but of a deepening satisfaction in their unique earth and climate and lush greenery and all that at first drew those courageous settlers southward. One should not dismiss out of hand either those glorious fortunes of the New South so intimately tied to the Old South. "The memory that we have treated our brother kindly, magnanimously, and generously will do to carry with us down the ragged path of life," so said surgeon Bedford Brown in 1893.[47]

CHAPTER THIRTEEN

A NEW SOUTH OR STILL THE OLD SOUTH?

> It would be impossible to express in exact terms the extent to which improved health could increase human happiness; but every observer of human misery among the poor reports that disease plays the leading role.
> —IRVING FISHER, *REPORT ON NATIONAL VITALITY*, 1909

By 1880 Reconstruction had collapsed. Lax supervision of integration and passive disregard of Black initiatives allowed southern white elites to once again rise in influence and political power. As a result, white supremacy gained hold. By 1890, the "Jim Crow" system of subordination and segregation relegated the Black man to second-class status, even lower than the poor whites struggling in the wake of total economic ruin. The labor system for freed Blacks was atrocious, with various measures taken to advantage white employers in stripping Blacks of any potential to enhance financial gain and security. One notable example was the lopsided sharecropping scheme of subjugating gullible and uneducated Black farmers. Defeat of Rebel armies and abject surrender had not really changed much. For the Union, emancipation of formerly enslaved people accomplished almost nothing, not for another one hundred years. Whites were forced to reorganize and adjust to recuperate even a fraction of the revenue seen antebellum. For the Blacks, their plight was, in the immediacy, worse. Poverty-stricken, ignorant, and corralled into a near-slave caste once again, there was little opportunity for any true equality on par with even the lowest white laborer.

In states of the Deep South, the situation remained grim. The sizeable proportions of African Americans, sometimes accounting for a third of the population, imposed a new kind of distinctiveness on southern medical practice: money. Poor Blacks—and there were vast numbers of them—had little of it. And money continued to be the motivator for providing health care. If money was not forthcoming, treatment was too often denied. One white Mississippi doctor told the *Boston Globe*, "If there is a n----r in my waiting room who doesn't have $3 in cash, he can sit there and die. I don't treat n----rs without money." Even Black doctors took a similar stance, afraid that an impoverished clientele would spell financial ruin for them. No money, no medicine was the refrain.[1] In Mississippi there were few Black physicians anyway before 1890, and not until 1900 was there even an association for the continued education of Black health professionals, the Mississippi Medical and Surgical Association.[2] It was one of the few ways Black physicians could share information. They were usually excluded from white medical societies.

Yet progress in the medical arts transformed health care following the Civil War, not only in the United States, but globally. Rapid growth of academic systems began in the United States in the 1860s. This surge of productivity in the sciences was a direct result of the influence of Germany's scholarly endeavor to decentralize educational and research institutions, creating an atmosphere of competition that fostered curiosity, initiative, and productivity. In the northern United States, relatively free of damage from the Civil War, educators went abroad, became enamored with the German system, and brought much of what they had learned back to America. With private endowments and federal money (such as the Land Grant Act of 1862) educational institutes and men of research flourished. Graduate schools in the sciences rose to the forefront, foremost among them the Johns Hopkins Medical School. As a result, in the latter half of the nineteenth century American scientific discoveries far outpaced even those of Germany. The twentieth century was to become the American Century of the Sciences, as northern universities led the charge to open new frontiers in human health.[3]

Expertise in healing skills became a science of hypotheses, experimentation, and of proofs—to be someday called "evidence-based medicine." No longer confined to the bedside in rationalistic bursts of clinical supposition, the practice of medicine began to rely instead on laboratory technology, measurements, and analytic outcomes. In the United States, this was noticeably apparent in universities of the North, where faculty, little affected by the wastage of war, fiddled in their laboratories and with their patients in manners that incorporated enlightened reports of the great anatomists and physiologists of the time: Rudolf Virchow, Claude Bernard, François Magendie, and Louis Pasteur. Miasmas gave way to microorganisms so tiny as to elude detection unless viewed microscopically. Dissecting diseases illuminated causative agents rather than bizarre mixtures of humors, air, soil, and sun. But in the South, devastated by war and impoverished, the southern practitioner, imbedded in bedside manners and stubborn theories of southern propensities, could not, at first, embrace contemporary ideas of pure scholarship. Besides, medical singularity, even though minimized by the war, held sway in framing not only academic purpose but also political justification. "Recognizing the sociopolitical utility of the notion of Southern medical distinctiveness in furthering Southern nationalism does not change the fact that as a scientific concept it was central to the [Southern] thinking physician's intellectual program for medicine," suggests historian John Harley Warner.[4] While of practical value perhaps, such medical insularity had less universal appeal to enhance understanding of basic mechanisms of diseases and therapeutics. Their grip on so-called sectional medicine became more of a curse than a cure. Could it be, though, that southern medicine, like southern society, was inexorably tied to the soil, the climate, and the air? Was not the agrarian nature of culture one of rural isolationism, intense self-discipline and labor, and therefore more dependent on personal—almost intimate—interactions rather than abstract reliance on industrial capitalism and mass production of manufactured goods—including therapeutics?

Without doubt, deprivations of war had totally derailed academic progress and scholarly activity in the South. Not until the delicate infrastructure of urban southern subsistence and commerce were rebuilt was it possible to extend social productivity to include the more theoretical pursuits of the natural sciences and medicine. The everyday physician of the South, once again returning to his country roots, did not necessarily consider himself a major cog in the grand cosmic world of scientific medicine. Instead, he featured a personal, intimate relationship with his suffering patients as much following the Civil War as his forbearers did following the Revolutionary War. Historian Bertram Wyatt-Brown typified this attitude thusly: "Southerners continued to admire the Revolutionary [War] rhetoric with its primal overtones that glorified ascriptions of power and race. That legacy of honor . . . broadened the basis of the ethic far beyond the limits of aristocracy or monarchy, most especially and most enduringly in the slave South."[5]

But southern medical sectionalism could not long withstand the advancement of medical science that burst onto the world stage with the industrialization of the Gilded Age. The peculiarities of those southern miasmas gave way to the ubiquitous pathogens of the microbial environment. It was not so much the air, soil, and decay as simply favorable breeding grounds for human misery. As for those endemic fevers of the South, solutions came. For the periodic distempers—the tertian and quartan fevers—the source of the illness escaped detection until the mosquito-borne protozoan pathogen was uncovered in 1880 by the French military surgeon Charles Laveran. He had painstakingly searched under primitive lenses through wet smears of fresh blood until one bleary-eyed morning he finally detected the waving *flagella* projecting from one of the pigmented spherical bodies—a living organism, a parasite. Sir William Osler in 1887 confirmed Laveran's findings and associated the liberated protozoa with the periodic fevers of the disease, referring to the "hematozoa of malaria" and attributing the ailment to action of the parasites on red blood corpuscles fostering the characteristic paroxysms of fever in addressing the Pathological Society of Philadelphia in 1886.[6] The British physician Ronald Ross painstakingly identified protozoa, the *Plasmodium* species, in the salivary glands of the mosquito that had fed on the blood of infected men, thus completing the life cycle.[7]

By 1900, yellow fever had reluctantly submitted to science and wise public health measures. American troops in Cuba had been severely stricken during the Spanish-American War of 1898. The time-honored method of quarantine had serious effects on commerce and travel and was not the hoped-for remedy for the disease. Climatic conditions without question played a role and, it was still thought, decomposing organic matter fueled dissemination. Southern cities like New Orleans with its ineffective sewer system were perfect breeding grounds for the illness. The surgeon general of the army, George Sternberg, advised, "During the season favorable for the epidemic prevalence of the disease its propagation without doubt depends largely upon local unsanitary conditions, and it is doubtful whether it could effect a lodgment in a clean and well paved city."[8] But physicians began to realize that bad air and poor sanitation were not the only problems. Yellow fever, doctors concluded, was not contagious in pure air.

In 1901 United States Army surgeon Walter Reed reported his research on transmissibility of yellow fever. He found, working on volunteers, that the human vector was the mosquito, identified by him as the *Culex* mosquito but later found to be the *Aedes* mosquito. The disease was transmitted by the bite of the insect. The best prevention, then, he concluded, was eradication of the mosquito population. He was still uncertain of the pathogen that caused illness in humans, but it was carried in human blood.[9] It was not until 1927 that the English pathologist Adrian Stokes identified a virus-like particle in the blood of infected subjects that caused the disease (Stokes himself was to die shortly thereafter of yellow fever). In 1938 Max Theiler of the Rockefeller Institute produced the first human vaccine against yellow fever. With efforts to control the *Aedes* mosquito and use of the vaccine, the dreaded epidemics in North America were over. The South was finally exonerated for its ailing miasmatic climate.[10]

Proper sanitation had a tremendous impact on disease. Effective sewage disposal, plumbing, and water treatment helped eliminate illnesses such as typhoid fever, dysentery, and cholera. What could not be corrected soon was poverty, the main determinant of sickness, death, and longevity. This, one could find in abundance in the urban South and elsewhere, remnants of an emancipation that was not freedom nor equality. Poor, underserved African Americans of necessity continued to inhabit the less-desirable dwellings and crowded neighborhoods of cities and even rural townships. And there disease festered. Tuberculosis, toxoplasmosis, rheumatic fever, protozoan dysenteries, and other diseases embedded into impoverished communities. "[A]mong the poorest populations living in the US there remains highly prevalent a group of serious parasitic and bacterial diseases," concluded epidemiologist Peter Hotez. This population, he found, centered on "people of color living in the Mississippi Delta and elsewhere in the American South."[11] By the turn of the century, it was clear that improvements in sanitation and an understanding of infectious diseases had radically altered societal abilities to enhance health and prevent disease. But this alteration was unevenly distributed among the urban inhabitants of the United States.

And what of the healing arts? Education of a future generation of doctors was vital to the health of the South. Abraham Flexner's revolutionary 1910 report on medical education in the United States upended the status quo and whittled away at southern education. Overall, he unabashedly encouraged the closing of 124 of 155 of the nation's medical schools. His detailed in-person surveys of most schools, particularly proprietary schools, were appalling, showing marginally trained faculty, inadequate resources, and scant patient exposure. Many of them were little more than jackleg trade schools, bleeding their enrollees of every sweat-soaked greenback and spitting out diplomas as worthless as the hack courses they held. Conversely, according to his report, a medical school should link closely with universities, already devoted to scholarly activity, and in large cities where there was an abundance of clinical material. State fiscal support was key. "The physician is a social instrument. If there were no disease, there would be no doctors," Flexner maintained, and, therefore, under social control. Medical training "is a public service corporation," he went on. "It is chartered by the state; it utilizes public hospitals on the ground of the social nature of its service."[12] Could there be proprietary holdings? Rarely, he felt. Vanderbilt University and Johns Hopkins Hospital were notable examples.

His report stressed the importance of medical education firmly grounded in the basic sciences, one that was part of a scholarly approach to academics, most certainly aligned with higher education. The ideal curriculum would be administered by a full-time faculty composed of physicians, scientists, scholars, and teachers with deep foundations in the essences of natural disciplines.

Unfortunately, that occurred uncommonly in the South. According to Flexner, every state in the South overflowed with doctors—emanating from schools of questionable integrity. Too many doctors—and too many schools. He insisted on university affiliation for proper training. In fact, Flexner believed that none of the southern state universities was "wisely placed." Even the revered

Medical College of the State of South Carolina received a caustic review: meager equipment, a trashy dissecting room, no access to laboratories, no museum, no library or other teaching aids, little obstetrical work, little emphasis on any clinical exposure.[13] As for Georgia, "The Augusta situation (Medical College of Georgia) is hopeless." Flexner urged tight control by the University of Georgia at Athens or "snap the slender thread" by which Augusta's illustrative Medical College was so tenuously university tied.[14] In fact, of the eleven southern states, just six schools should be able to handle output of needed physicians, he concluded. Flexner suggested the following: Tulane University (New Orleans), Vanderbilt University (Nashville), University of Virginia (Charlottesville or maybe Richmond), University of Georgia (amalgamation of Atlanta programs), University of Alabama (Birmingham), and the University of Texas (Galveston).[15]

For one, the citizens of Augusta rallied in response. The proud tradition of Augusta's medical education would not be so easily put to rest. Flexner's report was sobering but instructive. Dean of the Medical College William H. Doughty Jr. took the lead. His team of concerned individuals began a vigorous program of reconstruction. By 1915 a phoenix indeed had arisen from the ashes, a new Medical College with firm attachments to the University of Georgia and a brand-new city hospital for clinical experience.[16] Far from hopeless, the renewed Medical College of Georgia would be a beacon of medical education for the state of Georgia.

As for education of the Black physician, Flexner had little sympathy. "The practice of the negro doctor will be limited to his own race," Flexner wrote. The danger of ill health among Blacks, of course, was communication of such infections as tuberculosis and hookworm to their white neighbors. In this, the health of the African American assumes paramount importance, not so much as a humanitarian effort in and of its own. Flexner begrudgingly allowed, "[The African American] is, as far as the eye can see, a permanent factor in the nation. He has his rights and due and value as an individual; but he has, besides, the tremendous importance that belongs to a potential source of infection and contagion." "He must be educated not only for his sake, but for ours," Flexner concluded.[17] Yet medical training of Black doctors and nurses was also deplorable, he pointed out. Five of the seven predominately Black medical colleges should be immediately closed. The only two worth preserving were Howard University in Washington, DC, and Meharry Medical College in Nashville.

In terms of specialty training, opportunities for Black physicians were almost nonexistent. The first recognized residency program appeared at the new Johns Hopkins Hospital in the 1890s under the tutelage of medicine chief William Osler. He incorporated in his curriculum bedside rounding to acquaint his trainees with the nuances of clinical practice firsthand. When surgeon William Halsted arrived, he took up Osler's practices and applied them to the specialty of surgery, bringing into play basic sciences and progressive clinical responsibilities, modeled after the German programs he had visited.[18]

By the turn of the century, training curricula—many modeled after the Hopkins method of Osler and Halsted—had sprouted in other northern hospitals such as the Mayo Clinic in Rochester, Minnesota, and Harvard and Yale. It was no surprise that this new paradigm did not immediately penetrate the deeper South. In fact, most southern physicians in search of additional specialization would have to travel north, much as they did in the early days of the Union. There were simply no local opportunities. Of the few Black southern physicians wanting a specialty path, it was even worse. They were not solicited nor well received in the North. Segregation and Jim Crow took hold even there. When a young Black physician, a graduate of Meharry, arrived at the Chicago Postgraduate School of Medicine in 1892, the superintendent, seeing that he was Black, coldly announced that he did not know the new arrival was "colored." Blurting out that the laws of the state prohibited him from refusing to admit the young man, the pompous chief told him bluntly, "I can tell you that we had rather not have you, and further, there is not much we can do for you." The Black doctor, John Perry, was permitted to attend lectures but was shunned by his classmates and excluded from much of the bedside teaching.[19] The effect of segregation practices was disastrous for Black physicians, not allowed into many specialty programs and pushed aside when they were. White colleagues generally held them in disdain, and even many white patients—even some Black patients at that—refused their presence.

For those Black individuals fortunate enough to finish specialty training, problems persisted. Developing a focused practice was not easy, and many barely scraped together a livable wage. One white Nashville physician summed up their plight: "The Negro specialist must accept the fact that he is pioneering and must begin his specialty practice on a somewhat limited scale. By this I mean that Negroes cannot find it economically feasible to practice a specialty."[20] And so it was. It would be well into the twentieth century before any semblance of equal opportunity permitted Black doctors the same advantages for postgraduate training as their white brethren availed—even more so, of course, in the South. And even then, they struggled for credibility and for acceptance into white-dominated specialty societies. It was inconceivable, southerners might have presumptuously thought, that these "coloreds," a generation removed from captive field hands—indolent and illiterate—could rise to the level of intellectual sophistication that they claimed and that their profession deserved.

As a result, southern Blacks benefitted little. By 1906, according to Irving Fisher's sweeping health report of 1909, the death rate per 1,000 in cities having not less than 10 percent "colored" inhabitants was 17.2 for whites and 28.1 for blacks.[21] "These racial differences may be ascribed in part to different habits and conditions of life, but probably in part also to varying racial susceptibility to disease."[22] Indeed, there is truth in that. Unsanitary conditions and poor nutrition provided ample opportunity for infectious ailments that weaken constitutions and hamper efforts to achieve the vitality necessary for gainful employment and social interaction. Fisher went on: "It would be impossible to express in exact terms the extent to which improved health could increase human happiness; but every observer of human misery among the poor reports that disease plays the leading role."[23]

Inequities aside, by the dawn of the twentieth century, the myth of southern medical distinctiveness had largely been put to rest. For a time, it all had fit nicely with that insistence of southern uniqueness. Economy, society, morality, and behavior stemmed from an interplay of sun, earth, and even divine purpose. Yes, there were southerners, steeped in romance, autocratic civility, and gentility, who harkened back to those *Gone with the Wind* days of expansive plantations, lucrative commerce, and, yes, even workers in bondage. In those moments it was all so glorious, this proprietorship, this freedom to uphold a lifestyle and beliefs unquestionably unique to their part of America. But wiser sorts knew better.

As for health, ailments of the South, no doubt exaggerated by perturbations of climate and geography, were the same as found in northern cities and fields. It might have been largely the curse of slavery, in some regard, that subjected white southerners to the plagues of fever, mosquito-borne, and the horrors of filth and hovels in which Blacks were corralled. Agrarian temperaments resisted sanitary measures invoked by the urbanized North, populated by kinds so foreign as to be labeled "strangers" in the South. Rural health care did not lend itself to scientific discoveries. Simple matters of fevers, infections, farm injuries, and childbirth consumed the average country doctor's time and energy. Little could he probe the nuances of illness to the extent of his urbanized, academic colleagues. As noted by Rosemary Stevens, "The rural general practitioner ... could not hope to keep up with scientific improvements in medicine, however hard he tried; nor did he have the time to make his own scientific observations or to keep proper records. There was already a gap between the potential of medical science and the level of knowledge in the field."[24]

Then, was it all contrived? Some present-day scholars, essayist Orville Vernon Burton argues, insist that that southern exceptionalism is a myth, that this "otherness" distorts and hampers social and political reality. No doubt there are persistent claims of distinctiveness still. The South is friendlier, kinder, more hospitable, refined. There was an exaggerated sense of masculinity and femininity, all to the grander embodiment of Christian moral values. Sadly, such admirable characteristics were founded on the belief of white supremacy and applied only to those fortunate ones of the southern aristocracy. The Black South had a much different take on this exceptionalism—one borne of marginalization, disenfranchisement, and segregation. The genteel nature of southerners was closely allied to fits of violence against the sizeable faction of African American residents. "Separate but equal" soon became their battle cry. Burton's "otherness" still draped the South in perplexities. "The peculiar history of the South, of blacks and whites, of the mix and timing of folks' arrivals and the frictions along the way, made the South the 'Other,' and continues to do so," Burton concluded.[25]

But it is our history, our American history, as we continue that arduous journey toward an understanding of the human constitution and the enlightened comprehension that all men and women, inside and out, are indeed created equal and, by that very fact, entitled to the same health and happiness. Was it now a "New South," a term coined by that visionary nineteenth-century journalist and reformist Henry W. Grady? Was it what the medical profession hoped for, driven by technology and science, part of a global venture to better mankind? Was it now a changed country, industrialized, modernized, progressive, integrated? Or would it remain a more dire forecast, a stark reminder of the stubbornness of human behavior, what southern historian Robert S. Cotterill proclaimed it to be in 1948: "There is, in very fact, no Old South and no New. There is only The South. Fundamentally, as it was in the beginning it is now, and, if God please, it shall be evermore."[26] Will those sickly vapors of Dixie ever truly vanish?

ACKNOWLEDGMENTS

A work such as this cannot be done without the generous assistance of many supportive people. While the pioneers of "southern medicine" spoke in their own words and need not be interpreted or analyzed further, the context in which they lived has certainly been worthy of analysis and mitigation. Only time can show the true relevance—or irrelevance—of ideas and thoughts, but we must put those sometimes radical, progressive, or regressive notions as pieces of a mosaic to obtain a full picture of the advances of mankind in caring for our fellow humans. In that vein, I hold in gratitude the numbers of authors referenced in this work who shed light on the lives and times of many of these intrepid individuals who tried to make sense of the myriad health issues of southern people.

I would like to thank Emily Bundy and all the fine people at the University Press of Mississippi for deeming my work worthy of publication. Her staff of reviewers—anonymous though they may have been—added important critical commentary to my work and allowed me to amend passages for meaning and accuracy. In particular I would like to thank Elizabeth Farry for her meticulous editing. They all have helped produce a stronger manuscript. I would also like to thank my former literary agent and friend, Regina Ryan, for her thoughtful comments and guidance in forming this history.

While much archival information is readily available online, there were still records that needed research and copying. My thanks to Renée Bosman of the Davis Library at the University of North Carolina–Chapel Hill for material on Solomon Mordecai. In like fashion, my thanks to Renée A. Sharrock, curator, Historical Collections and Archives, Robert B. Greenblatt MD Library, Augusta University, on information about Milton Antony. My gratitude to Mary J. Holt, history librarian, Rudolph Matas Library of the Health Sciences, Tulane University, for her help in procuring archival information on the founding of the Medical College of Louisiana in 1834. I am deeply appreciative of the help of Ruth A. Riley, director of library services, School of Medicine, University of

South Carolina, for her help in procuring information concerning the Medical College of the University of South Carolina, 1868–1876.

As always, my thanks and appreciation to Suzette Robinson and the staff of the Rowland Medical Library of the University of Mississippi Medical Center for their tireless efforts to procure obscure literature and archival records. Suzette's team spares no effort in finding the arcane works that were important to completing this project.

NOTES

PREFACE

1. De Bow, "Future of the South," 6–16, quote 8.
2. Duffy, "Note on Ante-Bellum Southern Nationalism," 266–76.
3. Savitt and Young, *Disease and Distinctiveness*, 8.
4. Anderson, "Telling Stories, Making Selves," 21–38, quote 25.

CHAPTER ONE: THE CONGO IS NOT MORE DIFFERENT

1. Carpenter, *South as a Conscious Minority*, 7–8.
2. Ramsay, *History of South Carolina*, 56.
3. "Old South" generally refers to that southeastern part of colonial North America, incorporating the colonies/states of Virginia, North and South Carolina, and Georgia but eventually bringing in the agricultural territories of Louisiana, Alabama, and Mississippi—and their eventual statehood. While emphasizing antebellum history, the Old South in its customs and culture spans the post–Civil War years to include the early days of Reconstruction, as I have taken liberty to do in this history.
4. Wallerstein, "What Can One Mean by Southern Culture?," 1–13, containing Current's quotes, 10.
5. Best, *True Discourse of the Late Voyage of Discouverie*, 37.
6. Kupperman, "Puzzle of the American Climate," 1262–1289. For the early colonial English "climate" equated with "latitude."
7. Forry, *Climate of the United States*, 355, 360.
8. Arbuthnot, *Essay Concerning the Effects of Air on Human Bodies*, 151–52.
9. Wyatt-Brown, *Shaping of Southern Culture*, 89. A central theme throughout this work is that of "culture." What is culture? I have taken the definition as offered by Margaret S. Archer in *Culture and Agency: The Place of Culture in Social Theory*. Archer suggests that a dualism exists between a cultural system (the shared ideas, beliefs, available knowledge) and sociocultural interaction (how societal members draw on those elements of the cultural system). One might think of it as a meshing of structure and practice. While most of the South had conformity on their societal ideas, there was not uniform reaction to those. But despite

disagreement, the general flow of attitudes (structure) and behavior (practices) adhered to their shared beliefs and understanding—their cultural system.

10. Gray, *History of Agriculture*, 467. Gray went on to say, however, that enslaved Africans made remarkable progress in acquiring a variety of skills—even without structured education—that, in antebellum years, provided the necessary underpinnings for a vibrant agrarian economy. Nevertheless, the prevailing attitude in the South in the eighteenth century was that Black people were particularly suited to labor in subtropical climates. They were truly considered beasts of burden, relegated to a life of perpetual servitude and physical toil as typified in the bigoted and highly offensive controversial book *The Negro a Beast, or In the Image of God*, authored by the former enslaver Charles Carroll. He and like-minded southerners argued for a distinctly inferior heritage from the white man as a literal "beast." See also the vehement rebuttal of Carroll's work by the noted abolitionist Edward Atkinson in his publication "The Negro a Beast."

11. Of course, there were important differences. Property was not necessarily subdivided or bestowed with obligatory allegiances, nor was there the military component typically seen in traditional medieval feudal societies. Nevertheless, a strong planter class exercised considerable political authority, aimed at self-preservation. See Ganshof, *Feudalism*.

12. See Manning, *What This Cruel War Was Over*, particularly 19–51.

13. Charles Mason and Jeremiah Dixon surveyed a boundary line, defined by the border of Pennsylvania and Maryland in the mid-1700s. This soon became the informal boundary between the "North" and the "South."

14. Da Costa, "French School of Surgery," 77–79.

15. McCullough, *Greater Journey*, 24.

16. Morgan, *Discourse upon the Institution of Medical Schools*, x.

17. Stevens, *American Medicine and the Public Interest*, 15 fn.

18. Carmer, *Stars Fell on Alabama*, xxiv.

19. Warner, "Southern Medical Reform."

20. Fenner, "Reports from Mississippi."

21. See Cartwright, "Diseases and Physical Peculiarities."

22. Warner, *Therapeutic Perspective*, 78.

CHAPTER TWO: COLONIES OF PLENTY

1. Waterhouse, *Declaration of the State of the Colony*, 3–6, quote 3.

2. "Ague" was a colonial term signifying illness characterized by paroxysms of fever and shivering. Most illustrious was the periodic sickness of malaria.

3. Beverley, *History and Present State of Virginia*, 69. See also Daniel J. Boorstin, *The Americans*, 209–19.

4. Based on Andrews, *Colonial Period of American History*, 185.

5. Byrd, *Histories of the Dividing Line*, 87.

6. Hilton, "Relation of a Discovery," 44–45.

7. Joseph Dalton to Lord Ashley, January 20, 1671, in in *Collections of the South Carolina Historical Society*, 379.

8. It was not until after the Revolutionary War that the town was officially named Charleston.

9. Wilson, "Account of the Province of Carolina."

10. Harrison, "Pelatiah Webster's Journal," 146.

11. Letter, James Oglethorpe to the Honorable Trustees, Savannah, February 10, 1733, 14207, Hargrett Library, University of Georgia, Athens, GA.

12. See the comprehensive biography of Oglethorpe written by Thaddeus Mason Harris, *Biographical Memorials of James Oglethorpe*. Maybe the name stemmed from the Native American Taino tribe in the Caribbean whose word for "sheet" was *zabana*, adopted by the Spanish (*sabana*) for a wide-open plain.

13. Letter, James Oglethorpe to the Honorable Trustees, Savannah, August 12, 1733, 14207, Hargrett Library, University of Georgia, Athens, GA. See also Altschuler and Jobanputra, "What Was the Cause of the Epidemic?" The Carolinian Colonel William Bull from the Ashley Plantation, who was quite familiar with the Savannah River region, was sent by Governor Robert Johnson of Charleston to assist Oglethorpe. He brought four people he enslaved, who apparently were a great help in clearing and cultivating the land.

14. Fox-Genovese, "Antebellum Southern Households," 232–33.

15. de Villiers, *Histoire*, 10.

16. de Villiers, *Histoire*, 15.

17. Although the Acadians would come in much larger numbers after the Seven Years' War, vigorously expelled from their northern homelands by an intensified, if not a prosecutorial British rule.

18. Fortier, *A History of Louisiana*, 101.

19. Contained in du Pratz, *Histoire de la Louisiane*, 141.

20. Fortier, *A History of Louisiana*, 51; Dowler, *Tableau of the Yellow Fever*, 7.

21. Stange, *Vital Negotiations*, 147. The *Compagnie d'Occident*, or, more formally, the *Compagnie des Indes Occidentale* or simply the Mississippi Company, was founded by the entrepreneur rascal John Law in 1717, granting him almost complete sovereignty over the most fertile lands of North America, adjacent to the Mississippi River. See Lowry and McCardle, *A History of Mississippi*.

22. See Stange, "Urban Governance in French Colonial North America" and Lemann, "Problems of Founding a Viable Colony." The Ursuline nuns were delighted to travel to the New World. They were suitably impressed with New Orleans, reporting back to their superiors: "Our city [New Orleans] is very beautiful, well-constructed, and methodically designed, as far as I can know myself and as I saw the day of our arrival in this country, because since that day, we have always stayed in our country. fencing . . . The streets there are very wide and drawn in a line, the main street after a league in length, the houses very well built in timber and mortar . . . it suffices to tell you that a song is being sung here publicly, in which there is that this city has as much appearance as the city of Paris . . . Indeed it is very beautiful, but besides that I do not have enough eloquence to be able to convince you all the beauty of it in the song." "Lettre à la Nouvelle-Orléans, Ce Vingt-Quatrieme Avril 1728," in *Relation du Voyage des Dames Religieuse*, 3–4.

23. Claiborne, *Mississippi as a Province, Territory and State*, 91.

24. de Roulhac Hamilton, *Papers of Thomas Ruffin*, 77–78. Thomas Ruffin was a Supreme Court of North Carolina judge of immense reputation. Speculators of the Old South, of course, were intensely interested in the new lands to the west, particularly with rumors of fertile soil and remarkable capacity to cultivate bumper crops.

25. Drake, *A Systematic Treatise*, 10.

26. Drake, *A Systematic Treatise*, 130.

27. Perlee, "Account of the Yellow Fever of Natchez," 4. See also Lowry and McCardle, *A History of Mississippi*.

CHAPTER THREE: A PARADISE OF ILLS

1. "Southern Medical Schools—Southern Toadyism."
2. Drake, *A Systematic Treatise*, 1.
3. Cartwright, "Cartwright on Southern Medicine."
4. Fenner, "Introductory Address."
5. Mitchell, "Health and the Medical Profession."
6. See Bartlett, *Discourse on the Times*, 72.
7. Smith, *History of the Province of New-York*, 212.
8. Hoban, *Pennsylvania Archives*, 7196–200.
9. Bell, "Medical Practice in Colonial America."
10. Letter to Ebenezer Hazard, September 27, 1762, in Butterfield, *Letters of Benjamin Rush*, 5. Ebenezer Hazard was a prominent Philadelphia merchant, church elder, and later historian.
11. Shryock, *Development of Modern Medicine*, 51.
12. Aelius Galenus, simply known as Galen, was a first-century CE physician and philosopher whose extremely popular theories of illness prompted a firm commitment to his humoral theory: imbalances of the four innate humors: black bile, yellow bile, blood, and phlegm.
13. Nimura, *The Doctors Blackwell*, 53.
14. Rush, *Eulogium*.
15. See Shryock, "Eighteenth Century Medicine in America."
16. See Rush, *Sixteen Introductory Lectures*, 151, 153.
17. Rush, *Eulogium*, 8.
18. Milligen-Johnston, "Short Description of the Province," 154.
19. Rogers, *Life and Letters*, 181.
20. Quote taken from Numbers and Numbers, "Science in the Old South," 176.
21. Smith, *Selection of the Correspondence*, 519–20.
22. See Guerra, "Medical Almanacs."
23. As told by Ramsay, *History of South Carolina*, 109–10.

CHAPTER FOUR: CORRUPTED AIR, PUTREFIED EARTH

1. de la Motta, *Oration on the Causes*, 7.
2. Lind, *Two Papers*, 56–60.
3. Lind, *Essay on Diseases*, 37.
4. Lind, *Two Papers*, 93.
5. Honigsbaum and Wilcox, "Cinchona."
6. See Avellaneda, "Hernando de Soto."
7. Sallares, Bouwman, and Anderung, "Spread of Malaria."
8. Celsus, *De Medicina*, 3.3, 228.
9. Varro, *Rerum Rusticarum*, 12.2, 211.
10. From Russell, "Malaria and Its Influence."
11. Shakespeare, *The Tempest*, Act II, Scene II, 43–33.
12. Pringle, *Observations*, 6.
13. Markham, *Memoir of the Lady*, 73–89. For a discussion of the controversy concerning Countess Chinchon. See also Haggis, "Fundamental Errors."

14. Lind, *Essay on Diseases*, 232.
15. Lind, *Two Papers*, 67.
16. See Wilson, "Fevers and Science."
17. Mitchell, "Account of the Yellow Fever," 182–83. Colden Cadwallader was a respected physician and scientist who had devoted much time and energy to yellow fever, ascribing it, in part, to filthy living conditions so prevalent in New York City at the time.
18. See Crosby, *American Plague*, particularly 7–16.
19. Figures from Patterson, "Yellow Fever Epidemics."
20. McCrady, *History of South Carolina under the Proprietary Government*, 308–9.
21. Duffy, "Yellow Fever," 191.
22. Webster, *Brief History*, 230.
23. Webster, *Brief History*, 211.
24. See Bancroft, *Essay*, 122–205.
25. Ramsay, *History of South-Carolina*, 83–84. See also Blake, "Yellow Fever."
26. Bancroft, *Essay*, 245.
27. Rush, "Result of Observations," 262.
28. See Creighton, *History of Epidemics*, 98–140.
29. Thomson, *Works of William Cullen*, 467–676, quote 609–10.
30. See Lewis, *Experimental History*, 188–89.
31. Contained in Risse, "'Typhus' Fever," 191.
32. See Angelakis, Bechah, and Raoult, "History of Epidemic Typhus."
33. Willis, "Of the Putrid Fever," 553–54.
34. Willis, "Of the Putrid Fever," 567. In fact, it would be proven to be a corrosion of the intestines that was so blatantly fatal.
35. See Rolleston, "Bretonneau."
36. Although ancient Babylonian texts indicate that if the disease is prolonged and red liquid flows from the victim's anus, he will recover. See Cunha, "Prolonged and Perplexing Fevers."
37. See Smith, "Gerhard's Distinction."
38. Mather, *Angel of Bethesda*, 93.
39. "Smallpox," in Atkinson et al., *Epidemiology and Prevention*, 281–306. For a pictorial depiction of the lesions of smallpox, see the comprehensive illustrated compendium of cases in Ricketts, *Diagnosis of Smallpox*.
40. Cullen, *First Lines*, 222–23.
41. See Nutton, "Reception of Fracastoro's Theory."
42. See Mather, *Angel of Bethesda*, 94.
43. Cullen, *First Lines*, 217–35.
44. See Latham, *Works of Thomas Sydenham*, Vol. 2, 251–57.
45. Moore, *History of Smallpox*, 215; Cullen, *First Lines*, 217–35.
46. Smallpox was thought to encourage an acidic environment. The alkaline milk was meant to neutralize the acidity of the affliction. Why an ass's milk, however, defies explanation.
47. Frewen, *Practice and Theory*, 45–46. See also Halsband, "New Light."
48. Mather, *Angel of Bethesda*, 97.
49. Moore, *History of Smallpox*, 251–52.
50. Ramsay, *History South Carolina*, 42–43.
51. Hopkins, *Greatest Killer*, 244.
52. Horace, "Virginibus Puerisque Canto," *South Carolina Gazette*, February 16, 1760, 3.

53. Pinckney, *Letterbook*, 147.

54. See Krebsbach, "Great Charlestown Smallpox Epidemic."

55. "A Proclamation," *Georgia Gazette*, October 6, 1763, 1.

56. Telamon Cuyler Historical Manuscripts, University of Georgia, Athens, GA, Box 12, Folder 33.

57. See Maxwell, "True State."

58. From Becker, "Smallpox in Washington's Army," 420.

59. Pringle, *Observations*, 262.

60. Currie, *Historical Account*, 403–4. Currie, himself, was a surgeon in Samuel Atlee's Pennsylvania Musket Battalion but had to resign his commission because of ill health.

61. Pringle, *Observations*, 233.

62. Moseley, *Treatise on Tropical Diseases*, 367.

63. For Sydenham's description of dysentery, see Dewhurst, "Sydenham."

64. Rush, *Works of Thomas Sydenham*, 443.

65. Now, of course, classic cholera is due to a specific bacterium, *Vibrio cholerae*. It was first known as Asiatic cholera and was not introduced in Europe until 1831. The disease is transmitted via spoiled food, contaminated water, and in living conditions of abject poverty. While a form of dysentery, that is, a gastrointestinal ailment, its virulence sets it apart as more lethal. The former term *cholera morbus* simply indicated a severe form of dysentery that often was fatal.

66. Howard-Jones, "Choleranomalies."

67. Pringle, *Observations*, 245.

68. Rush, "Result of Observations," 261.

CHAPTER FIVE: DOCTORING IN THE COLONIAL SOUTH

1. Brickell, *Natural History of North-Carolina*, 251–53. Consumption was a dreaded preoccupation in the eighteenth century, an illness that seemed to inexorably do in its victims and lacked the remotest of explanations.

2. Randolph, "Letter to the Board of Trade."

3. Harrison, "Pelatiah Webster's Journal," 146.

4. See Hirsch, *Huguenots*, 28–29. Quotes from Purry, *Memorial*, 21; Purry, *A Description of the Province of South Carolina*, 10.

5. Hayne, "Biographical Memoir," 207.

6. *Population of the United States*, 8.

7. Letter to Benjamin Rush, February 3, 1779, in Brunhouse and Ramsay, "David Ramsay," 58–59. Yet his feelings apparently wavered. In a later communication Ramsay lamented: "They are dastardly to a great degree. When they have been employed in servile labor near scenes of action, they have shown a most extravagant fear of danger. Slavery has annihilated every generous sentiment. That abject submission, which is inculcated on slaves at the first, & most necessary duty tends to destroy every spark of courage in their breasts. They might be learnt the manual exercise; but, it would be hard to learn a slave to despise danger." (Letter to Benjamin Rush, June 20, 1779, in Brunhouse and Ramsay, "David Ramsay," 60–61.

8. Letter to Benjamin Rush, July 29, 1772, in Brunhouse and Ramsay, "David Ramsay," 51.

9. See Ramsay, *Review of the Improvements*.

10. Ramsay "Dissertation on the Means of Preserving Health."

11. David Ramsay, *History of the American Revolution*, Vol. 1, 37.
12. *South Carolina Gazette*, Monday, February 13, 1775.
13. Letter to Benjamin Rush, August 6, 1776, in Brunhouse and Ramsay, "David Ramsay," 53.
14. See Ramsay, *Memoirs*, 112–13. See also Gillespie, "1795."
15. Letter to Benjamin Rush, December 14, 1785, in Brunhouse and Ramsay, "David Ramsay," 94. Ramsay felt that slavery was the leading problem in South Carolina, outdistancing even his pet concern about climate and health.
16. Ramsay, *History of South Carolina*, 89.
17. See Hayne, "Biographical Memoir." All quotes are from that article. Multi-barrel flintlock "horseman's pistols" were available in 1815. More common were the "over and under" two-barrel varieties, although a triple barrel pistol did exist. It is likely that only two shots were fired from the more accessible two-barrel pistol.
18. Davidson, *Friend of the People*, 10–11.
19. *Statutes at Large of South Carolina*, Vol. 4, No. 881, IX, 82.
20. One might notice a similarity with the twenty-first-century coronavirus pandemic. Not a few were reluctant to take the vaccine despite compelling evidence of its efficacy.
21. Ramsay, *History of South Carolina*, 65.
22. Latham, *Works of Thomas Sydenham*, Vol. 1, 32 and 34.
23. Currie, *Historical Account*, 2, 382.
24. Lind, *Essay on Diseases*, 37.
25. Lining, "Letter from Dr. John Lining."
26. Chalmers, *Account of the Weather*, 41.
27. White, "Topography of Savannah," 241.
28. See two descriptions of colonial Georgia in Krafka, "Medicine in Colonial Georgia" and Weaver, "Early Medical History of Georgia," 89–112, quote 90.
29. Figures from Bell, "Rice, Resistance."
30. "Extract from the Writings of Rev. John Wesley," in Cooper, *Experienced Botanist*, xi. See also Maddox, "John Wesley."
31. Vanderpool, "Wesleyan-Methodist Tradition."
32. Wesley, *Primitive Physic*, iii–iv and viii. See also Rogal, "Pills for the Poor" and Georgian, "Medicine and Politics."

CHAPTER SIX: REVOLUTION: THE GLORIOUS ALLY OF DISEASE

1. Sandy, "Divided Loyalties."
2. Holman, "William Gilmore Simm's Picture," 449.
3. McCandless, *Slavery, Disease, and Suffering*, 85–86. See Professor McCandless's comments about Revolutionary Fever in "Revolutionary Fever: Disease and War in the Lower South, 1776–1783."
4. Pringle, *Observations*, 4.
5. Pringle, *Observations*, 6.
6. Pringle, *Observations*, 8.
7. Archibald Campbell deftly reestablished British government in Savannah and all of Georgia so that it was the only state in the union that, after the Declaration of Independence, continued to convene a legislative body under the crown of Great Britain.

8. Dexter, *Estimates of Population*.

9. Moultrie, *Memoirs*, 44.

10. Searcy, "1779."

11. Grimké, "Journal of the Campaign."

12. "Official Letters of Major General James Pattison." Thomas Townshend (1733–1800) was an influential parliamentarian and briefly secretary at war in 1782.

13. Figures cited in Kopperman, "Medical Dimension."

14. Moultrie, *Memoirs*, letter to General Lincoln, November 17, 1779, 43.

15. Moultrie, *Memoirs*, 44.

16. Moultrie, *Memoirs*, 49.

17. Ramsay to Benjamin Rush, July 18, 1779, in Brunhouse and Ramsay, "David Ramsay," 62.

18. Ramsay to Benjamin Rush, March 21, 1780, in Brunhouse and Ramsay, "David Ramsay," 65.

19. Letter from Lord Campbell to Lord Dartmouth, October 19, 1775, in Wallace, *History of South Carolina*, 154–55.

20. Ramsay to Benjamin Rush, February 3, 1779, in Brunhouse and Ramsay, "David Ramsay," 58.

21. See Gibson, "Costume and Fashion."

22. Davidson, *Friend of the People*, 25 and 34. See also Johnson, *Traditions and Reminiscences*, 263–72.

23. McCandless, "Revolutionary Fever."

24. See "David Oliphant Report of Sick and Wounded at Continental Hospital," MSS 68, Waring Historical Library, Medical University of South Carolina, Charleston, SC.

25. Hayne, "Biographical Memoir," 209.

26. Ramsay, *History of the American Revolution*, Vol. 2, 223.

27. McCrady, *History of South Carolina in the Revolution*, 726.

28. Smith and Webber, "Josiah Smith's Diary."

29. Sullivan's Island was a spit of sand at the entrance to Charles Towne harbor. On June 28, 1776, Moultrie's band of determined marksmen destroyed British warships seeking to land an expeditionary force of troops to capture Charles Towne. This is referred to as the "first" siege of Charles Towne. See Russell, *American Revolution*, particularly chapter 7 "Sullivan's Island," 87–89.

30. Waring, "Report from the Continental General Hospital."

31. Davidson, *Friend of the People*, 39.

32. James, *Sketch of the Life*, appendix 1–7.

33. Casualty figures from Tarleton, *History of the Campaigns*, 86.

34. Meacham, *American Lion*, 11.

35. Letter from Moultrie to General Patterson, June 15, 1780, Moultrie, *Memoirs*, 112.

36. Letter from Dr. Oliphant to Moultrie, November 14, 1780, Moultrie, *Memoirs*, 142.

37. Ramsay, *History of the American Revolution* Vol. 2, 213.

38. Tiffany, *Sketch of the Life and Services*, 14 and 12.

39. Ross, *Correspondence of Charles*, Letter Earl Cornwallis to Sir Henry Clinton, August 10, 1780, 55.

40. Tarleton, *History of the Campaigns*, 111.

41. See Johnson, *Sketches of the Life and Correspondence*, Vol. 1, 498.

42. Letter from Hugh Williamson to Thomas Benbury, Edenton, December 1, 1780, *Colonial and State Records of North Carolina*, Vol. 15, 168.

43. Davidson, *Friend of the People*, 42.

44. Davidson, *Friend of the People*, 45.

45. Duncan, *Medical Men*, 311.

46. Jackson, *Treatise of the Fevers*, 301 and 299. "Dropsy" probably referred to the findings of generalized swelling (or edema). It very likely could have been nutritional in cause.

47. Ewald, *Diary of the American War*, 328.

48. Mather, *Angel of Bethesda*, 212.

49. "Letter Earl Cornwallis to Lord George Germain," Camden, South Carolina, August 20, 1780, *Colonial and State Records of North Carolina*, Vol. 15, 266.

50. Tarleton, *History of the Campaigns*, 155–56.

51. Lee, *Memoirs of the War*, 202.

52. Blanton, *Medicine in Virginia in the Eighteenth Century*, 253.

53. Figures from Foster and Putnam, "Battle of King's Mountain."

54. Foster and Putnam, "Battle of King's Mountain."

55. Draper, *King's Mountain*, 306.

56. Lord Cornwallis to Sir Henry Clinton, December 3, 1780, *Colonial Records of North Carolina*, Vol. 15, 302.

57. Ross, *Correspondence of Charles*, "Earl Cornwallis to Lord George Germain, April 18, 1781," 89–90.

58. Nathaniel Greene to George Washington, December 7, 1781, Papers of George Washington, Library of Congress, 99-01-02-04138.

59. Nathaniel Green to George Washington, December 7, 1781.

60. See Haw, "'Every Thing Here.'"

61. Hannah and his partner Saunders remain obscure individuals, likely Loyalists, who pastured their cattle on this tract of open pasture. Their identity beyond last names is unknown.

62. See Rankin, "Cowpens." See also Myers, *Cowpens Papers*, 24–30, quote 26.

63. Cornwallis to Rawdon, January 21, 1781, Folio 78, 30/11/84, Public Record Office, London, UK.

64. Ross, *Correspondence of Charles*, "Earl Cornwallis to Sir Henry Clinton, July 27, 1781," 106.

65. Ewald, *Diary of the American War*, 314.

66. Smyth, *Writings of Benjamin Franklin*, 111.

67. Ross, *Correspondence of Charles*, "Earl Cornwallis to Sir Henry Clinton, October 15, 1781," 124.

68. Ewald, *Diary of the American War*, 338.

69. Ewald, *Diary of the American War*, 338–39.

70. See Kopperman, "Medical Dimension."

71. Duncan, *Medical Men*, 353.

72. Thatcher, *Military Journal*, 343.

73. Thatcher, *Military Journal*, 337.

74. Duncan, *Medical Men*, 355.

75. Tilton, *Economical Observations*, 29. See also Duncan, *Medical Men*, 354.

76. "Doctor Robert Wharry to Doctor Reading Beatty, Then Stationed at Lancaster, Pennsylvania," in Horne et al., "Letters from Continental Officers."

77. "Journal of Lieut. William McDowell," *Pennsylvania Archives*, Second Series, Vol. 15 (Harrisburg: E. K. Meyers, 1890), 295–334, quotes 323, 328, and 329.
78. Johnson, *Sketches of the Life and Correspondence*, Vol. 2, 242–43.
79. Johnson, *Sketches of the Life and Correspondence*, Vol. 2, 247.
80. Nathaniel Greene to George Washington, March 9, 1782, *George Washington Papers*, Series 4, General Correspondence, Library of Congress, Washington, DC.
81. See Kyte, "General Greene's Plans."
82. Jones, *Plain Concise Practical Remarks*, 1. For a brief biography of John Jones, see Griesemer et al., "John Jones, M.D."
83. Jones, *Plain Concise Practical Remarks*, 13.
84. Referring to Winston Groom's famous 1986 novel *Forrest Gump*, about a likable character who, in all innocence, bumbles his way through sentinel events in American history.
85. Jones, *Plain Concise Practical Remarks*, 81.
86. Letter from Benjamin Rush to George Washington, December 26, 1777, in Lengel, *Papers of George Washington*, 7–9.
87. Gibbs, *Documentary History*, 269.
88. The Battle of Stono Ferry was a rearguard action around Charles Towne between Prévost's retreating British troops and General Lincoln's arriving Continentals in June 1779. Continentals failed to dislodge and overtake the British forces. So tempting a victory was not to be. Prévost got away.
89. Gibbs, *Documentary History*, 269.
90. Gibbs, *Documentary History*, 271.
91. Gibbs, *Documentary History*, 280.
92. Gibbs, *Documentary History*, 282.
93. Simms, *The Scout*, 295 and 297–98.
94. Thatcher, *Military Journal*, 426.
95. Duncan, *Medical Men*, 370–71.

CHAPTER SEVEN: THE ILLS OF SLAVERY

1. Jefferson, *Notes*, 174–75.
2. Kingsbury, *Virginia Company*, 243.
3. Smith, *Generall Historie*, 247. See also Sluiter, "New Light."
4. Sainsbury, *Calendar*, 57.
5. Gray, *History of Agriculture*, 344–48. See also Nicholson, "Legal Borrowing."
6. Colonists were eager to find a malleable and durable workforce immune to the rigors of southern climate. These laborers would truly become indentured "beasts of burden" for an affluent aristocracy. See chapter 1, note 10.
7. Davis, *Christian Slaves*, 3–26.
8. In rare cases, though, there were indentured servants—white and otherwise—whose limit of service had been negotiated as indefinite.
9. For concepts of indentured servitude and slavery see Jordan, *White over Black*, 44–98. The topic is also well covered in Thomas, *Slave Trade*.
10. de Tocqueville, *Democracy in America*, 349.
11. de Tocqueville, *Democracy in America*, 344.

12. "An Act for the Better Ordering and Governing of Negroes, Barbados, 1661," in Engerman, Drescher, and Paquette, *Slavery*, 105. See Sirmans, "Legal Status."

13. Coombs, "'Others Not Christians,'" 230.

14. Morgan, "Virginia Slavery." See also Menard, "From Servants to Slaves."

15. Hening, *Statutes at Large*, Vol. 1, 257, 539.

16. Durand of Dauphiné, *Frenchman in Virginia*, 95–96.

17. Newby-Alexander, "The 'Twenty and Odd.'"

18. Hening, *Statutes at Large*, Vol. 3, 447–48.

19. Hesseltine, *History of the South*, 46.

20. Hening, *Statutes at Large*, Vol. 3, 453–54. I prefer to use the term *ethnicity* but will use "race" or "racist" in the context of attributed behavior or direct quotes from other authors. Both African and European ancestry are part of *Homo sapiens*, colloquially known as the human race. In that sense, all are part of the same species. "Ethnicity" is a more appropriate term reflecting geo-cultural differences in heritage, attitudes, customs, and behavior by grouped members of *Homo sapiens*.

21. Thomas, *Slave Trade*, 244.

22. Byrd and Clayton, *American Health Dilemma*, 195.

23. Thomas, *Slave Trade*, 258.

24. Donnan, *Documents*, 126.

25. Salley, *Narratives of Early Carolina*, 103–4. See also Edelson, "Clearing Swamps."

26. Donnan, *Documents* 267–68, 296.

27. Donnan, *Documents*, 313.

28. Donnan, *Documents*, 415.

29. "Minutes of the Privy Council" of April 3, 1735, in Donnan, *Documents*, 587–88.

30. Donnan, *Documents*, 590–91, 608–9. From 1751 to 1780, well over twelve thousand enslaved Africans were imported, some from neighboring South Carolina and the Caribbean, but many directly from Africa (see Harris and Berry, *Slavery and Freedom*, 20.

31. Donnan, *Documents*, 414.

32. One must remember that the term *heathen* in those contemporary times meant one not yet aware of the Christian God—a "pagan." This applied to non-Christian whites, Asians, and Native Americans, as well as Blacks. See Lum, *Heathen*.

33. See Byrd and Clayton, *American Heath Dilemma*, 189.

34. See Garrigus, *Le Code Noir*. See also Stovall, "Race and the Making of the Nation," 205.

35. Donnan, *Documents*, 635, 641.

36. See "Minutes of the Council of Commerce of Louisiana" for September 6, 1719, in Dunbar Rowland, ed., *Mississippi Provincial Archives 1704–1743*, Vol. 3 (Jackson: Press of Mississippi Department of Archives and History, 1932), 255. Dauphine Island served as the major port of entry for French commerce to their southern Louisiana territory. Nearby Mobile Bay was too shallow and plagued by numerous sandbars as was the mouth of the Mississippi River.

37. Rowland, *Mississippi Archives*, 321.

38. du Manoir, "Concession," 168.

39. Figures cited from de La Harpe, *Journal Historique*, 246–57; and Burton and Smith, "Slavery in the Colonial Louisiana Backcountry."

40. Figures from Leglaunec, "Slave Migration."

41. Usner, *Indians, Settlers*, 37. One must remember that conditions for the crew were hardly better. Death rates for crewmen sometimes reached one in five as well, and their treatment and discipline could be even harsher than their human cargo. See Thomas, *Slave Trade*, 306–11.

42. du Manoir, "Concession."

43. Rowland, *Mississippi Archives*, 659–60.

44. For a more complete discussion, see Genovese, "Negro Laborer."

45. Tidyman, "Sketch of the Most Remarkable Diseases," 307.

46. Sydnor, "Life Span."

47. Cobb, *Most Southern Place*, 13.

48. Lutz, *Autobiography and Reminiscences*, 17–18.

49. Katz, *Negro Population*, 57. Overall, about 20 percent of the population of Africans were designated "free." Obviously, the vast majority of these individuals were in Maryland, Delaware, the middle Atlantic, and New England states. A rarity indeed was the free Negro in the South.

50. de Tocqueville, *Democracy in America*, 338.

51. Nott, "Statistics."

52. Sydnor, "Life Span."

53. See Dusinberre, *Slavemaster President*, 90–99. See also Scarborough, *Masters of the Big House*, 175–216. At the Touro Infirmary in New Orleans from 1855 to 1860 there were a total of 1,405 admissions, almost equally divided between enslaved Blacks (701) and whites (704). Surprisingly, overall, the death rate was dramatically skewed to the white patients: 23 percent died compared to just over 7 percent of Blacks. Yellow fever by far dominated the illnesses for which whites were admitted (331 cases). It was an uncommon cause for Blacks (just 20 cases). As might be expected, of those whites admitted with yellow fever almost three-quarters died. None of the 20 slaves died. (From Pritchett and Yun, "In-Hospital Mortality Rates.").

54. Fenner, "On the Hygiene," 433. He had moved to New Orleans in 1840.

55. Shryock, "Medical Practice."

56. Davenport, "Observations." See also Drake, "Diseases of the Negro Population" and Nott, "Statistics."

57. New, "On the Treatment," 211–13.

58. See Grier, "The Negro and His Diseases," 757.

59. Cartwright, "Diseases of Negroes," 210.

60. Brickell, "Epidemic Typhoid Pneumonia."

61. Cartwright, "Diseases of Negroes," 212.

62. Yandell, "Remarks," 93.

63. Savitt, *Medicine and Slavery*, 43–46.

64. Tidyman, "Sketch of the Most Remarkable Diseases," 316–18.

65. Beverly Robinson as quoted in Bankole-Medina, *Slavery and Medicine*, 159.

66. See Kenny, "'A Dictate of Both Interest and Mercy'?"

67. See Cartwright, "Report on the Diseases," "whipping the devil out of them" quote 708.

68. Cartwright, "Diseases and Physical Peculiarities."

69. Cartwright, "Remarks on Dysentery," 146, 156.

70. Duvallon, *Travels*, 81–82, 89, 93.

71. Fenner, "On the Hygiene," 434.

72. Ramsay, "Physiological Differences," I, 286–94 and II, 411–18.

73. Bankole, "Human/Subhuman Issue," 9.

74. See Pessen, "The Workingmen's Movement."

75. Pessen, "How Different."
76. Shapiro, *Last Great Season*, 79.
77. See Bousfield, "Account of Physicians of Color." See also Falk, "Black Abolitionist Doctors."
78. Miller, "Historic Background."
79. Byrd and Clayton, *American Health Dilemma*, 329.

CHAPTER EIGHT: NATIVE HEALING IN COLONIAL TIMES

1. For general reference, see Shryock, *Development of Modern Medicine*; Arikha, *Passions and Tempers*; Friedenbery, *Doctor in Colonial American*; Vogel, *American Indian Medicine*; and Terkel, *Colonial American Medicine*. The four humors as defined by Hippocrates and Galen were blood, yellow bile, phlegm, and black bile. For an elaboration of the four temperaments, see Lloyd, "The Hot and the Cold."
2. Salley, *Narratives of Early Carolina*, 142–45.
3. Ehle, *Trail of Tears*.
4. Starr, *History of the Cherokee Indians*.
5. Berkeley and Berkeley, *Reverend John Clayton*, 21–39.
6. Berkeley and Berkeley, *Reverend John Clayton*, 21–22.
7. Dixon, "Some Aspects."
8. Berkeley and Berkeley, *Reverend John Clayton*, 34.
9. Cooper, *Experienced Botanist*, v.
10. As du Pratz explained in his chronicles, a native jongleur was a combination surgeon, diviner, and sorcerer, corresponding to typical native roles for so-called healers (du Pratz, *Histoire de la Louisiane*, 137).
11. du Pratz, *Histoire de la Louisiane*, 137.
12. du Pratz, *Histoire de la Louisiane*, 209.
13. du Pratz, *Histoire de la Louisiane*, 211.
14. de Montigny, *Mémoires Historiques*, Vol. 1, 173–74.
15. Benjamin Rush, "An Inquiry into the Natural History of Medicine among the Indians of North-America," read before the American Philosophical Society, Philadelphia, February 4, 1774, in Rush, *Medical Inquiries*, 105. Before Rush, there are numerous references to "*sauvages*" pertaining to Native Americans in early French texts of Mississippi Valley explorations. See, for example, descriptions of the adventures of Pierre Lemoyne, Sieur d'Iberville along the Mississippi River in 1699 in Chevalier, *Voyage d'Iberville*. In this context, the meaning of *sauvages* was not so much primitive, ferocious, or subhuman but rather unspoiled and living in the wilderness.
16. Rush, *Medical Inquiries*, 105.
17. Rush, *Medical Inquiries*, 129.
18. Rush, *Medical Inquiries*, 46.
19. Cabanis, *Du Degre de Certitude*, 117.
20. Mooney, *Swimmer Manuscript*, 71–72. See also Ackerknecht, "Primitive Surgery."
21. See Bigelow, *American Medical Botany*.
22. Morgan and Perry, "Traditional Medicinal Plant Use."
23. Speck, "Catawba Herbals."

24. From Hutton, "Comparative Study."
25. Barton, *Collections for an Essay*, 37.
26. See Robinson, "New Worlds."
27. Rafinesque, *Medical Flora*, ii.
28. Smith, *Indian Doctor's Dispensary*, xii.
29. Josselyn, *New-England's Rarities Discovered* as reprinted in *Trans Am Antiquarian Soc* 4 (1860): 137–238, quotes 183, 185, 194, 196–98. See Bartram and Harper, "Diary of a Journey." See also in translated form Kalm, *Travels*.
30. Cowan, "Impact of the Materia Medica."
31. Thomson, *New Guide to Health*, 5. See also Haller, *The People's Doctor*. For the impact of botanical advocates like Thomson on rural Mississippi, see Bridgforth, "Medicine in Antebellum Mississippi."

CHAPTER NINE: SOUTHERN MEDICINE FOR SOUTHERN SICKNESS

1. Fenner, "Introductory Address."
2. Fenner, "Introductory Address," 8, 12.
3. Fenner, "Reports from Mississippi," 354.
4. Shryock, "Medical Practice," 166.
5. Eve, "Medical Education."
6. Mott, *Travels*, 45.
7. Warner, *Against the Spirit*, 258.
8. Warner, "Selective Transport," 217.
9. Osler, *Alabama Student*, 1–18, quote 8. Osler had been chair of clinical medicine at the University of Pennsylvania and physician-in-chief of the Johns Hopkins Hospital before accepting the Regius Professor of Medicine at Oxford, England.
10. Osler, *Alabama Student*, 11–12. The industrious, thoughtful, and dedicated John Bassett died of tuberculosis at age forty-six.
11. See Morgan, *Discourse upon the Institution of Medical Schools* and Nitzsche, *University of Pennsylvania*.
12. See D. Kilbride, "Southern Medical Students."
13. "University of Pennsylvania Medical Department."
14. Ezell, "A Southern Education," 310.
15. Kilbride, "Southern Medical Students," 701. See also Gayley, *History of the Jefferson Medical College*.
16. Hospitality to southerners as quoted in Abrahams, "Secession from Northern Medical Schools." Long-haired students as quoted in Corner, "Apprenticed to Aesculapius," 254.
17. The almshouse opened in 1732 as the first facility for the care of the poor in America. The Pennsylvania Hospital first opened in 1752, also designated for the care the poor.
18. Solomon Mordecai to Ellen Mordecai, November 6, 1819, Mordecai Family Papers (University of North Carolina Library, Chapel Hill), Reel 2.
19. Solomon Mordecai to Ellen Mordecai, April 29, 1821, Mordecai Family Papers (University of North Carolina Library, Chapel Hill), Reel 2.
20. See Barlow and Powell, "Dedicated Medical Student." See also Nuermberger, "Some Notes." During the antebellum period, Mobile had become the center of Jewish life in Alabama.

Their influx, however, did not begin until Mobile passed from French hands to British, Spanish, and then United States governing. While part of French Louisiana, Jews had been expelled by edict of the 1685 *Code Noir*.

21. See Rothstein, *American Physicians*, 26–40.
22. See Warner "Southern Medical Reform."
23. Wells, "Professionalization."
24. *Centennial Memorial of the Medical College*, 11–12.
25. Russell, "'An Ornament to Our City.'"
26. *Acts and Resolutions*, 74–75.
27. Dickson, *Introductory Lecture*, 16–17.
28. Moultrie, *Introductory Address*, 20. Thomas Cooper had similarly advocated for salaries and longer courses of instruction in 1821, recommendations that were largely ignored. Moultrie's life would be one of devotion to the medical profession, a true visionary ahead of his time regarding medical education. He eventually served as a founding member and vice president of the new American Medical Association.
29. Byrd, "First Charles Town Workhouse," 38.
30. Klebaner, "Public Poor Relief," 219.
31. Edwards, *Ordinances*, 46.
32. Ramsay, "Clinical Report," 47–48. See also Waring, "Marine Hospitals of Charleston."
33. "Infirmary," *Charleston Daily Courier*, November 14, 1839, 3.
34. See McCrady, "Historical Address," 386–424. See also Waring, "Charleston Medicine."
35. Quote from Waring, *History of Medicine*, 78.
36. Waring, "Charleston Medicine."
37. Jacob, *Anthony Roots and Branches*. See also Spalding, *History of the Medical College*; Coleman and Gurr, *Dictionary*; and Moores, "Exegit Monumentum Aere Perennius."
38. Jacob, *Anthony Roots and Branches*, 76–77.
39. Antony, "Case of Extensive Caries."
40. "Mr. Editor," *Augusta Chronicle and Georgia Advertiser*, December 28, 1822, 2.
41. "Introduction," *South Med Surg J*, 2. In June 1836 the first edition of the *Southern Medical and Surgical Journal* was published by Milton Antony, Louis Alexander Dugas, Joseph Adams Eve, and others, another milestone in Antony's crusade to develop local medical excellence.
42. Delony, "Letter to the Editors," 259.
43. "Medical College of Georgia," *Augusta Chronicle*, October 24, 1835, 2.
44. See "Milton Antony," in Coleman and Gurr, *Georgia Biography*, 33.
45. James Moultrie had proposed a similar extension at the Medical College of the State of South Carolina in 1834 amid, at first, similar resistance.
46. See "Medical Intelligence" *South Med Surg J*.
47. "Health of Augusta," *Georgian Constitutionalist*, September 26, 1839, 2. See also *Report on the Origin and Cause*, 22–23.
48. Letter, Thomas Jefferson to Joseph Cabell, November 28, 1820, in Cabell, *Early History*, 185.
49. "An Act Appropriating Part of the Revenue of the Library Fund, and for Other Purposes," February 21, 1818, in Cabell, *Early History*, 427–32, quote 430.
50. "Report of the Board of Commissioners," 334. The meeting of commissioners, including, besides Jefferson, former president James Madison and eighteen other dignitaries, was held at the Mountain Top Tavern in Rockfish Gap in Virginia.

51. Letter, Thomas Jefferson to Joseph Cabell, January 11, 1825, Cabell, *Early History*, 330–32, quote 331.

52. Letter, Thomas Jefferson to Joseph Cabell, May 16, 1824, Cabell, *Early History*, 308–12, quote 310.

53. Indeed, as Jefferson suggested, most well-to-do shunned hospitals as literal dens of odious plague and flagging ailments where halls were strewn with suffering and death, patients bereft of family and attention.

54. Letter, Thomas Jefferson to Joseph Cabell, May 16, 1824, Cabell, *Early History*, 308–12, quote 310.

55. Blanton, *Medicine in Virginia in the Nineteenth Century*, 5–68.

56. Letter, Joseph Cabell to Thomas Jefferson, December 17, 1824, Cabell, *Early History*, 316–18, quote 317.

57. See Radbill, "Autobiographical Ana," 23.

58. Chapman, "American Medicine," 404, 408. In fact, all the professors at Virginia were foreign born.

59. Information on John Emmet primarily from Emmet, *Memoir*.

60. Emmet, *Memoir*, 24. Emmet, as it turned out, married not a southerner but one Mary Byrd Farley Tucker of Bermuda. And he never moved to the North.

61. Letter, Thomas Jefferson to John Patten Emmet, March 6, 1825, *The Thomas Jefferson Papers*, Library of Congress, Series 1: General Correspondence 1651 to 1827, Washington, DC.

62. Emmet, *Memoir*, 27.

63. Emmet, *Memoir*, 30.

64. Bruce, *History of the University of Virginia*, Vol. 2, 112. See also a biographical sketch of Alfred Magill in "Magill, Alfred Thurston, M.D.," *Alumni Bulletin University of Virginia* 16 (1923): 319.

65. See Bruce, *History of the University of Virginia*, Vol. 2, 105–16.

66. Harrison, "Prospects of Letters," 28.

67. "Richmond Medical School," *Richmond Enquirer*, October 9, 1835, 4.

68. Quote taken from Blanton, "Augustus Lockman Warner."

69. Warner was aided in these efforts by John Cullen, Thomas Johnson, R. L Bohannan, Socrates Maupin, L. W. Chamberlayne, and Robert Munford, described as "all young men of good training and enthusiasm." See Blanton, "Augustus Lockman Warner."

70. Quoted in Blanton, *Medicine in Virginia in the Nineteenth Century*, 38–39.

71. "Medical College at Richmond," 827. The Richmond Almshouse or Poor and Work House opened in 1806 just outside the city limits, serving paupers, criminals, the insane, orphans, and dissolute homeless. The Almshouse, Capitol building, and the penitentiary were the largest buildings in the city. The City Hospital was first mentioned in conjunction with the Hampden-Sydney Medical Department and probably was built for indigent care in times of contagion or epidemics. Both the almshouse and city hospital were probably dingy affairs with a minimum of cleanliness or nursing care. See Blanton, *Medicine in Virginia in the Nineteenth Century*, 211–21. See also Gibson Worsham, "The Richmond Almshouse and Hospital: Early Provisions for the Poor and Infirm," *Urban Scale Richmond*, November 29, 2016, http://urbanscalerichmondvirginia.blogspot.com/2016/11/the-richmond-almhouse-and-hospital.html.

72. From Smith, "First 125 Years," quote from "Excerpt, first catalogue, 1839."

73. See Savitt, "Use of Blacks."

74. "Medical College at Richmond."

75. See Dabney, *Richmond*, 148. The various medical factions around Richmond raised quite a stir in choosing the chairman of the Medical Department, so much so that trustees of Hampden-Sydney College became so disgusted that they severed relationships with their medical wing.

76. Don Andreas Almonester was quite the philanthropist. He was listed as the "founder" of the cathedral, the hospital, the lazaretto (quarantine station), and the convent of the Ursuline nuns. He died in 1798 and was interred in the Saint Louis Cathedral.

77. Pope, *Tour*, 37.

78. Figure from Fossier, "Charity Hospital," 795.

79. Fossier, "Charity Hospital," 75: 795.

80. Fossier "Charity Hospital," 76: 30.

81. Fenner, "Historical Sketch," 73.

82. Reference for the lives of Warren Stone and Thomas Hunt can be found in Duffy, *Tulane University Medical Center*; Miles, "Memorial Address," *NO Med Surg J* (this is an identical address in honor of Dr. Warren Stone that Dr. Miles of New Orleans delivered to the Southern Surgical and Gynecological Association the year before, in 1894); "Thomas Hunt, M.D.," *NO Med Surg J*; "Tulane Medical Department," *NO Med Surg J*; Gross, *Autobiography*, 103–9; Waring, "Asiatic Cholera."

83. Found in Miles, "Memorial Address," 771.

84. *Registre du Comité Médical de La Nouvelle Orléans*, courtesy of the Rudolph Matas Library of the Health Sciences, New Orleans, LA.

85. Duffy, *Tulane University Medical Center*, 12.

86. *Registre du Comité Médical*.

87. It may have been a question of remuneration. Salaries at the Charity Hospital were paltry. Private enterprises such as those of Stone's might have been for the simple purpose of providing a livable income. As for Stone's hospital, he turned over management to the Sisters of Charity.

88. Gross, *Autobiography*, 108.

89. *Trial and Expulsion*, 25.

90. Miles, "Memorial Address," 774.

91. Editorial, [New Orleans] *Bee*, September 29, 1834.

92. *First Prospectus of the Medical College of Louisiana, 1834*, courtesy of the Rudolph Matas Library of the Health Sciences, New Orleans, LA.

93. Fossier, "History of Medical Education."

94. "Réflexions sur le Collège Médical," *L'Abeille* [New Orleans], October 21, 1834, 1.

95. "Du Collège Médical de la Louisiana," *L'Abeille* [New Orleans], October 1, 1834, 1.

96. Fossier, "History of Medical Education."

97. Barton, *Introductory Lecture*, 17, 21.

98. "Medical College of Louisiana," [New Orleans] *Bee*, April 29, 1835, 2.

99. The state legislature passed an act during the first session of the Twelfth Legislature in 1835 that established the Medical College of New Orleans, listing seven Creole physicians as charter members. John Duffy, ed., *The Rudolph Matas History of Medicine in Louisiana* Vol. 2 (Baton Rouge: Louisiana State University Press, 1962), 244.

100. See Olschner, "Medical Journals," 3. The first Louisiana medical journal was published in 1839 by the Société Médicale de la Nouvelle-Orléans and titled *Journal de la*

Société Médicale de la Nouvelle-Orléans. Little is known of its circulation except that by the end of that year it was defunct.

101. Quotes (excepting "Young Turks") from: "New Orleans School of Medicine" *NO Med News Hosp Gaz*, 489–90 and 620. See also Fossier, "History of Medical Education." Biography of Erasmus Fenner can be found in Duffy, "Erasmus Darwin Fenner."

102. Figures also from Fossier, "History of Medical Education."

103. "Medical Sectionalism."

104. "Medical Schools, No. 1."

105. "Southern Medical Schools—Southern Toadyism," *Georgia Blister and Critic* 1 (1854): 34–35.

106. Marshall, "Home Education," 430, 431.

CHAPTER TEN: SECESSION'S VULGAR SCOURGES

1. Richardson, *Compilation*, 104–5.

2. Matthews, *The Statutes at Large*, 39.

3. Actually, Moore was the third physician to fill that role. He was preceded by Drs. David DeLeon and Charles Smith, each of whom held office only a matter of months.

4. See Wiese, "Life and Times," 916–22, from where these figures were obtained. See also Purcell and Hummel, "Samuel Preston Moore."

5. Blanton, *Medicine in Virginia in the Nineteenth Century*, 272. This number may even be misleading. Some doctors, despite their training, preferred to join the army as common infantrymen. As of January 1861, the entire Medical Corps of the United States Army consisted of the surgeon general, thirty surgeons, and eighty-three assistant surgeons. With the start of hostilities, three surgeons and twenty-one assistant surgeons resigned to join the Confederate Army. See Brown, *Medical Department*, 215.

6. Figures from Waring, *History of Medicine*, 123; and dress code and pay scale from Cunningham, "Organization and Administration."

7. "Salutatory," *Confed Med Surg J*, 13.

8. Nash, "Some Reminiscences," 128, 129.

9. Daniel, *Recollections*, 13, 14.

10. Daniel, *Recollections*, 75.

11. Blanton, *Medicine in Virginia in the Nineteenth Century*, 282–83.

12. Browning and Silver, *Environmental History*, 133–59.

13. Day, *Down South*, 103.

14. Matthews, *Public Laws*, 63–64. See also Cunningham, "Organization and Administration."

15. See Cunningham, "Confederate General Hospitals." Moore's hut design may have, in fact, been a remedy for hospital-acquired infections, the agents of which prospered in the rich environment of packed bodies, poor hygiene, and sluggish ventilation.

16. Chancellor, "Memoir." See also Nightingale, *Notes on Hospitals*, 56; and Cook, "Henry Curry." Yankee doctors subscribed as well, as was detailed in Smart, *Medical and Surgical History*, 899–966.

17. Hume, "Chimborazo Hospital."

18. See Gildersleeve, "History of Chimborazo Hospital." See also Blanton, *Medicine in Virginia in the Nineteenth Century*, 301–2.

19. Figures from Blanton, *Medicine in Virginia in the Nineteenth Century*, 302.

20. See W. A. Carrington, "Report of the Apportionment of the General Hospitals In and Around Richmond," February 13, 1864, Rare Books Collection, Library of Congress, Washington, DC; "From the North Carolina Soldiers," *Fayetteville Observer*, June 26, 1862, 3. See also Simkins and Patton, "The Work of Southern Women."

21. P. Y. Pember, "Reminiscences of a Southern Hospital," *The Cosmopolite* I (1866): 297–309, quote 297.

22. Pember, "Reminiscences," 307.

23. Bruce, *History of the University of Virginia 1819–1919*, Vol. 3, 314, 322.

24. "Charleston Wayside Hospital and Soldiers' Depot," *Charleston Mercury*, January 4, 1862, 2. Hopley, *Life in the South*, 93.

25. Bryce, *Reminiscences*. See also Waring, *History of Medicine*, 131–42.

26. Letter, N. H. Whitfield to John W. Ellis, July 1, 1861, Papers of John Willis Ellis, Vol. 2, 877–78, North Carolina Office of Archives and History, Raleigh, NC.

27. Whitfield to Ellis.

28. Whitfield to Ellis.

29. See *General Military Hospital*, 1.

30. See Norris, "'For the Benefit of Our Gallant Volunteers.'"

31. Hospital Committee, "An Appeal for the Sick and Wounded Soldiers," May 7, 1863, Documenting the American South. University Library, University of North Carolina at Chapel Hill, 2002.

32. See Cunningham, "Edmund Burke Haywood," 160.

33. Butler, *Autobiography*, 415–53.

34. Miles, "Memorial Address," *Trans South Surg Gynecol Assoc*. This address was identical to the one Miles published in the *New Orleans Medical and Surgical Journal* the following year (previously cited). See also "The Negroes in New-Orleans," *New York Times*, December 7, 1862, 2.

35. Denney, *Civil War Medicine*, 78–79.

36. Cumming, *Journal of Hospital Life*, 18.

37. Quote from Cumming, *Journal of Hospital Life*, 16.

38. Groom, *Vicksburg, 1863*, 390–91. See also Freemon, "Medical Care."

39. Denney, *Civil War Medicine*, 298.

40. Armes, *Autobiography*, 225–27.

41. Figures from Breeden, "Medical History."

42. The Savannah Medical College formed in 1853, bringing in Savannah's Poor House and Marine Hospital for clinical material. It never really thrived and closed during the Civil War.

43. Jones, "Original and Eclectic."

44. Figures from Breeden, *Joseph Jones*, 104 and 107.

45. Blanton, *Medicine in Virginia in the Nineteenth Century*, 296. The Confederate Army of the Potomac, almost fifty thousand strong, reported over thirty-six thousand cases of diarrhea and dysentery between July 1861 and March 1862.

46. Quoted in Breeden, *Joseph Jones*, 123.

47. Jones, *Medical and Surgical Memoirs*, 271.

48. See Watson, "Biographical Sketch," 594.

49. Information and quotes from Jones, "Investigations upon the Nature," 152, 167–68, 284.

50. Keen, "Military Surgery."

51. J. Jones, "Diseases Dependent upon the Action of Specific Poisons and Supposed to Arise from Crowding and Foul Exhalations," in Flint, *Contributions*, 600–618, quote 600.

52. J. Jones, "General Conclusions Drawn from the Preceding Investigations upon the Diseases of the Federal Prisoners Confined at Andersonville," in Flint, *Contributions*, 642–55, quote 643. See also Humphreys, "Stranger to Our Camps."

53. S. P. Moore, Confederate States of America, War Department, Surgeon-General's Office, Richmond, VA, July 15,1863; Watson, "Biographical Sketch."

54. See Helling and McNabney, "Role of Amputation." Civil War historians Laurann Figg and Jane Ferrell-Beck calculated that sixty thousand amputations were done during the war, which is very likely an underestimate as many Confederate records were lost. Figg and Farrell-Beck, "Amputations in the Civil War."

55. See Gross, *Manual of Military Surgery*. This was apparently a pirated edition of Gross's *Manual*, first published in Philadelphia (J. B. Lippincott, 1861). Gross composed his manual in just nine days and published it within fourteen days. See Patina and Moran, "Civil War Manuals."

56. Chisolm, *Manual of Military Surgery* (1861), 16–61, quote 47.

57. Chisolm, *Manual of Military Surgery* (1864), 1–2. This is the second edition of Chisolm's expansive work on military surgery.

58. Chisolm, *A Manual of Military Surgery* (1861), quotes 276, 301–2. "Damage control" was not a term used during the Civil War, but in general terms, this was surgery that could be done at once to control life-threatening bleeding or to prevent later infections, including so-called hospital gangrene. This usually referred to early amputation for mangled limbs hopelessly destroyed beyond repair. Chisolm's manual contained accepted therapeutics, much of which were gathered from the Crimean War of 1853–1856 and could be found in various texts, like Macleod, *Notes on the Surgery of War*.

59. See "Julian John Chisolm," in Waring, *History of Medicine*, 212–14. His name is actually John Julian Chisolm, not Julian John. See also *In Honor of Julian John Chisolm, M.D., Published on the One Hundredth Anniversary of His Birth, 1930*, by members of his family (Archives, University of Maryland at Baltimore).

60. Nash, "Some Reminiscences."

61. Ainsworth and Kirkley, *War of the Rebellion*, 1041.

62. Porcher, *Resources*, iii. This manuscript was apparently written at the suggestion of Surgeon-General Samuel Moore. See also Townsend, "Francis Peyre Porcher."

63. "Indigenous Remedies."

64. Hasegawa and Hambrecht, "Confederate Medical Laboratories."

65. Davis, *Rise and Fall*, 310.

66. W. H. Prioleau, "To the Ladies of Georgia," Medical Purveyor's Office, Savannah, Geogria. March 31, 1863. The *Charleston Mercury* also advertised for the "Garden Poppy" and gave careful instruction for its cultivation and harvest of the gum opium. See Thomas Lining, "Cultivation of the Garden Poppy," *Charleston Mercury*, April 20, 1863, 4–5.

67. Daniel, *Recollections*, 208.

68. "Salutatory," 13.

69. See a detailed review of the history of the Journal in Sharpe, "Confederate States Medical and Surgical Journal."

70. The Association of Army and Navy Surgeons continued on after the war. "For the advancement of science—to rescue from oblivion all the important medical and surgical facts developed within the armies of the Confederate States during the late war," read advertisements for the meeting of 1874 in Atlanta. Sometime in the 1880s the association disbanded (Circular, S. P. Moore, "Convention of Confederate Surgeons, 1874," Georgia Historical Society).

71. "Medicine in the Confederate States."

72. Breeden, *Joseph Jones*, 217. The balance presumably surrendered or could not be found at war's end.

73. See Faust, "Rhetoric and Ritual."

74. Andrews, *War-Time Journal*, 198.

75. Edmondson quote taken from Levine, *Fall of the House of Dixie*, 289.

76. Kean, *Inside the Confederate Government*, 208.

77. Jones, "Medical History," 119.

78. Stowe, *Doctoring the South*, 261.

79. Kean, *Inside the Confederate Government*, 210.

80. Figures from Somers, *Southern States*, 52.

81. Downs, *Sick from Freedom*, 41.

82. In fact, for many enslaved people, nothing had changed. Many were kept in chains long after the South capitulated, their enslavers deceiving them by hiding the fact that the war had emancipated them.

83. Eaton, *Grant, Lincoln*, 2.

84. See Legan, "Disease and the Freedmen."

85. Taken from Franklin, "Public Welfare." See also Taylor, *The Negro in South Carolina*, 19–39.

86. Pike, *Prostrate State*, 77–78.

CHAPTER ELEVEN: AN ABOMINATION OF HEALTH: RECONSTRUCTION OF THE SOUTH

1. Henry Ward Beecher, "Centennial Review," in *Patriotic Addresses* (New York: Fords, Howard, and Hulbert, 1887), 779.

2. Fleming, *Documentary History*, 11–12.

3. Du Bois, "Reconstruction and Its Benefits."

4. Fleming, *Documentary History*, 20.

5. Fleming, *Documentary History*, 43–44.

6. *Carpetbagger* was a derogatory term used by southerners for any person from the northern states who appeared to exploit their local communities for profit or political gain. Of course, there were many from the North whose intentions were admirable and who, in fact, sought a true resurrection of southern society.

7. Buck, *Road to Reunion*, 12. See also Moore, "One Hundred Years of Reconstruction," 153–80, particularly 154.

8. Buck, *Road to Reunion*, 25.

9. Bierce, *Phantoms*, 293.

10. Lee, "The South since the War," 315.

11. Temin, "Patterns of Cotton Agriculture."

12. Stetar, "In Search of a Direction," 344.

13. See Dunning, *Reconstruction*, 85–123. There were four major programs instituted by the bureau: rations distribution, health care, education, and judicial. See Colby, "Freedmen's Bureau," from which expenditure figures were taken.

14. From Waring, *History of Medicine*, 144.

15. Bullock, *History of Emory University*, 149–50.

16. See Calhoun, "Founding and the Early History."

17. Editorial, *Atlanta Med Surg J* 7 (1866): 85–86. The Medical College would eventually morph into the Emory University School of Medicine.

18. Editorial, *Atlanta Med Surg J* 7 (1866): 43–45.

19. Stout, "An Address."

20. Spalding, *History of the Medical College*, 79–80.

21. "Southern Medical and Surgical Journal."

22. See "Catalogue of the University of Virginia."

23. Taken from Trowbridge, *The South*, 546.

24. "Memorial, of the Dean and Faculty of the Medical College of the State of South Carolina," January 6, 1869, courtesy of the Medical Library, School of Medicine, University of South Carolina, Columbia, SC. Also referenced, Lange and McGowan, "Brief History."

25. Lange and McGowan, "Brief History," 634.

26. Hunter, "Late to the Dance," including quote taken from Tunnell, *Crucible of Reconstruction*, 19.

27. See Duffy, "Sectional Conflict."

28. Brickell, "Biographical Sketch."

29. See Downs, *Sick from Freedom*, 66–94.

30. See Waring, *History of Medicine*, 161–72, quote 169.

31. Somers, *Southern States*, 54.

32. Walton, "Comparative Mortality."

33. See Foster, "Limitations."

34. Foster, "Limitations."

35. Howard, *Autobiography*, 390. Stanton was an abolitionist and supporter of vigorous reconstruction. He rankled at Andrew Johnson's mealy treatment of the rebellious southern states.

36. Dyson, *Founding of Howard University*, 7–16.

37. Dr. Augusta (1825–1890) received his medical training in Toronto, having been denied admission to the University of Pennsylvania. In 1863 he wrote President Lincoln about an appointment as a surgeon for one of the Black regiments and received a commission as a surgeon at Camp Barker in Washington, DC, as the Union Army's first Black physician. It was likely there that he met Howard, who appointed him to the faculty of his new school. See Butts, "Alexander Thomas Augusta."

38. Cobb, "Progress and Portents," 119.

39. Bousfield, "Account of Physicians of Color."

40. Figures from Pierce, *Freedmen's Bureau*, 91. See also Howard, *Autobiography*, particularly 445–55.

41. Summerville, *Educating Black Doctors*, 12.

42. Morais, *History of the Negro in Medicine*, 44.

43. Central Tennessee College was partially financed by the Freedmen's Bureau but struggled to find proper housing as white Nashville residents blocked the sale of land in their locale.

44. See Gordon, "William J. Sneed." See also Poinsett, "Meharry Medical College." Samuel Meharry's rich endowment was a debt of gratitude for freed Africans. As a teenager, freedmen had rescued him when his loaded salt wagon, stuck in mud, teetered on ruin. They gave him food and shelter and helped retrieve his embedded cargo. For that, he had promised someday to pay them back. Meharry, now prosperous beyond his wildest imagination, made good his promise. See also Riley, "History of America's Premier Independent Black Medical School." The Methodist Freedman's Aid Society and the John E. Slater Fund contributed heavily to the success of the school.

45. Summerville, *Black Doctors*, 18. See Cobb, "Progress and Portents."

46. Figures from Cobb, "Progress and Portents," 119.

47. See Hume, "Carpetbaggers."

CHAPTER TWELVE: SURGERY AS SOUTHERN MEDICAL REDEMPTION

1. Warner, *Therapeutic Perspective*, 83–102. See also Sullivan, "Sanguine Practices," 211–12.

2. Conkin, "The South in Southern Agrarianism." See Warner, "Southern Medical Reform," 367.

3. Cartwright, "Cartwright on Southern Medicine."

4. "Southern Medical Schools—Southern Toadyism." The *Blister and Critic* was purported to be a monthly journal "devoted to the development of Southern medical literature and the exposition of the diseases and physical peculiarities of the negro race."

5. See Blanton, *Medicine in Virginia in the Eighteenth Century*, 11.

6. Tilton, *Economic Observations*, 19.

7. Cartwright, "Cartwright on Southern Medicine," 263.

8. Bailey, "Surgical Cases."

9. Cartwright, "Some Account."

10. Gross, "Century of American Medicine."

11. Fourcroy, *Rapport et Projet*, 11–12.

12. Gelfand, *Professionalizing Modern Medicine*. It should be noted that eighteenth-century English physicians and surgeons historically had distinctive roles, one being university educated, intellectually grounded, and officially sanctioned to practice physic and the other an offshoot of the company of barbers, considered more of a tradesman than true natural philosopher. Surgery was hardly considered a branch of medicine at that time.

13. Shryock, "Interplay of Social and Internal Factors."

14. Jones, *Plain Concise Practical Remarks*, v.

15. McDowell, "Three Cases."

16. See Sims, "On the Treatment." See also Sims, *Story of My Life*, 236–46, quote 209. See also Wall, "Medical Ethics." For an in-depth and relatively contemporary discussion of bladder fistulas see Pozzi, *Treatise*, 297–347.

17. In fact, Eve was captured in the process. He finally was released through the efforts of a family friend, one Marie-Joseph Paul Yves Roch Gilbert du Motier, better known as the Marquis de Lafayette.

18. Eve, "Address to the Class."

19. See Haller, "The Negro and the Southern Physician."

20. Eve, "Case of Excision."

21. Eve, *Collection of Remarkable Cases*, particularly 218–19, quote vi. See also Miller, Thweatt, and Geevarghese, "Surgeon's Duty to Serve."

22. Eve proved to be a much better technician than administrator. His efforts at the Gate City Hospital fell far short of acceptable. Samuel Stout, director of the Army of Tennessee's hospitals, observed on touring the place in 1863 that it had turned into a "veritable Augean stable . . . [he] had often to tiptoe to keep from stepping on filth, sputa, excrement, & urine." Eve was eventually transferred to a smaller hospital in Augusta. (Davis, "Another Look," 15).

23. Battey, "Conditions of Success." He called his operations "ovariotomy," but in reality, he completely removed the ovary, a procedure more properly called "oophorectomy." See Battey, "Normal Ovariotomy."

24. Battey, "Castration in Nervous Diseases," 484.

25. See Van de Warker, "The Fetich."

26. Eve, "A Sketch of the Life and Labors"; Longo, "Rise and Fall."

27. McMurtry, "Plea for Progressive Surgery."

28. Longo, "Rise and Fall," 266.

29. For the impact of military medicine on therapeutic progress in the North, see Devine, *Learning from the Wounded*. For a description of surgical practices up to the Civil War, see Hall, "Rise of Professional Surgery."

30. Long, "Wisdom of the Past."

31. Cash, *Mind of the South*, particularly 148–89, quote 183. See also Woodman, "Sequel to Slavery."

32. McGuire, "Annual Address."

33. Stout, "An Address."

34. "What Science Has to Settle."

35. Matas, "The Surgical Peculiarities," 125–26. See also Legan, "Disease and the Freedmen," 257–67. See also Pohl, "African American Southerners."

36. Figures from Bonner, *American Doctors and German Universities*, 23. As it evolved, however, the American system differed in important ways from the German. More egalitarian than the rigid hierarchical German institutions, American universities, while more structured than antebellum years, were more flexible and open to curricular innovation. See also Bonner, "German Model" and Carroll, "Creating the Modern Physician."

37. Shrady, "Specialism as a Practice."

38. As quoted by Graham, "Samuel Gross Looks In."

39. "Fellows of the American Surgical Association."

40. Davis, "Annual Address."

41. Davis, "Annual Address." See also Bland, "Founding Fathers vs Jerome Cochran."

42. McGuire, "Annual Address," 1–12.

43. Brown, "The Southern Surgical and Gynecological Association."

44. Brown, "The Southern Surgical and Gynecological Association," 11, 21.

45. Davis, "Annual Address," 11.

46. Douglas, "In Memoriam," 466 and 470. Richard "Dixie" Douglas was a colorful character in his own right. A renowned southern gynecological and abdominal surgeon at Vanderbilt University, Douglas was named "Dixie" by his father, as he was born on the day South Carolina seceded from the Union. Among his clinical accomplishments, though, "Dixie" Douglas helped engineer the merger of the University of Nashville with Vanderbilt University.

47. Brown, "The Southern Surgical and Gynecological Association."

CHAPTER THIRTEEN: A NEW SOUTH OR STILL THE OLD SOUTH?

1. Quote taken from Ward, *Out in the Rural*, 14.
2. See McMillen, *Dark Journey*, 169.
3. See Ben-David, "Scientific Productivity."
4. Warner, "Science in Medicine."
5. Wyatt-Brown, *Shaping of Southern Culture*, 55.
6. Tigertt, "Osler on Malaria."
7. Bruce-Chwatt, "Transmission of Malaria."
8. Doty, "Scientific Prevention," 684.
9. Reed, Carroll, and Agramonte, "The Etiology of Yellow Fever."
10. See Bryan, "Discovery of the Yellow Fever Virus." See also Norrby, "Yellow Fever and Max Theiler."
11. Hotez, "Neglected Infections," 237–38.
12. Flexner, *Medical Education*, 154.
13. Flexner, *Medical Education*, 301.
14. Flexner, *Medical Education*, 206.
15. Flexner, *Medical Education*, 148.
16. Spalding, *History of the Medical College*, 118–29.
17. All quotes here from Flexner, *Medical Education*, 180.
18. Polavarapu et al., "100 Years of Surgical Education."
19. Ward, *Black Physicians*, 72.
20. Quoted from Reitzes, *Negroes and Medicine*, 321 in Ward, *Black Physicians*, 81.
21. Fisher, *Report on National Vitality*.
22. Fisher, *Report on National Vitality*, 22.
23. Fisher, *Report on National Vitality*, 124.
24. Stevens, *American Medicine and the Public Interest*, 44.
25. Burton, "The South as 'Other,'" 50.
26. Cotterill, "The Old South to the New."

BIBLIOGRAPHY

Abrahams, H. J. "Secession from Northern Medical Schools." *Trans Stud Coll Physicians Phila* 36 (1968): 29–45.

Ackerknecht, E. H. "Primitive Surgery." *Am Anthrop* 49 (1947): 25–45.

Acts and Resolutions of the General Assembly of the State of South Carolina. Columbia, SC: D. and J. M. Faust, 1824.

Adair, James. *The History of the American Indians.* London: Edward and Charles Dilly, 1776.

Ainsworth, Fred C., and Joseph W. Kirkley, eds. *The War of the Rebellion: A Compilation of the Official Records of the Union and Confederate Armies.* Vol. 1. Washington, DC: Government Printing Office, 1900.

Altschuler, E. L., and A. Jobanputra. "What Was the Cause of the Epidemic in Savannah in 1733?" *J R Soc Med* 107 (2014): 468–73.

Anderson, D. "Telling Stories, Making Selves: Nostalgia, the Lost Cause, and Postbellum Plantation Memoirs and Reminiscences." In *Civil War and Narrative: Testimony, Historiography, Memory,* edited by Karine Deslandes, Fabrice Mourlon, and Bruno Tribout, 21–38. Cham: Palgrave, 2017.

Anderson, Fred. *Crucible of War.* New York: Vintage Books, 2001.

Andrews, Charles M. *The Colonial Period of American History: The Settlements.* Vol. 3. New Haven, CT: Yale University Press, 1937.

Andrews, D. M. "De Soto's Route from Cofitachequi in Georgia to Cosa, in Alabama." *Am Anthrop* 19 (1917): 55–67.

Andrews, Eliza Frances. *The War-Time Journal of a Georgia Girl 1864–1865.* New York: D. Appleton, 1908.

Angelakis, E., Y. Bechah, and D. Raoult. "The History of Epidemic Typhus." *Microbiol Spectr* 4 (2016): 1–9.

Antony, M. "Case of Extensive Caries of the Fifth and Sixth Ribs, and Disorganization of the Greater Part of the Right Lobe of Lungs, with a Description of the Operation for the Same." *Phil J Med Phys Sci* 6 (1823): 108–17.

Arbuthnot, John. *An Essay Concerning the Effects of Air on Human Bodies.* London: J. Tonson, 1733.

Archer, Margaret S. *Culture and Agency: The Place of Culture in Social Theory.* New York: Cambridge University Press, 1996.

Arikha, Noga. *Passions and Tempers.* New York: HarperCollins, 2007.

Armes, William Dallam, ed. *The Autobiography of Joseph Le Conte.* New York: D. Appleton, 1903.

Armitage, D. "John Locke, Carolina, and the Two Treatises of Government." *Pol Theory* 32 (2004): 602–27.
Atkinson, E. "The Negro a Beast." *North American Review* 181 (1905): 202–15.
Atkinson, William, Jennifer Hamborsky, Lynne McIntyre, and Charles Wolfe, eds. *Epidemiology and Prevention of Vaccine-Preventable Diseases*. Washington, DC: Public Health Foundation, 2005.
Avellaneda, I. "Hernando de Soto and His Florida Fantasy." In *The Hernando de Soto Expedition: History, Historiography, and "Discovery" in the Southeast*, edited by Patricia Kay Galloway, 207–18. Lincoln: University of Nebraska Press, 2006.
Bailey, T. P. "Surgical Cases." *Charleston Med J & Review* 14 (1859): 740–45.
Bancroft, Edward Nathaniel. *Essay on the Disease Called Yellow Fever*. Baltimore: Cushing and Jewett, 1821.
Bankole, K. "The Human/Subhuman Issue and Slave Medicine in Louisiana." *Race, Gender, Class* 5 (1998): 3–11.
Bankole-Medina, Katherine. *Slavery and Medicine*. Washington, DC: Liberated Scholars Press, 2017.
Barlow, W., and D. O. Powell. "A Dedicated Medical Student: Solomon Mordecai, 1819–1822." *J Earlyl Rep* 7 (1987): 377–97.
Bartlett, Elisha. *Discourse on the Times, Character, and Writings of Hippocrates*. New York: H. Bailliere, 1852.
Barton, Benjamin Smith. *Collections for an Essaay Towards a Materia Medica of the United States*. Philadelphia: Edward Earle, 1810.
Barton, Edward H. *Introductory Lecture: Climate and Salubrity*. New Orleans: E. Johns, 1835.
Bartram, John, and Francis Harper. "Diary of a Journey through the Carolinas, Georgia, and Florida from July 1, 1756 to April 10, 1766." *Transactions of the American Philosophical Society* 33 (1942): 1–120.
Basanier, M. *L'Historie Notable de la Floride Située en Indes Occidentales Contenant*. Paris: Guilliaume Avuray, 1586.
Battey, R. "Castration in Nervous Diseases." *Am J Med Sci* 92 (1886): 483–90.
Battey, R. "Conditions of Success in Ovariotomy." *Atlanta Med Surg J* 2 (1885): 1–7.
Battey, R. "Normal Ovariotomy—Case." *Atlanta Med Surg J* 10 (1872): 321–39.
Becker, A. M. "Smallpox in Washington's Army: Strategic Implications of the Disease during the American Revolutionary War." *J Mil Hist* 68 (2004): 381–430.
Bell, K. B. "Rice, Resistance, and Forced Transatlantic Communities: (Re)envisioning the African Diaspora in Low Country Georgia, 1750–1800." *J African Am Hist* 95 (2010): 157–82.
Bell, W. J. "Medical Practice in Colonial America." *Bull Hist Med* 31 (1957): 442–53.
Ben-David, J. "Scientific Productivity and Academic Organization in Nineteenth Century Medicine." *Am Soc Rev* 25 (1960): 828–43.
Berkeley, Edmund, and Dorothy Smith Berkeley. *The Reverend John Clayton: A Parson with a Scientific Mind*. Charlottesville: University Press of Virginia, 1965.
Best, George. *A True Discourse of the Late Voyage of Discouverie, for the Finding of a Passage to Cathaya*. London: Henry Bynnyman, 1578.
Beverley, Robert. *The History and Present State of Virginia*. London: R. Parker, 1705.
Bierce, Ambrose. *Phantoms of a Blood-Stained Period*. Edited by Russell Duncan and David J. Klosser. Amherst: University of Massachusetts Press, 2002.

Bigelow, Jacob. *American Medical Botany*. Boston: Cummings and Hilliard, 1820.
Bigelow, John, ed. *The Complete Works of Benjamin Franklin Vol. 1 1706–1744*. New York: G. P. Putnam's Sons, 1887.
Blake, J. B. "Yellow Fever in Eighteenth Century America." *Bull NY Acad Med* 44 (1968): 673–86.
Bland, K. I. "The Founding Fathers vs Jerome Cochran: Organization and Development of the Southern Surgical and Gynecological Association in Birmingham." *J Am Coll Surg* 226 (2018): 696–713.
Blanton, W. B. "Augustus Lockman Warner, 1807–1847." *Ann Med Hist* 4 (1942): 1–9.
Blanton, W. B. "Epidemics, Real and Imaginary, and Other Factors Influencing Seventeenth Century Virginia's Population." *Bull Hist Med* 31 (1957): 454–62.
Blanton, Wyndham B. *Medicine in Virginia in the Eighteenth Century*. Richmond: Garrett and Massie, 1931.
Blanton, Wyndham B. *Medicine in Virginia in the Nineteenth Century*. Richmond: Garrett and Massie, 1933.
Boerhaave, Hermann. *Institutiones Medicae, Pars I*. Madrid: Villalpandea, 1796.
Bonner, T. N. "The German Model of Training Physicians in the United States, 1870–1914: How Closely Was It Followed?" *Bull Hist Med* 64 (1990): 18–34.
Bonner, Thomas N. *American Doctors and German Universities*. Lincoln: University of Nebraska Press, 1963.
Boorstin, Daniel J. *The Americans: The Colonial Experience*. Bombay: Allied Publishers, 1958.
Bousfield, M. O. "An Account of Physicians of Color in the United States." *Bull Hist Med* 17 (1945): 61–84.
Bowers, Claude G. *The Tragic Era: The Revolution after Lincoln*. Cambridge, MA: Houghton Mifflin, 1929.
Breeden, James O. *Joseph Jones, M.D.* Lexington: University of Kentucky Press, 2014.
Breeden, J. O. "A Medical History of the Later Stages of the Atlanta Campaign." *J South Hist* 35 (1969): 31–59.
Brickell, D. W. "Biographical Sketch of Erasmus Darwin Fenner, M.D." *South J Med Sci* 1 (1866): 401–23.
Brickell, D. W. "Epidemic Typhoid Pneumonia amongst Negroes." *NO Med News Hosp Gaz* 2 (1856): 531–48.
Brickell, John. *The Natural History of North-Carolina*. Dublin: James Carson, 1737.
Bridgforth, L. R. "Medicine in Antebellum Mississippi." *J Miss State Med Assoc* 38 (1997): 367–77.
Brown, B. "The Southern Surgical and Gynecological Association—Its Origin, Objects, and Aims." *Trans Surg Gynecol Assoc* 6 (1893): 1–21.
Brown, Harvey E. *The Medical Department of the United States Army from 1775–1873*. Washington, DC: Surgeon General's Office, 1873.
Browning, Judkin, and Timothy Silver. *An Environmental History of the Civil War*. Chapel Hill: University of North Carolina Press, 2020.
Bruce, Philip Alexander. *History of the University of Virginia, 1819–1919*. Vol. 2. New York: Macmillan, 1920.
Bruce, Philip Alexancer. *History of the University of Virginia, 1819–1919*. Vol. 3. New York: Macmillan, 1921.
Bruce-Chwatt, L. J. "Transmission of Malaria: 75th Anniversary of Ronald Ross's Great Discovery." *Br Med J* 3 (1972): 464–66.

Brunhouse, Robert L., and David Ramsay. "David Ramsay, 1749–1815, Selections from His Writing." *Trans Am Phil Soc* 55 (1965): 58–59.
Bryan, C. S. "Discovery of the Yellow Fever Virus." *Int J Inf Dis* 2 (1997): 52–54.
Bryce, Campbell. *Reiminiscences of the Hospitals of Columbia, S.C.* Philadelphia: J. B. Lippincott Company, 1897.
Buck, Paul H. *The Road to Reunion 1865–1900*. Boston: Little, Brown, 1937.
Bullock, Henry M. *A History of Emory University*. Nashville: Parthenon Press, 1936.
Burton, H. S., and F. T. Smith. "Slavery in the Colonial Louisiana Backcountry: Natchitoches, 1714–1803." *Louisiana Hist* 52 (2011): 133–88.
Burton, O. V. "The South as 'Other,' the South as 'Stranger.'" *J South Hist* 79 (2013): 7–50.
Butler, Benjamin F. *Autobiography and Personal Reminiscences of Major-General Benj. F. Butler: Butler's Book: A Review of His Legal, Political, and Military Career*. Boston: A. M. Thayer, 1892.
Butterfield, L. H., ed. *Letters of Benjamin Rush, Vol. 1, 1761–1792*. Princeton, NJ: Princeton University Press, 1951.
Butts, H. M. "Alexander Thomas Augusta—Physician, Teacher and Human Rights Activist." *J Natl Med Assoc* 97 (2005): 106–9.
Byrd, M. D. "The First Charles Town Workhouse, 1738–1775: A Deterrent to White Pauperism?" *SC Hist Mag* 110 (2009): 35–52.
Byrd, Michael, and Linda A. Clayton. *An American Health Dilemma*. New York: Routledge, 2000.
Byrd, William. *Histories of the Dividing Line Betwixt Virginia and North Carolina, with Introduction and Notes*. Raleigh: North Carolina Historical Commission, 1929.
Cabanis, Pierre Jean Georges. *Du Degre de Certitude de la Médecine*. Paris: Firmin Didot, 1798.
Cabell, Nathaniel, ed. *Early History of the University of Virginia as Contained in the Letters of Thomas Jefferson and Joseph Cabell*. Richmond: J. W. Randolph, 1856.
Calhoun, F. P. "The Founding and the Early History of the Atlanta Medical College, 1854–1885." *Georgia Hist Q* 9 (1925): 34–54.
Carmer, Carl. *Stars Fell on Alabama*. New York: Farrar and Rinehart, 1934.
Carpenter, Jesse T. *The South as a Conscious Minority, 1789–1861*. New York: New York University Press, 1930.
Carroll, Charles. *The Negro a Beast, or In the Image of God*. Saint Louis, MO: American Book and Bible House, 1900.
Carroll, K. L. "Creating the Modern Physician." *J Soc Arch Hist* 75 (2016): 48–73.
Cartwright, S. A. "The Diseases and Physical Peculiarities of the Negro Race." *South Med Rep* 2 (1859): 421–29.
Cartwright, S. A. "The Diseases of Negroes—Pulmonary Congestions, Pneumonia, &c." *De Bow's Rev* 11 (1851): 209–13.
Cartwright, S. A. "Cartwright on Southern Medicine." *NO Med Surg J* 3 (1846/1847): 259–72.
Cartwright, S. A. "Remarks on Dysentery among Negroes." *NO Med Surg J* 11 (1854): 145–63.
Cartwright, S. A. "Report on the Diseases and Physical Peculiarities of the Negro Race." *NO Med Surg J* 7 (1851): 691–715.
Cartwright, S. A. "Some Account of a New Method of Reducing Dislocations, Applicable both to Recent and Ancient Times." *New Orleans Med Surg J* 1 (1844): 43–56.
Cash, W. J. *The Mind of the South*. New York: Vintage Books, 1941.
"Catalogue of the University of Virginia, 1865–66." *South Med Surg J* 21 (1866): 354–56.

Celsus. *De Medicina*. Translated by W. G. Spencer. Cambridge, MA: Harvard University Press, 1971.

Centennial Memorial of the Medical College of the State of South Carolina 1824-1924. Charleston: Medical College of South Carolina, 1924.

Chalmers, Lionel. *An Account of the Weather and Diseases of South-Carolina*. Vol. 1. London: Edward and Charles Dilly, 1776.

Chancellor, C. W. "A Memoir of the Late Samuel Preston Moore, M.D., Surgeon General of the Confederate States Army." *South Pract* 25 (1903): 634-39.

Chapman, N. "American Medicine." *Phila J Med Phys Sci* 9 (1824): 404-9.

Chevalier, M. E. *Voyage d'Iberville: Journal du Voyage Fait Par Deux Fregates du Roi, La Badine, Commandee par M. d'Iberville, et Le Marin*. Montreal: E. Senegal, 1871.

Chisolm, J. Julian. *A Manual of Military Surgery*. Richmond: West and Johnston, 1861.

Chisolm, J. Julian. *A Manual of Military Surgery*. Columbia, SC: Evans and Cogswell, 1864.

Claiborne, J. F. H. *Mississippi as a Province, Territory and State*. Vol. 1. Jackson: Power and Barksdale, 1880.

Cobb, James C. *The Most Southern Place on Earth: The Mississippi Delta and the Roots of Regional Identity*. New York: Oxford University Press, 1992.

Cobb, W. M. "Progress and Portents for the Negro in Medicine." *The Crisis* 55 (1948): 107-22.

Colby, I. C. "The Freedmen's Bureau: From Social Welfare to Segregation." *Phylon* 46 (1985): 219-30.

Coleman, Kenneth, and Charles Stephen Gurr. *Dictionary of Georgia Biography*. Vol. 1. Athens: University of Georgia Press, 1983.

Collections of the South Carolina Historical Society. Vol. 5. Charleston: South Carolina Historical Society, 1897.

The Colonial Records of Georgia, 1735-1737, Vol. 21. Atlanta: Chas. P. Byrd, 1910.

The Colonial Records of the State of Georgia, 1737-1740, Vol. 22. Atlanta: Chas. P. Byrd, 1913.

Conkin, P. K. "The South in Southern Agrarianism." In *The Evolution of Southern Culture*, edited by Numan V. Bartley, 131-45. Athens: University of Georgia Press, 1988.

Cook, G. C. "Henry Curry FRIBA (1820-1900): Leading Victorian Hospital Architect, and Early Exponent of the 'Pavilion Principle.'" *Postgrad Med* (2002) 352-50.

Cook, H. J. "Boerhaave and the Flight from Reason in Medicine." *Bull Hist Med* 74 (2000): 221-40.

Coombs, J. C. "'Others Not Christians in the Service of the English': Interpreting the Status of Africans and African Americans in Early Virginia." *Virg Mag Hist Bio* 127 (2019): 212-38.

Cooper, J. W. *The Experienced Botanist or Indian Physician*. Ebensburg, PA: Canan and Scott, 1833.

Corner, G. W. "Apprenticed to Aesculapius: The American Medical Student, 1765-1965." *Proc Am Phil Soc* 109 (1965): 249-58.

Cotterill, R. S. "The Old South to the New." *J South Hist* 15 (1949): 3-8.

Cowan, D. L. "The Impact of the Materia Medica of the North American Indians on Professional Practice." *Veroff Int Ges Gesch Pharm* 53 (1984): 51-63.

Creighton, Charles. *A History of Epidemics in Britain*. Cambridge: Cambridge University Press, 1894.

Crockett, David. *Col Crockett's Exploits and Adventures in Texas*. Philadelphia: T. K. and P. G. Collins, 1836.

Crosby, Molly Caldwell. *American Plague*. New York: Berkley Books, 2006.
Cullen, William. *First Lines of the Practice of Physic*. Vol. 1. Philadelphia: T. Dobson, 1816.
Cumming, Kate. *A Journal of Hospital Life in the Confederate Army of Tennessee*. Louisville, KY: John P. Morton, 1869.
Cunha, C. B. "Prolonged and Perplexing Fevers in Antiquity: Malaria and Typhoid Fever." *Infect Dis Clin N Am* 21 (2007): 857–66.
Cunningham, H. H. "Confederate General Hospitals: Establishment and Organization." *J South Hist* 20 (1954): 376–94.
Cunningham, H. H. "Edmund Burke Haywood and Raleigh's Confederate Hospitals." *NC Hist Rev* 35 (1958): 153–66.
Cunningham, H. H. "Organization and Administration of the Confederate Medical Department." *NC Hist Rev* 31 (1954): 385–409.
Currie, William. *An Historical Account of the Climates and Diseases of the United States of America*. Philadelphia: T. Dobson, 1792.
Curtin, P. D. "Epidemiology and the Slave Trade." *Pol Sci Q* 83 (1968): 190–216.
Cushing, Harvey. *The Life of Sir William Osler*. London: Clarendon Press, 1925.
Da Costa, J. C. "The French School of Surgery during the Reign of Louis Philippe." *Ann Med Hist* 4 (1922): 77–79.
Dabney, Virginius. *Richmond: The Story of a City*. New York: Doubleday, 1976.
Daniel, F. E. *Recollections of a Rebel Surgeon*. Austin, TX: Von Boekmann, Schutze, 1899.
Davenport, H. G. "Observations on Typhoid Fever." *NO Med Surg J* 8 (1851–52): 580–90.
Davidson, Chalmers G. *Friend of the People: The Life of Dr. Peter Fayssoux*. Columbia: Medical Association of South Carolina, 1950.
Davis, Jefferson. *The Rise and Fall of the Confederate Government*. Vol. 1. New York: D. Appleton, 1912.
Davis, Robert C. *Christian Slaves, Muslim Masters*. New York: Palgrave, 2003.
Davis, Steve. "Another Look at Civil War Medical Care: Atlanta's Confederate Hospitals." *Journal of the Medical Association of Georgia* 88 (1999): 9–23.
Davis, W. E. B. "Annual Address of the President." *Trans South Surg Gynecol Assoc* 15 (1902): 1–20.
Day, Samuel Phillips. *Down South, Or, An Englishman's Experience at the Seat of the American War*. Vol. 2. Bedford, MA: Applewood Books, 1862.
De Bow, J. D. B. "The Future of the South." *De Bow's Review* 1 (1866): 6–16.
de Chastellux, Marquis. *Travels in North-America in the Years 1780–81–82*. New York, 1828.
de La Harpe, Bénard. *Journal Historique de l'Établissement des Française a la Louisiane*. Paris: A.-L. Boimare, 1831.
de la Harpe, B. "Memoir on the Importance of Colonizing Louisiana." In *Historical Collections of Louisiana, Part III*, edited by B. F. French, 112–13. New York: D. Appleton, 1851.
de la Motta, Jacob. *An Oration on the Causes of the Mortality among Strangers during the Late Summer and Fall*. Savannah, GA: Kappel and Bartlet, 1820.
Delony, E. "A Letter to the Editors." *South Med Surg J* 1 (1836): 257–61.
de Montigny, Jean-François-Benjamin Dumont. *Mémoires Historiques sur la Louisiane*. Vol. 1. Paris: Claude Jean Baptiste Bauche, 1753.
de Montigny, Jean François-Benjamin Dumont. *Mémoires Historiques sur la Louisiane*. Vol. 2. Paris: Claude Jean Baptiste Bauche, 1753.

Denney, Robert E. *Civil War Medicine: Care and Comfort of the Wounded.* New York: Sterling, 1995.
de Roulhac Hamilton, J. G., ed. *The Papers of Thomas Ruffin.* Vol. 2. Raleigh, NC: Edwards and Broughton, 1918.
de Tocqueville, Alexis. *Democracy in America.* Vol. 1. Translated by Henry Reeve. New York: George Adlard, 1838.
de Villiers, Marc. *Histoire de la Fondation de la Nouvelle-Orléans.* Paris: Imprimerie Nationale, 1916.
Devine, Shauna. *Learning from the Wounded: The Civil War and the Rise of American Medical Science.* Chapel Hill: University of North Carolina Press, 2014.
Devine, S. "'To Make Something Out of the Dying in This War': The Civil War and the Rise of American Medical Science." *J Civil War Era* 6 (2016): 149–63.
Dewhurst, K. "Sydenham on 'A Dysentery.'" *Bull Hist Med* 29 (1955): 393–400.
Dexter, Franklin Bowditch. *Estimates of Population in the American Colonies.* Worcester, MA: Charles Hamilton, 1887.
Diary of Viscount Percival, First Earl of Egmont, Vol. 1 1730–1733. London: His Majesty's Stationery Office, 1920.
Dickson, Samuel Henry. *Introductory Lecture, Delivered at the Commencement of the Second Session of the Medical College of South-Carolina.* Charleston, SC: W. Riley, 1826.
Dixon, R. B. "Some Aspects of the American Shaman." *J Am Folklore* 21 (1908): 1–12.
Dock, G. "The 'Primitive Physic' of Rev. John Wesley." *JAMA* 64 (1915): 629–38.
Donnan, Elizabeth. *Documents Illustrative of the History of the Slave Trade.* Vol. 4. Washington, DC: Carnegie Institute, 1935.
Doty, A. H. "The Scientific Prevention of Yellow Fever." *North Am Rev* 167 (1898): 681–89.
Douglas, R. "In Memoriam: William Elias Brownlee Davis, M.D." *Trans South Surg Gynecol Assoc* 16 (1903): 465–71.
Dowler, Bennet. *Tableau of the Yellow Fever of 1853: With Topographical, Chronologica, and Historical Sketches of the Epidemics of New Orleans Since Their Origin in 1796.* New Orleans: Office of the Picayune, 1854.
Downs, Jim. *Sick from Freedom.* New York: Oxford University Press, 2012.
Drake, D. "Diseases of the Negro Population." *South Med Surg J* 1 (1845): 341–43.
Drake, Daniel. *A Systematic Treatise of the Principal Diseases of the Interior Valley of North America.* Cincinnati, OH: Winthrop B. Smith, 1850.
Draper, Lyman C. *King's Mountain and Its Heroes.* New York: Dauber and Pine, 1929.
Du Bois, W. E. B. "Reconstruction and Its Benefits." *Am Hist Rev* 15 (1910): 781–99.
Du Bois, W. E. B. *The Suppression of the African Slave-Trade to the United States of America 1638–1870.* New York: Longmans, Green, 1896.
Duffy, John. "Eighteenth-Century Carolina Health Conditions." *J South Hist* 18 (1952): 289–302.
Duffy, John. "Erasmus Darwin Fenner (1807–1866) Journalist, Educator, and Sanitarian." *J Med Ed* 35 (1960): 819–31.
Duffy, John. "A Note on Ante-Bellum Southern Nationalism and Medical Practice." *J South Hist* 34 (1968): 266–76.
Duffy, John. "Sectional Conflict and Medical Education in Louisiana." *J South Hist* 23 (1957): 289–306.

Duffy, John. *The Tulane University Medical Center: One Hundred and Fifty Years of Medical Education.* Baton Rouge: Louisiana State University Press, 1984.
Duffy, John. "Yellow Fever in Colonial Charleston." *SC Hist Gen Mag* 52 (1951): 189–97.
du Manoir, F. "Concession of Ste Catherine at the Natchez." *Louisiana Hist Q* 2 (1919): 164–73.
Duncan, Louis C. *Medical Men in the American Revolution 1775–1783.* Carlisle Barracks, PA: Medical Field Service School, 1931.
Dunning, William Archibald. *Reconstruction, Political and Economic.* New York: Harper and Brothers, 1907.
du Pratz, Antoine-Simon Le Page. *Histoire de la Louisiane, Tome I.* Paris: de Bure, 1758.
Durand of Dauphiné. *A Frenchman in Virginia, Being the Memoirs of a Huguenot Refugee in 1686.* Richmond: private printing, 1923.
Dusinberre, William. *Slavemaster President: The Double Career of James Polk.* Oxford: Oxford University Press, 2007.
Duvallon, Pierre-Louis Berquin. *Travels in Louisiana and Florida, in the Year 1802, Giving a Correct Picture of Those Countries.* Translated by John Davis. New York: J. Riley, 1806.
Dyson, Walter. *The Founding of Howard University.* Vol. 1. Washington, DC: Howard University Studies in History, 1921.
Earle, C. "Environment, Disease and Mortality in Early Virginia." *J Hist Geo* 4 (1979): 365–90.
Eaton, John. *Grant, Lincoln and the Freedmen.* New York: Longmans, Green, 1907.
Edelson, S. M. "Clearing Swamps, Harvesting Forests: Trees and the Making of a Plantation Landscape in the Colonial South Carolina Lowcountry." *Ag Hist* 81 (2007): 381–406.
Edwards, Alexander, ed. *Ordinances of the City Council of Charleston.* Charleston, SC: W. P. Young, 1802.
Ehle, John. *Trail of Tears.* New York: Anchor Books, 1989.
Emmet, Thomas Addis. *A Memoir of John Patton Emmet M.D.* New York: privately printed, 1898.
Engerman, Stanley, Seymour Drescher, and Robert Paquette, eds. *Slavery.* Oxford: Oxford University Press, 2001.
Eve, J. A. "Medical Education." *South Med Surg J* 1 (1836): 216–23.
Eve, J. A. "A Sketch of the Life and Labors of Dr. Robert Battey of Rome, Georgia." *Virginia Med Monthly* 5 (1878): 1–8.
Eve, P. F. "Address to the Class on Opening the Course of Lectures in the Medical College of Georgia." *South Med J* 3 (1838): 1–12.
Eve, P. F. "Case of Excision of the Uterus." *Am J Med Sci* 19 (1850): 395–400.
Eve, Paul F. *A Collection of Remarkable Cases in Surgery.* Philadelphia: J. B. Lippincott, 1857.
Ewald, Johann. *Diary of the American War: A Hessian Journal.* Translated by Joseph P. Tustin. New Haven, CT: Yale University Press, 1979.
Ezell, J. S. "A Southern Education for Southrons." *J South Hist* 17 (1951): 303–27.
Falk, L. A. "Black Abolitionist Doctors and Healers." *Bull Hist Med* 54 (1980): 258–72.
Farrar, S. C. "General Report on the Topography, Meterology and Diseases of Jackson, the Capital of Mississippi." *South Med Reports* 1 (1849): 345–59.
Faust, D. G. "The Rhetoric and Ritual of Agriculture in Antebellum South Carolina." *J South Hist* 45 (1979): 541–68.
"Fellows of the American Surgical Association." *Trans Am Surg Assoc* 2 (1885): v–xiv.
Fenner, E., ed. "Historical Sketch of the Charity Hospital." *NO Med J* 1 (1844): 66–77.
Fenner, E. D. "Introductory Address." *South Med Reports* 1 (1849): 7–13.

Fenner, E. D. "On the Hygiene of Cotton Plantations and the Management of Negro Slaves." *South Med Rep* 2 (1850): 430–36.

Fenner, E. D. "Reports from Mississippi." *South Med Reports* 1 (1849): 354.

Figg, L., and J. Farrell-Beck. "Amputations in the Civil War: Physical and Social Dimensions." *J Hist Allied Sci* 48 (1993): 454–75.

Fisher, Irving. *Report on National Vitality, Its Wastes and Conservation*. Washington, DC: Government Printing Office, 1909.

Fleming, Walter L. *Documentary History of Reconstruction*. Vol. 1. New York: Peter Smith, 1950.

Flexner, Abraham. *Medical Education in the United States and Canada*. New York: Carnegie Foundation, 1910.

Flint, Austin. *Contributions Relating to the Causation and Prevention of Disease and to Camp Diseases*. New York: US Sanitary Commission, 1867.

Forry, Samuel. *The Climate of the United States and the Endemic Influences*. New York: J. and H. G. Langley, 1842.

Fortier, Alcée. *A History of Louisiana*. Vol. 1. Paris: Goupil, 1904.

Fossier, A. E. "The Charity Hospital of Louisiana." *NO Med Surg J* 75/76 (1923): 728–30; 791–98; 24–31; 67–74; 128–38; 188–96.

Fossier, A. E. "History of Medical Education in New Orleans." *Ann Med Hist* 6 (1935): 320–52.

Foster, G. M. "The Limitations of Federal Health Care for Freedmen, 1862–1868." *J South Hist* 48 (1982): 349–72.

Foster, S., and A. W. Putnam. "The Battle of King's Mountain." *Am Hist Rev* 1 (1896): 22–47.

Fourcroy, Antoine-François. *Rapport et Projet de Décret sur l'Etablissment d'une École Central de Santé à Paris*. Paris: Convention Nationale, 1794.

Fox-Genovese, Elizabeth. "Antebellum Southern Households: A New Perspective on a Familiar Question." *Review* 7 (1983): 232–33.

Franklin, J. H. "Public Welfare in the South during the Reconstruction Era, 1865–80." *Soc Serv Rev* 44 (1970): 379–92.

Freeman, F. R. "American Colonial Scientists Who Published in the 'Philosophical Transactions' of the Royal Society." *Notes Rec R Soc London* 39 (1985): 191–206.

Freemon, F. R. "Medical Care at the Siege of Vicksburg, 1863." *Bull NY Acad Med* 67 (1991): 429–38.

Frewen, Thomas. *The Practice and Theory of Inoculation*. London: S. Austen, 1749.

Friedenbery, Zachary B. *The Doctor in Colonial America*. Danbury, CT: Routledge, 1998.

Ganshof, F. L. *Feudalism*. Translated by Philip Greirson. Toronto: University of Toronto Press, 1996.

Garrigus, John, trans. *Le Code Noir Ou Recueil des Reglements Rendus Jusqu'a Present*. Paris: Prault, 1767.

Gaspar, David Barry, and David Patrick Geggus. *A Turbulent Time: The French Revolution and the Greater Caribbean*. Bloomington: Indiana University Press, 1997.

Gayley, James F. *A History of the Jefferson Medical College of Philadelphia*. Philadelphia: Joseph M. Wilson, 1858.

Gelfand, Toby. *Professionalizing Modern Medicine: Paris Surgeons and Medical Science and Institutions in the 18th Century*. Westport CT: Greenwood Press, 1980.

General Military Hospital for the North Carolina Troops in Petersburg Virginia. Raleigh, NC: Strother and Marcom, 1861.

Genovese, E. D. "The Negro Laborer in Africa and the Slave South." *Phylon* 21 (1960): 343–50.

George II. "Charter of the Colony." In *Colonial Records of the State of Georgia, Vol. 1*, edited by Allen D. Candler. Atlanta: Franklin Printing and Publishing, 1904.

Georgian, E. A. "Medicine and Politics: The Primitive Physic and Early American Medicine." *Wesley and Methodist Studies* 8 (2016): 35–51.

Gibbs, R. W. *Documentary History of the American Revolution*. Vol. 2. New York: D. Appleton, 1857.

Gibson, G. "Costume and Fashion in Charleston 1769–1782." *SC Hist Mag* 82 (1981): 225–47.

Gildersleeve, J. R. "History of Chimborazo Hospital, C.S.A." *South Hist Soc Papers* 36 (1908): 86–94.

Gillespie, J. B. "1795: Martha Laurens Ramsay's 'Dark Night of the Soul.'" *William and Mary Q* 48 (1991): 68–92.

Gordon, R. C. "William J. Sneed: Surgeon, Humanist, and Educator." *Journal of Investigative Surgery* 18 (2005): 5–6.

Graham, E. A. "Samuel Gross Looks In on the American Surgical Association." *Ann Surg* 106 (1937): 481–91.

Gray, Lewis Cecil. *History of Agriculture in the Southern United States*. Vol. 1. Washington, DC: Carnegie Institute, 1933.

Greenhill, William Alexander, ed. *Thomas Sydenham, M.D., Opera Omnia*. London: Sydenham Society, 1844.

Grier, S. L. "The Negro and His Diseases." *NO Med Surg J* 9 (1853): 752–61.

Griesemer, A. D., W. D. Widman, K. A. Forde, and M. A. Hardy. "John Jones, M.D.: Pioneer, Patriot, and Founder of American Surgery." *World J Surg* 34 (2010): 605–9.

Grimké, J. F. "Journal of the Campaign to the Southward, May 9th to July 14th, 1778." *SC Hist Gen Mag* 12 (1911): 190–206.

Groom, Winston. *Forrest Gump*. New York: Doubleday, 1986.

Groom, Winston. *Vicksburg, 1863*. New York: Alfred A. Knopf, 2009.

Gross, Samuel D. *Autobiography of Samuel D. Gross, M.D.* Vol. 2. Philadelphia: George Barrie, 1887.

Gross, S. D. "A Century of American Medicine, 1776–1876." *Am J Med Sci* 71 (1876): 431–84.

Gross, S. D. *A Manual of Military Surgery*. Richmond: C. H. Wynne, 1862.

Guerra, F. "Medical Almanacs of the American Colonial Period." *J Hist Allied Sci* 36 (1961): 234–55.

Haggard, W. D. "The President's Annual Address." *Trans Southern Surg Gynecol Assoc* 1 (1889): 27–32.

Haggis, A. W. "Fundamental Errors in the Early History of Cinchona." *Bull Hist Med* 10 (1941): 568–92.

Hall, C. R. "The Rise of Professional Surgery in the United States." *Bull Hist Med* 26 (1952): 231–62.

Haller, J. S. "The Negro and the Southern Physician: A Study of Medical and Racial Attitudes, 1800–1860." *Med Hist* 16 (1972): 238–53.

Haller, John S. *The People's Doctor: Samuel Thomson and the American Botanical Movement 1790–1860*. Carbondale: Southern Illinois University Press, 2001.

Halsband, R. "New Light on Lady Mary Wortley Montagu's Contribution to Inoculation." *J Hist Med Allied Sci* (1953): 390–405.

Hamilton, W. B. "Mississippi 1817: A Sociological and Economic Analysis." *J Miss Hist* 20 (1967): 270–92.

Hammond, J. C. "Slavery, Settlement, and Empire: The Expansion and Growth of Slavery in the Interior of the North American Continent, 1770–1820." *J Early Rep* 32 (2012): 175–206.

Harris, Leslie M., and Daina Ramey Berry. *Slavery and Freedom in Savannah*. Athens: University of Georgia Press, 2014.

Harris, Thaddeus Mason. *Biographical Memorials of James Oglethorpe*. Boston: Freeman and Bolles, 1841.

Harrison, J. B. "The Prospects of Letters and Taste in Virginia." In *Six Addresses on the State of Letters and Science in Virginia*, edited by A. J. Morrison, 21–30. Roanoke, VA: Stone Printing and Manufacturing, 1917.

Harrison, T. P. "Pelatiah Webster's Journal of a Voyage to Charlestown." In *Publications of the Southern History Association*. Vol. 2. Washington, DC: The Association, 1898, 131–48.

Hasegawa, G. R., and F. T. Hambrecht. "The Confederate Medical Laboratories." *South Med J* 96 (2003): 1221–1230.

Haw, J. "'Every Thing Here Depends upon Opinion': Nathaniel Greene and Public Support in the Southern Campaigns of the American Revolution." *SC Hist Mag* 109 (2008): 212–31.

Hayne, R. Y. "Biographical Memoir of David Ramsay, M.D." *Analectic Mag* 6 (1815): 204–24.

Haywood, John. *The Natural and Aboriginal History of Tennessee*. Nashville: George Wilson, 1823.

Helling, T. S., and W. K. McNabney. "The Role of Amputation in the Management of Battlefield Casualties: A History of Two Millenia." *J Trauma* 49 (2000): 930–39.

Hening, William Waller. *The Statutes at Large (Virginia)*. Vol. 1. New York: R and W and G Bartow, 1823.

Hening, William Waller. *The Statutes at Large (Virginia)*. Vol. 3. New York: R and W and G Bartow, 1823.

Hesseltine, William B. *A History of the South 1607–1936*. New York: Prentice-Hall, 1936.

Hilton, William. "A Relation of a Discovery." In *Narratives of Early Carolina*, edited by Alexander S. Salley, 37–61. New York: Charles Scribner's Sons, 1911.

Hinshelwood, B. "The Carolinian Context of John Locke's Theory of Slavery." *Political Theory* 41 (2013): 562–90.

Hirsch, Arthur Henry. *The Huguenots of Colonial South Carolina*. Durham, NC: Duke University Press, 1928.

Historical Statistics of the United States: Colonial Times to 1970, Part 1. Washington, DC: Government Printing Office, 1975.

Hoban, Charles F., ed. *Pennsylvania Archives, Eighth Series, Vol. 8, 1771–1776*. Harrisburg, PA: State Library, 1935.

Holman, C. H. "William Gilmore Simm's Picture of the Revolution as a Civil Conflict." *J South Hist* 15 (1949): 441–64.

Honigsbaum, M., and M. Wilcox. "Cinchona." In *Traditional Medicinal Plants and Malaria*, edited by Merlin Wilcox, Gerard Bodeker, Philippe Rasoanaivo, and Jonathan Addae-Kyereme, 22–47. Boca Raton, FL: CRC Press, 2004.

Hopkins, Donald. *The Greatest Killer: Smallpox in History*. 1983. Chicago: University of Chicago Press, 2002.

Hopley, Catherine Cooper. *Life in the South; From the Commencement of the War.* London: Chapman and Hall, 1863.

Horne, I. V., R. Wharry, J. Fithian, et al. "Letters from Continental Officers to Doctor Reading Beatty, 1781–1788." *Penn Mag Hist Bio* 54 (1930): 155–74.

Hotez, Peter J. "Neglected Infections of Poverty in the United States of America." In *The Causes and Impacts of Neglected Tropical and Zoonotic Diseases: Opportunities for Integrated Intervention Strategies*, edited by Eileen R. Choffnes and David A. Relman, 237–64. Washington, DC: National Academies Press, 2011.

Howard, Oliver Otis. *Autobiography of Oliver Otis Howard.* New York: Baker and Taylor, 1908.

Howard-Jones, Norman. "Choleranomalies: The Unhistory of Medicine as Exemplified by Cholera." *Perspect Bio Med* 15 (1972): 422–34.

Hudson, Charles. *The Southeastern Indians.* Knoxville: University of Tennessee Press, 1976.

Hume, Edgar Erskine. "Chimborazo Hospital, Confederate States Army, America's Largest Military Hospital." *Virginia Med Monthly* 61 (1934): 189–95.

Hume, R. L. "Carpetbaggers in the Reconstruction South: A Group Portrait of Outside Whites in the 'Black and Tan' Constitutional Convention." *J Am Hist* 64 (1977): 313–30.

Humphreys, M. "A Stranger to Our Camps: Typhus in American History." *Bull Hist Med* 80 (2006): 269–90.

Hunter, G. H. "Late to the Dance: New Orleans and the Emergence of a Confederate City." *J Louisiana Hist Assoc* 57 (2016): 297–322.

Hutton, Kimberly. "A Comparative Study of the Plants Used for Medicinal Purposes by the Creek and Seminoles Tribes." Master's dissertation. University of South Florida, 2010.

Huxham, John. *An Essay on Fevers.* London: S. Austen, 1750.

"Indigenous Remedies of the South." *Confed Med Surg J* 1 (1864): 106–8.

"Introduction." *South Med Surg J* 1 (1836): 1–4.

Irwin, L. "Cherokee Healing: Myth, Dreams, and Medicine." *Am Indian Q* 16 (1992): 237–57.

Jackson, Robert. *A Treatise of the Fevers of Jamaica.* London: J. Murray, 1791.

Jacob, Nancy Vashti Anthony. *Anthony Roots and Branches.* Shreveport, LA: N. V. A. Jacob, 1971.

James, William Dobein. *A Sketch of the Life of Brig. Gen. Francis Marion and a History of His Brigade.* Marietta, GA: Continental Book Company, 1948.

Jefferson, Thomas. *Notes of the State of Virginia.* Richmond: J. W. Randolph, 1853.

Johnson, Joseph. *Traditions and Reminiscences Chiefly of the American Revolution in the South.* Charleston, SC: Walker and James, 1851.

Johnson, William. *Sketches of the Life and Correspondence of Nathaniel Green.* Vol. 1. Charleston, SC: A. E. Miller, 1822.

Johnson, William. *Sketches of the Life and Correspondence of Nathaniel Greene.* Vol. 2. Charleston, SC: A. E. Miller, 1822.

Jones, J. "Investigations upon the Nature, Causes and Treatment of Hospital Gangrene as it Prevailed in the Confederate Armies, 1861–1865." In *Surgical Memoirs of the War of the Rebellion*, edited by Frank Hastings Hamilton, 143–548. New York: US Sanitary Commission, 1871.

Jones, J. "The Medical History of the Confederate States Army and Navy." *South Hist Soc* 20 (1892): 109–66.

Jones, J. "Original and Eclectic." *South Med Surg J* 17 (1861): 593–614.

Jones, John. *Plain Concise Practical Remarks on the Treatment of Wounds and Fractures.* New York: John Holt, 1775.
Jones, Joseph. *Medical and Surgical Memoirs.* Vol. 1. New Orleans: Clark and Hofeline, 1876.
Jordan, Winthrop D. *White over Black: American Attitudes towards the Negro, 1550-1812.* Chapel Hill: University of North Carolina Press, 2012.
Josselyn, John. *New-England's Rarities Discovered.* London: G. Widdowes, 1672.
Kalm, Peter. *Travels into North America.* London: T. Lowndes, 1772.
Katz, William Loren. *Negro Population in the United States, 1790-1915.* New York: Arno Press, 1968.
Kean, Robert Garlick Hill. *Inside the Confederate Government: The Diary of Robert Garlick Hill Kean.* New York: Oxford University Press, 1957.
Keen, W. W. "Military Surgery in 1861 and 1918." *Ann Am Pol Soc Sci* 80 (1918): 11-22.
Kelton, P. "The Great Southeastern Smallpox Epidemic, 1696-1760: The Region's First Major Epidemic?" In *The Transformation of the Southeastern Indians, 1540-1760*, by Marvin T. Smith, 21-38. Jackson: University Press of Mississippi, 2002.
Kenny, S. C. "'A Dictate of Both Interest and Mercy'? Slave Hospitals in the Antebellum South." *J Hist Med Allied Sci* 65 (2009): 1-47.
Kilbride, D. "Southern Medical Students in Philadelphia, 1800-1861: Science and Sociability in the 'Republic of Medicine.'" *J South Hist* 65 (1999): 697-732.
Kingsbury, Susan Myra, ed. *The Records of the Virginia Company of London.* Vol. 3. Washington, DC: United States Printing Office, 1933.
Kiple, V. H. "Black Tongue and Black Men: Pellagra and Slavery in the Antebellum South." *J South Hist* 43 (1977): 411-28.
Klebaner, B. J. "Public Poor Relief in Charleston, 1800-1860." *SC Hist Mag* 55 (1954): 210-20.
Kopperman, P. E. "The Medical Dimension in Cornwallis' Army 1780-1781." *NC Hist Rev* 89 (2012): 367-98.
Kousoulis, A. A. "Etymology of Cholera." *Emerg Infect Dis* 540 (2012).
Krafka, J., Jr. "Medicine in Colonial Georgia." *Georgia Hist Q* 20 (1936): 326-44.
Krebsbach, S. "The Great Charlestown Smallpox Epidemic of 1760." *SC Hist Mag* 97 (1996): 30-37.
Kupperman, K. O. "The Puzzle of the American Climate in the Early Colonial Period." *Am Hist Rev* 87 (1982): 1262-1289.
Kyte, G. W. "General Greene's Plans for the Capture of Charleston, 1781-1782." *SC Hist Mag* 62 (1961): 96-106.
Lane, N. "The Unseen World: Reflections on Leeuenhoek (1677) 'Concerning Little Animals.'" *Phil Trans R Soc B* 370 (2015): 1-10.
Lange, R. T., and J. J. McGowan. "A Brief History of the School of Medicine University of South Carolina." *J SC Med Assoc* 83 (1987): 632-36.
Langlois, G.-A. "Deux Fondations Scientifiques à la Nouvelle-Orléans (1728-30): La Connaissance à l'Épreuve de la Réalité Coloniale." *Fr Col Hist* 4 (2003): 99-115.
Latham, R. G., trans. *The Works of Thomas Sydenham, M.D.* Vol. 1. London: Sydenham Society, 1848.
Latham, R. G., trans. *The Works of Thomas Sydenham, M.D.* Vol. 2. London: Sydenham Society, 1848.
Latzko, D. A. "Mapping the Short-Run Impact of the Civil War and Emancipation on the South Carolina Economy." *SC Hist Mag* 116 (2015): 258-79.

Lee, Harry. *Memoirs of the War in the Southern Department of the United States.* New York: University Publishing Company, 1869.
Lee, S. D. "The South since the War." In *Confederate Military History, Vol. 12*, edited by Clement A. Evans, 267–368. Atlanta: Confederate Publishing Company, 1899.
Legan, M. S. "Disease and the Freedmen in Mississippi during Reconstruction." *J Hist Med Allied Sci* 28 (1973): 257–67.
Leglaunec, J.-P. "Slave Migration in Spanish and Early American Louisiana: New Sources and New Estimates." *Louisiana Hist* 46 (2005): 185–209.
Lemann, S. G. "The Problems of Founding a Viable Colony: The Military in Early French Louisiana." *Proc Fr Col Hist Soc* 6/7 (1982): 27–35.
Lengel, Edward G., ed. *The Papers of George Washington, Revolutionary War Series, Vol. 13.* Charlottesville: University of Virginia Press, 2003.
Letters of Joseph Clay Merchant of Savannah 1776–1793. Vol. 8. Savannah: Georgia Historical Society, 1913.
Levine, Bruce. *The Fall of the House of Dixie.* New York: Random House, 2013.
Lewis, William. *An Experimental History of the Materia Medica.* London: J. Johnson and R. Baldwin, 1784.
Lind, James. *An Essay on Diseases Incidental to Europeans in Hot Climates.* London: T. Becket and P. A. De Hondt, 1768.
Lind, James. *Two Papers on Fevers and Infections.* London: D. Wilson, 1763.
Lining, J. "A Letter From Dr. John Lining at Charles-Town in South Carolina, to James Jurin, M.D." *Phil Trans* 43 (1744–1745): 318–30.
Lloyd, G. E. R. "The Hot and the Cold, the Dry and the Wet in Greek Philosophy." *J Hellenic Studies* 84 (1964): 92–106.
Long, J. W. "The Wisdom of the Past, A Prophecy of the Future." *Surg Gynecol Obstet* 20 (1915): 277–84.
Longo, L. D. "The Rise and Fall of Battey's Operation: A Fashion in Surgery." *Bull Hist Med* 53 (1979): 244–67.
Lowry, Robert, and William H. McCardle. *A History of Mississippi.* Jackson, MS: R. H. Henry, 1891.
Lum, Kathryn Gin. *Heathen: Religion and Race in American History.* Cambridge, MA: Harvard University Press, 2022.
Lutz, Frank J., ed. *The Autobiography and Reminiscences of S. Pollack, M.D.* Saint Louis, MO: Saint Louis Medical Review, 1904.
MacDonald, F. W. *The Journal of the Rev. John Wesley.* Vol. 1. 1906. London: J. M. Dent and Sons, 1921.
MacLeod, George H. B. *Notes on the Surgery of War in the Crimea.* Philadelphia: J. B. Lippincott, 1862.
Maddox, R. L. "John Wesley on Holistic Health and Healing." *Methodist Hist* 46 (2007): 4–33.
"Management of Negroes upon Southern Estates." *De Bow's Rev*, 1851, 621–25.
Mandle, J. R. "The Economic Underdevelopment of the United States South in the Post-Bellum Era." In *Disparities in Economic Development Since the Industrial Revolution*, edited by Paul Bairoch and Maurice Lévy-Leboyer, 86–97. London: Macmillan, 1981.
Manning, Chandra. *What This Cruel War Was Over.* New York: Random House, 2007.
Margry, Pierre. *Découvertes et Établissements des Français dans l'Ouest et dans le Sud.* Vol. 4. Paris: D. Jouaust, 1880.

Markham, Clements R. *A Memoir of the Lady Ana de Osorio, Countess of Chinchon and Vice-Queen of Peru*. London: Trubner, 1874.
Marshall, C. K. "Home Education at the South." *De Bow's Rev* 18 (1855): 430–32.
Matas, R. "The Surgical Peculiarities of the American Negro." *Trans Am Surg Assoc* 15 (1896): 3–126.
Matas, Rudolph. *History of Medicine in Louisiana*. Vol. 2. Baton Rouge: Louisiana State University Press, 1962.
Mather, Cotton. *The Angel of Bethesda*. Barre, MA: American Antiquarian Society, 1972.
Matthews, James M., ed. *Public Laws of the Confederate States of America, First Congress, 1862*. Richmond: R. M. Smith, 1862.
Matthews, James M. *The Statutes at Large of the Provisional Government of the Confederate States of America*. Richmond: R. M. Smith, 1864.
Maxwell, W. Q. "A True State of the Smallpox in Williamsburg, February 22, 1748." *Virg Mag Hist Bio* 63 (1955): 269–74.
McCandless, P. "Revolutionary Fever: Disease and War in the Lower South." *Trans Am Clin Clim Assoc* 118 (2007): 225–49.
McCandless, Peter. *Slavery, Disease, and Suffering in the Southern Lowcountry*. Cambridge: Cambridge University Press, 2011.
McCord, David J., ed. *The Statutes at Large of South Carolina*. Vol. 7. Columbia, SC: A. S. Johnston, 1840.
McCrady, E. "An Historical Address before the Graduating Class of the Medical College of the State of South Carolina, 1885." In *Year Book—1895, City of Charleston*, 386–424. Charleston, SC: Walker, Evans and Cogswell, 1895.
McCrady, Edward. *The History of South Carolina in the Revolution 1775-1780*. New York: Macmillan, 1901.
McCrady, Edward. *The History of South Carolina under the Proprietary Government 1670-1719*. New York: Macmillan, 1897.
McCrady, Edward. *Slavery in the Province of South Carolina, 1670-1770*. Charleston, SC: American Historical Association, 1895.
McCullough, David. *The Greater Journey: Americans in Paris*. New York: Simon and Schuster, 2011.
McDowell, E. "Three Cases of Extirpation of Diseased Ovaria." *Eclectic Repertory and Analytical Review* 7 (1817): 242–44.
McGuire, H. "Annual Address of the President." *Trans Southern Surg Gynecol Assoc* 2 (1890): 1–12.
McMillen, Neil R. *Dark Journey: Black Mississippians in the Age of Jim Crow*. Urbana: University of Illinois Press, 1989.
McMurtry, L. "A Plea for Progressive Surgery." *Trans South Surg Gynecol Assoc* 5 (1892): 1–7.
McNeill, J. R. "Yellow Jack and Geopolitics." *Review* 27 (2004): 343–64.
Meacham, Jon. *American Lion: Andrew Jackson in the White House*. New York: Random House, 2009.
"Medical College at Richmond, Va." *South Lit Messenger* 5 (1839): 827–28.
"Medical Intelligence." *South Med Surg J* 2 (1838): 449–50.
"Medical Schools, No. 1." *NO Med News Hosp Gaz* 3 (1857): 676–79
"Medical Sectionalism." *NO Med News Hosp Gaz* 4 (1857): 156–58.
"Medicine in the Confederate States." *Lancet* 1 (1864): 445–46.

Menard, R. "From Servants to Slaves: The Transformation of the Chesapeake Labor System." *Southern Studies* 16 (1977): 355–90.
Miles, A. B. "Memorial Address on Dr. Warren Stone." *NO Med Surg J* 22 (1895): 769–88.
Miles, A. B. "Memorial Address on Dr. Warren Stone." *Trans South Surg Gynecol Assoc* 7 (1894): 6–14.
Miller, B. T., J. J. Thweatt, and S. K. Geevarghese. "The Surgeon's Duty to Serve: The Forgotten Life of Paul F. Eve." *J Am Coll Surg* 223 (2016): 537–41.
Miller, K. "The Historic Background of the Negro Physician." *J Negro Hist* 1 (1916): 99–109.
Milligen-Johnston, George. "A Short Description of the Province of South-Carolina." In *Colonial South Carolina: Two Contemporary Descriptions*, edited by Chapman J. Milling, 111–81. Columbia: University of South Carolina Press, 1951.
Mitchel, J. "Account of the Yellow Fever Which Prevailed in Virginia in the Years 1737, 1741, and 1742." *Am Med Phil Reg* 4 (1814): 181–215.
Mitchell, M. C. "Health and the Medical Profession in the Lower South, 1845–1860." *J South Hist* 10 (1944): 424–46.
Mooney, J. "Cherokee Theory and Practice of Medicine." *J Am Folklore* 3 (1890): 44–50.
Mooney, James. *The Sacred Formulas of the Cherokees*. Washington, DC, 1891.
Mooney, James. *The Swimmer Manuscript*. Washington, DC: Government Printing Office, 1932.
Moore, A. B. "One Hundred Years of Reconstruction of the South." *J South Hist* 9 (1943): 153–80.
Moore, James. *The History of Smallpox*. London: Longman, Hurst, Rees, Orme, and Brown, 1815.
Moores, R. R. "Exegit Monumentum Aere Perennius." *Richmond County Hist* 9 (1977): 10–17.
Morais, Herbert M. *The History of the Negro in Medicine*. New York: Publishers Company, 1967.
Morgan, E. E., and J. E. Perry. "Traditional Medicinal Plant Use among Virginia's Powhatan Indians." *Banisteria* 35 (2010): 11–31.
Morgan, John. *A Discourse upon the Institution of Medical Schools in America*. Philadelphia: William Bradford, 1765.
Morgan, P. D. "Virginia Slavery in Atlantic Context, 1550–1650." In *Virginia 1619: Slavery and Freedom in the Making of English America*, edited by Paul Musselwhite, Peter C. Mancall, and James Horn, 85–107. Chapel Hill: University of North Carolina Press, 2019.
Morris, C. "Impenetrable but Easy: The French Transformation of the Lower Mississippi Valley and the Founding of New Orleans." In *Transforming New Orleans and Its Environs: Centuries of Change*, edited by Craig E. Colten, 22–42. Pittsburgh, PA: University of Pittsburgh Press, 2014.
Moseley, Benjamin. *A Treatise on Tropical Diseases on Military Operations and on the Climate of the West-Indies*. London: T. Cadell, 1792.
Moses, L. G. *The Indian Man: A Biography of James Mooney*. Lincoln: University of Nebraska Press, 2002.
Mott, Valentine. *Travels in Europe and the East*. New York: Harper and Brothers, 1845.
Moultrie, James. *Introductory Address Delivered at the Opening of the Medical College of the State of South Carolina*. Charleston, SC: J. S. Burges, 1834.
Moultrie, William. *Memoirs of the American Revolution*. Vol. 2. New York: David Longworth, 1802.
Myers, Theodorus Bailey, ed. *Cowpens Papers*. Charleston, SC: News and Courier, 1881.
Nash, H. M. "Some Reminiscences of a Confederate Surgeon." *Trans Coll Phys Phil* 28 (1906): 122–44.

New, C. B. "On the Treatment of Cholera on Plantations." *NO Med Surg J* 7 (1850): 211–13.
"New Orleans School of Medicine." *NO Med News Hosp Gaz* 3 (1856–1857): 489–90.
Newby-Alexander, C. L. "The 'Twenty and Odd.'" *Phylon* 57 (1960): 25–36.
Nicholson, B. J. "Legal Borrowing and the Origins of Slave Law in the British Colonies." *Am J Legal Hist* 38 (1994): 38–54.
Nightingale, Florence. *Notes on Hospitals*. London: Longman, Green, 1863.
Nimura, Janice P. *The Doctors Blackwell*. New York: W. W. Norton, 2021.
Nitzsche, George Erasmus. *University of Pennsylvania: Its History, Traditions, Buildings, and Memorials*. Philadelphia: International Printing Company, 1918.
Norrby, E. "Yellow Fever and Max Theiler: The Only Nobel Prize for a Virus Vaccine." *J Exp Med* 204 (2007): 2779–2784.
Norris, D. A. "'For the Benefit of Our Gallant Volunteers': North Carolina's State Medical Department and Civilian Volunteer Efforts, 1861–1862." *NC Hist Rev* 75 (1998): 297–326.
Nott, J. C. "Statistics of Southern Slave Population." *De Bow's Rev* 4 (1847): 275–87.
Nuermberger, R. K. "Some Notes on the Mordecai Family." *Virginia Mag Hist Bio* 49 (1941): 364–73.
Numbers, R. L., and J. S. Numbers. "Science in the Old South." *J South Hist* 48 (1982): 163–84.
Nutton, V. "The Reception of Fracastoro's Theory of Contagion: The Seed That Fell among Thorns." *Osiris* 6 (1990): 196–234.
"Official Letters of Major General James Pattison, Part I." *Collections NY Hist Soc* 8 (1876): 120–21.
Olschner, K. "Medical Journals in Louisiana before the Civil War." *Bulletin of the Medical Library Association* 60 (1972): 1–13.
Olwell, R. A. "'Domestick Enemies': Slavery and Political Independence in South Carolina, May 1775–March 1776." *J South Hist* 55 (1989): 21–48.
Osler, William. *An Alabama Student and Other Biographical Essays*. New York: Oxford University Press, 1909.
"Our Salutatory." *South J Med Sci* 1 (1866): 187–89.
Patina, M., and M. Moran. "Civil War Manuals of Military Surgery—Samuel D. Gross vs. Julian J. Chisolm." *J Urology* 203 (Suppl) (2020): e284.
Patterson, K. D. "Yellow Fever Epidemics and Mortality in the United States, 1693–1905." *Soc Sci Med* 34 (1992): 855–65.
Perlee, A. "An Account of the Yellow Fever of Natchez, as it Prevailed in the Autumn of 1817 and 1819." *Phil J Med Phys Sci* 3 (1821): 1–17.
Pessen, E. "How Different from Each Other Were the Antebellum North and South?" *Am Hist Rev* 85 (1980): 1119–149.
Pessen, E. "The Workingmen's Movement of the Jacksonian Era." *Mississippi Valley Hist Rev* 43 (1956): 428–43.
Pierce, Paul Skeels. *The Freedmen's Bureau*. Vol. 3. Iowa City: University of Iowa, 1904.
Pike, James S. *The Prostrate State*. New York: D. Appleton, 1874.
Pinckney, Elise, ed. *The Letterbook of Eliza Pinckney 1739–1962*. Columbia: University of South Carolina Press, 1972.
Pohl, L. M. "African American Southerners and White Physicians: Medical Care at the Turn of the Twentieth Century." *Bull Hist Med* 86 (2012): 178–205.
Poinsett, A. "Meharry Medical College Celebrates Its 100th Anniversary." *Ebony* 31 (1976): 31–39.

Polavarapu, H. V., A. N. Kulaylat, S. Sun, and O. Hamed. "100 Years of Surgical Education: The Past, Present, and Future." *Bull Am Coll Surg* 98 (2013): 22–27.

Pope, John. *A Tour through the Southern and Western Territories of the United States of North-America; The Spanish Dominions on the River Mississippi and the Floridas*. Richmond: John Dixon, 1792.

Population of the United States as Returned at the First Census, by State, 1790. Washington, DC: Government Printing Office, 1908.

Porcher, Francis Peyre. *Resources of the Southern Fields and Forests*. Charleston, SC: Stram-Power Press, 1863.

Pozzi, S. *Treatise on Gynecology Medical and Surgical*. Vol. 2. Translated by Brooks H. Wells. New York: William Wood, 1892.

Practical Rules for the Management and Medical Treatment of Negro Slaves in the Sugar Colonies. London: J. Barfield, 1803.

Pringle, John. *Observations on the Diseases of the Army*. London: A. Millar, D. Wilson, T. Durham, 1764.

Pritchett, J., and M.-S. Yun. "The In-Hospital Mortality Rates of Slaves and Freemen: Evidence from Touro Infirmary, New Orleans, Louisiana." *Expl Econ Hist* 46 (2009): 241–52.

Purcell, P. N., and R. P. Hummel Jr. "Samuel Preston Moore: Surgeon-General of the Confederacy." *Am J Surg* 164 (1992): 361–65.

Purry, Jean Pierre. *A Description of the Province of South Carolina, Drawn Up at Charles Town, in September, 1731*. Washington, DC: Peter Force, 1837.

Purry, Jean Pierre. *Memorial Presented to His Grace My Lord the Duke of Newcastle . . . Upon the Present Condition of Carolina*. Augusta, GA: privately printed, 1880.

Radbill, S. X. "The Autobiographical Ana of Robley Dunglison, M.D." *Trans Amer Phil Soc* 53 (1963): 3–185.

Rafinesque, C. S. *Medical Flora; or, Manual of the Medical Botany of the United States of North America*. Philadelphia: Atkinson and Alexander, 1828.

Ramsay, David. "A Dissertation on the Means of Preserving Health, in Charleston, and the Adjacent Low Country." Read before the Medical Society of South-Carolina, on the 29th of May, 1790. Charleston, SC: Markland and McIver, 1790, 3–34.

Ramsay, David. *History of South Carolina from Its First Settlement in 1670 to the Year 1808*. Vol. 2. Newberry, SC: W. J. Duffie, 1858.

Ramsay, David. *History of the American Revolution*. Vol. 1. Philadelphia: R. Aitken and Son, 1789.

Ramsay, David. *The History of the American Revolution*. Vol. 2. Trenton, NJ: James J. Wilson, 1811.

Ramsay, David. *Memoirs of the Life of Martha Laurens Ramsay*. Boston: Crocker and Brewster, 1827.

Ramsay, David. *A Review of the Improvements, Progress, and State of Medicine in the XVIIIth Century*. Charleston, SC: W. P. Young, 1801.

Ramsay, W. G. "Clinical Report of Cases Treated in the Marine Hospital, Charleston." *Am J Med Sci* 18 (1836): 47–53.

Ramsay, W. G. "The Physiological Differences between the Euopeans (or White Man) and the Negro." *South Agriculturalist* 12 (1839): 411–18.

Randolph, E. "Letter to the Board of Trade, 1699." In *Narratives of Early Carolina*, edited by Alexander S. Salley, 208–9. New York: Charles Scribner's Sons, 1911.

Rankin, H. F. "Cowpens: Prelude to Yorktown." *NC Hist Rev* 31 (1954): 336–69.
Reed, W., J. Carroll, and A. Agramonte. "The Etiology of Yellow Fever." *J Am Med Assoc* 36 (1901): 431–40.
Regan, E. "Le Moyne d'Iberville (1661–1706)." *Records Am Cath Hist Soc Phil* 49 (1938): 193–213.
Reitzes, Dietrich C. *Negroes and Medicine*. Cambridge, MA: Harvard University Press, 1959.
Relation du Voyage des Dames Religieuse: Ursulines de Rouen, à la Nouvelle Orléans. Rouen: Antoine le Prevost, 1728.
"Report of the Board of Commissioners for the University of Virginia to the Virgina General Assembly, August 4, 1818." In *The Papers of James Madison, Retirement Series, Vol. 1, 4 March 1817—31 January 1820*, edited by David B. Mattern, 326–40. Charlottesville: University of Virginia Press, 2009.
A Report on the Origin and Cause of the Late Epidemic in Augusta, Ga. Augusta, GA: Browne, Cushney, and McCafferty, 1839.
Richardson, James. *A Compilation of the Messages and Papers of the Confederacy*. Vol. 1. Nashville: United States Publishing Company, 1906.
Ricketts, T. F. *The Diagnosis of Smallpox*. New York: Funk and Wagnalls, 1910.
Riley, J. "Smallpox and American Indians Revisited." *J Hist Med Allied Sci* 65 (2010): 445–77.
Riley, W. J. "The History of America's Premier Independent Black Medical School." *J Blacks Higher Ed* 60 (2008): 74–76.
Risse, G. B. "'Typhus' Fever in Eighteenth-Century Hospitals: New Approaches to Medical Treatment." *Bull Hist Med* 59 (1985): 176–95.
Robertson, Robert. *Observations on the Jail, Hospital, or Ship Fever*. London: J. Murray, 1783.
Robinson, M. "New Worlds, New Medicines: Indian Remedies and English Medicine in Early America." *Early Am Studies* 3 (2005): 94–110.
Rogal, S. J. "Pills for the Poor: John Wesley's Primitive Physick." *Yale J Biol Med* 51 (1978): 81–90.
Rogers, Emma, ed. *Life and Letters of William Barton Rogers*. Boston: Houghton, Mifflin, 1896.
Rolleston, J. D. "Bretonneau: His Life and Work." *Proc R Soc Med* 18 (1925): 1–12.
Roper, L. H. "The 1701 'Act for the Better Ordering of Slaves': Reconsidering the History of Slavery in Proprietary South Carolina." *William Mary Q* 64 (2007): 395–418.
Ross, Charles, ed. *Correspondence of Charles, First Marquis Cornwallis*. Vol. 1. London: John Murray, 1859.
Rothstein, William G. *American Physicians in the Nineteenth Century: From Sects to Science*. Baltimore: Johns Hopkins University Press, 1985.
Rowland, L. S. "'Alone on the River': The Rise and Fall of the Savannah River Rice Plantations of St. Peter's Paris, South Carolina." *SC Hist Mag* 88 (1987): 121–50.
Rush, Benjamin. *An Eulogium in Honor of the Late Dr. William Cullen*. Philadelphia: Thomas Dobson, 1790.
Rush, Benjamin. *Medical Inquiries and Observations*. Vol. 1. Philadelphia: Hopkins and Earle, 1809.
Rush, B. "The Result of Observations Made upon the Diseases Which Occurred in the Military Hospitals of the United States." In *Medical Inquiries and Observations, Vol. 1*, edited by Benjamin Rush, 255–62. Philadelphia: T. Dobson, 1794.
Rush, Benjamin. *Sixteen Introductory Lectures to Courses of Lectures upon the Institutes and Practice of Medicine*. Philadelphia: Bradford and Innskeep, 1811.

Rush, Benjamin, ed. *The Works of Thomas Sydenham, M.D. on Acute and Chronic Diseases.* Philadelphia: Benjamin and Thomas Kite, 1809.
Russell, David Lee. *The American Revolution in the Southern Colonies.* Jefferson, NC: McFarland, 2000.
Russell, P. F. "Malaria and Its Influence on World Health." *Bull NY Acad Med* 19 (1943): 599–630.
Russell, R. "'An Ornament to Our City': The Creation and Recreation of the College of Charleston's Campus, 1785–1861." *South Carolina Historical Magazine* 107 (2006): 124–46.
Sainsbury, W. Noel, ed. *Calendar of State Papers, Colonial Series 1574–1660.* Vol. 1. London: Longman, Green, Longman and Roberts, 1860.
Sallares, R., A. Bouwman, and C. Anderung. "The Spread of Malaria to Southern Europe in Antiquity: New Approaches to Old Problems." *Med Hist* 48 (2004): 311–28.
Salley, Alexander S., Jr. *Narratives of Early Carolina 1650–1708.* New York: Charles Scribner's Sons, 1911.
"Salutatory." *Confed Med Surg J* 1 (1864): 13–15.
Sandy, L. "Divided Loyalties in a 'Predatory War': Plantation Overseers and Slavery during the American Revolution." *J Am Studies* 48 (2014): 357–92.
Sargent, Winthrop. *Sargent's Code: A Collection of the Original Laws of the Mississippi Territory Enacted 1799–1800.* Jackson, MS: Historical Records Survey, 1939.
Savitt, Todd L. *Medicine and Slavery: The Diseases and Health Care of Blacks in Antebellum Virginia.* Champaign: University of Illinois Press, 1978.
Savitt, Todd L. "The Use of Blacks for Medical Experimentation and Demonstration in the Old South." *J South Hist* 48 (1982): 331–48.
Savitt, Todd L., and James Harvey Young. *Disease and Distinctiveness in the American South.* Knoxville: University of Tennessee Press, 1988.
Scarborough, William Kauffman. *Masters of the Big House.* Baton Rouge: Louisiana State University Press, 2003.
Searcy, M. C. "1779: The First Year of the British Occupation of Georgia." *Georgia Hist Soc* 67 (1983): 168–88.
Shaffer, A. H. "Between Two Worlds: David Ramsay and the Politics of Slavery." *J South Hist* 50 (1984): 175–96.
Shakespeare, William. *The Tempest.* Edited by Joseph Wayne Barley. New York: American Book Company, 1917.
Shapiro, Michael. *The Last Great Season.* New York: Doubleday, 2003.
Sharpe, W. D. "The Confederate States Medical and Surgical Journal: 1864–1865." *Bull NY Acad Med* 52 (1976): 373–418.
Shipp, Barnard. *The History of Hernando De Soto and Florida.* Philadelphia: Robert M. Lindsay, 1881.
Shrady, G. F. "Specialism as a Practice." *Med Record* 10 (1875): 489–90.
Shryock, Richard Harrison. *The Development of Modern Medicine: An Interpretation of the Social and Scientific Factors Involved.* 1936. Madison: University of Wisconsin Press, 1974.
Shryock, R. H. "Eighteenth Century Medicine in America." *Amer Antiquarian Soc* 59 (1949): 275–92.
Shryock, R. H. "The Interplay of Social and Internal Factors in the History of Modern Medicine." *Scientific Monthly* 76 (1953): 221–30.
Shryock, R. H. "Medical Practice in the Old South." *South Atlantic Q* 29 (1930): 160–78.

Shugerman, J. H. "The Louisiana Purchase and South Carolina's Reopening of the Slave Trade in 1803." *J Early Rep* 22 (2002): 263–90.
Simkins, F. B., and J. W. Patton. "The Work of Southern Women among the Sick and Wounded of the Confederate Armies." *J South Hist* 1 (1935): 475–96.
Simms, William Gilmore. *The Scout, or The Black Riders of Congaree*. New York: Butler Bros., 1888.
Sims, J. M. "On the Treatment of Vesico-Vaginal Fistula." *Am J Med Sci* 23 (1852): 59–82.
Sims, J. Marion. *The Story of My Life*. New York: D. Appleton, 1884.
Sirmans, M. E. "The Legal Status of the Slave in South Carolina." *J South Hist* 28 (1962): 462–73.
Sluiter, E. "New Light on the '20 and Odd Negroes' Arriving in Virginia, August 1619." *William Mary Q* 54 (1997): 395–98.
Smart, Charles, ed. *Medical and Surgical History of the War of the Rebellion*. Vol. 1 Part III. Washington, DC: Government Printing Office, 1888.
Smith, B. A. "Impatient and Pestilent: Public Health and the Reopening of the Slave Trade in Early National Charleston." *SC Hist Mag* 114 (2013): 29–58.
Smith, D. C. "Gerhard's Distinction between Typhoid and Typhus and Its Reception in America, 1833–1860." *Bull Hist Med* 54 (1980): 368–85.
Smith, H. A. M. "Old Charles Town and Its Vicinity, Accabee and Wappoo Where Indigo Was First Cultivated." *SC Hist Gen Mag* 16 (1915): 1–15.
Smith, J., and M. L. Webber. "Josiah Smith's Diary, 1780–1781." *SC Hist Gen Mag* 34 (1933): 31–39.
Smith, James Edward. *A Selection of the Correspondence of Linnaeus and Other Naturalists*. Vol. 1. London: Longman, Hurst, 1821.
Smith, John. *The Generall Historie of Virginia, New England and The Summer Isles*. Vol. 1. New York: Macmillan, 1907.
Smith, Peter. *The Indian Doctor's Dispensary*. Cincinnati, OH: Browne and Looker, 1813.
Smith, R. B. "The First 125 Years." *Bull Med College Virginia* 61 (1963): 5–96.
Smith, William. *The History of the Province of New-York*. London: Thomas Wilcox, 1757.
Smyth, Albert Henry, ed. *The Writings of Benjamin Franklin*. Vol. 10. New York: Macmillan, 1907.
Snydor, C. S. "Life Span of Mississippi Slaves." *Am Hist Rev* 35 (1930): 566–74.
Somers, Robert. *The Southern States since the War 1870–1*. New York: Macmillan, 1871.
South, S. "Exploratory Archeology at the Site of 1670–1680 Charles Towne on Albemarle Point in South Carolina." *University of South Carolina Research Manuscript Series* 137 (1969): 1–57.
"Southern Medical and Surgical Journal." *South Med Surg J* 21 (1866): 164–65.
"Southern Medical Schools—Southern Toadyism." *Georgia Blister and Critic* 1 (1854): 34–35.
Spalding, Phinizy. *The History of the Medical College of Georgia*. Athens: University of Georgia Press, 2011.
Speck, F. G. "Catawba Herbals and Curative Practices." *J Am Folklore* 57 (1944): 37–50.
Stange, Marion. "Urban Governance in French Colonial North America: Hospital Care in Québec and Nouvelle-Orléans in the Seventeenth and Eighteenth Centuries." *Zeitschrift für Kanada-Studien* 29 (2009): 108–19.
Stange, Marion. *Vital Negotiations: Protecting Settlers' Health in Colonial Louisiana and South Carolina, 1720–1763*. Göttingen: Vandenhoeck and Ruprecht, 2012.
Starr, Emmet. *History of the Cherokee Indians and Their Legends and Folk Lore*. 1921. Oklahoma City, OK: Warden Company, 1969.
Statutes at Large of South Carolina, Vol. 4 No. 881. Columbia, SC: A. S. Johnston, 1838.

Stetar, J. M. "In Search of a Direction: Southern Higher Education after the Civil War." *Hist Ed Q* 25 (1985): 341–67.
Stevens, Rosemary. *American Medicine and the Public Interest*. Berkeley: University of California Press, 1971.
Stout, S. H. "An Address, Introductory to the Eighth Regular Summer Course of Lectures in the Atlanta Medical College." *Atlanta Med Surg J* 7 (1866): 196–211.
Stovall, T. "Race and the Making of the Nation: Blacks in Modern France." In *Diasporic Africa: A Reader*, edited by Michael Gomez, 200–216. New York: New York University Press, 2006.
Stowe, Steven M. *Doctoring the South*. Chapel Hill: University of North Carolina Press, 2004.
Sullivan, R. B. "Sanguine Practices: A Historical and Historiographic Reconsideration of Heroic Therapy in the Age of Rush." *Bulletin of the History of Medicine* 69 (1994): 211–34.
Summerville, James. *Educating Black Doctors: A History of Meharry Medical College*. Tuscaloosa: University of Alabama Press, 1983.
Sydnor, Charles S. "Life Span of Mississippi Slaves." *Am Hist Rev* 35 (1930): 566–74.
Sydnor, Charles Sackett. *Slavery in Mississippi*. New York: D. Appleton-Century Company, 1933.
Tarleton, Banastre. *A History of the Campaigns of 1780 and 1781 in the Southern Provinces of North America*. London: T. Cadell, 1787.
Taylor, Alrutheus Ambush. *The Negro in South Carolina during Reconstruction*. Washington, DC: Association for the Study of Negro Life and History, 1924.
Temin, P. "Patterns of Cotton Agriculture in Post-Bellum Georgia." *J Econ Hist* 43 (1983): 661–74.
Terkel, Susan Neiburg. *Colonial American Medicine*. London: Franklin Watts, 1993.
Thatcher, James. *American Medical Biography*. New York: Milford House, 1828, 1967.
Thatcher, James. *A Military Journal during the American Revolutionary War from 1775 to 1783*. Boston: Richardson and Lord, 1823.
Thomas, Hugh. *The Slave Trade*. New York: Simon and Schuster, 1997.
"Thomas Hunt, M.D." *NO Med Surg J* 22 (1867): 40–42.
Thomson, John. *The Works of William Cullen*. Vol. 1. Edinburgh: William Blackwood, 1827.
Thomson, Samuel. *New Guide to Health: Or, Botanic Family Physician*. Boston: E. G. House, 1822.
Tidyman, P. "A Sketch of the Most Remarkable Diseases of the Negroes of the Southern States, with an Account of the Method of Treating Them, Accompanied by Physiological Observations." *Phila J Med Phys Sci* 12 (1826): 306–38.
Tiffany, Osmond. *A Sketch of the Life and Services of Gen. Otho Holland Williams*. Baltimore: John Murphy, 1851.
Tigertt, W. D. "Osler on Malaria." *Can Med Assoc J* 131 (1984): 1282–1284.
Tilton, James. *Economical Observations on Military Hospitals*. Wilmington, DE: J. Wilson, 1813.
Townsend, J. F. "Francis Peyre Porcher, M.D. (1824–1895)." *Ann Med Hist* 1 (1939): 177–88.
Trial and Expulsion of Charles A. Luzenberg. New Orleans: Physico Medical Society of New Orleans, 1838.
Trowbridge, J. T. *The South: A Tour of Its Battle-Fields and Ruined Cities, a Journey through the Desolated States, and Talks with the People*. Hartford, CT: L. Stebbins, 1866.
True, R. H. "Folk Materia Medica." *J Am Folklore* 14 (1901): 105–14.
Trustees. *An Account Shewing the Progress of the Colony of Georgia in America from Its First Establishment*. 1742. Washington, DC: Peter Force, 1835.
"Tulane Medical Department." *NO Med Surg J* 54 (1902): 680–90.

Tunnell, Ted. *Crucible of Reconstruction: War, Radicalism, and Race in Louisiana, 1862–1877.* Baton Rouge: Louisiana State University Press, 1984.
"University of Pennsylvania Medical Department." *Am J Med Sci* 22 (1838): 259–63.
Usner, Daniel H., Jr. "American Indians on the Cotton Frontier: Changing Economic Relations with Citizens and Slaves in the Mississippi Territory." *J Am Hist* 72 (1985): 297–317.
Usner, Daniel H., Jr. *Indians, Settlers, and Slaves in a Frontier Exchange Economy: The Lower Mississippi Valley Before 1783.* Chapel Hill: University of North Carolina Press, 1992.
Vanderpool, H. Y. "The Wesleyan-Methodist Tradition." In *Caring and Curing,* edited by Ronald L. Numbers and Darnel W. Amundsen, 317–53. Baltimore: Johns Hopkins University Press, 1986.
Van de Warker, E. "The Fetich [sic] of the Ovary." *Am J Obstet Dis Women Children* 52 (1906): 366–73.
Varro, Marcus Terentius. *Rerum Rusticarum.* Translated by W. D. Hooper. Cambridge, MA: Harvard University Press, 1934.
Villiers, Marc, and Gabriel Hanotaux. *Histoire de la Fondation de la Nouvelle-Orleans.* Paris: Imprimerie Nationale, 1917.
Vogel, Virgil J. *American Indian Medicine.* Norman: University of Oklahoma Press, 1970.
Wall, L. L. "The Medical Ethics of Dr. J. Marion Sims: A Fresh Look at the Historical Record." *J Med Ethics* 32 (2006): 346–50.
Wallace, David Duncan. *The History of South Carolina.* Vol. 2. New York: American Historical Society, 1934.
Wallerstein, E. "What Can One Mean by Southern Culture?" In *The Evolution of Southern Culture,* edited by Numan V. Bartley, 1–13. Athens: University of Georgia Press, 1988.
Walton, J. T. "The Comparative Mortality of the White and Colored Races in the South." *Charlotte Med J* 10 (1897): 291–94.
Ward, Thomas J. *Black Physicians in the Jim Crow South.* Fayetteville: University of Arkansas Press, 2003.
Ward, Thomas J., Jr. *Out in the Rural.* New York: Oxford University Press, 2017.
Waring, J. I. "Asiatic Cholera in South Carolina." *Bull Hist Med* 40 (1966): 459–66.
Waring, J. I. "Charleston Medicine 1800–1860." *J Hist Med Allied Sci* 31 (1976): 320–42.
Waring, Joseph Ioor. *A History of Medicine in South Carolina 1825–1900.* Columbia: South Carolina Medical Society, 1967.
Waring, J. I. "The Marine Hospitals of Charleston." *Bull Hist Med* 10 (1941): 651–65.
Waring, J. I. "A Report from the Continental General Hospital in 1780." *SC Hist Gen Mag* 42 (1941): 147–48.
Warner, John Harley. *Against the Spirit of System.* Baltimore: Johns Hopkins University Press, 1998.
Warner, John Harley. "Science in Medicine." *Osiris* 1 (1985): 37–58.
Warner, John Harley. "The Selective Transport of Medical Knowledge: Antebellum American Physicians and Parisian Medical Therpeutics." *Bulletin of the History of Medicine* 59 (1985): 213–31.
Warner, J. H. "A Southern Medical Reform: The Meaning of the Antebellum Argument for Southern Medical Education." *Bull Hist Med* 57 (1983): 364–81.
Warner, John Harley. *The Therapeutic Perspective: Medical Practice, Knowledge, and Identity in America, 1820–1855.* Cambridge, MA: Harvard University Press, 1986.

Waterhouse, Edward. *A Declaration of the State of the Colony and Affaires in Virginia.* London: G. Eld, 1622.

Watson, Irving A. "Biographical Sketch of Dr. Joseph Jones." In *Physicians and Surgeons of America*, edited by Irving A. Watson, 593–97. Concord, NH: Republican Free Press, 1896.

Weaver, J. C. "Early Medical History of Georgia." *J Med Assoc Georgia* 29 (1940): 89–112.

Webster, Noah. *A Brief History of Epidemic and Pestilential Diseases.* Vol. 1. Hartford, CT: Hudson and Goodwin, 1799.

Wells, J. D. "Professionalization and the Southern Middle Class." In *Southern Society and Its Transformations 1790–1860*, edited by Susanna Delfino, Michele Gillespie, and Louis M. Kyriakoudes, 157–78. Columbia: University of Missouri Press, 2011.

Wesley, John. *Primitive Physic: Or an Easy and Natural Method of Curing Most Diseases.* Edinburgh: Thornton and Collie, 1846.

"What Science Has to Settle." *Atlanta Med Surg J* 8 (1868): 517–19.

White, J. E. "Topography of Savannah and Its Vicinity: A Report to the Georgia Medical Society, May 3, 1806." *Georgia Hist Q* 1 (1917): 236–42.

Wiese, E. R. "Life and Times of Samuel Preston Moore, Surgeon-General of the Confederate States of America." *South Med J* 23 (1930): 916–22.

Williamson, H. "An Attempt to Account for the Change of Climate, Which Has Been Observed in the Middle Colonies in North-America." *Trans Am Phil Soc* 1 (1771): 272–80.

Willis, Thomas. "Of the Putrid Fever." In *The London Practice of Physick*, 552–70. London: Thomas Baffet, 1685.

Wilson, L. G. "Fevers and Science in Early Nineteenth Century Medicine." *J Hist Med Allied Sci* 33 (1978): 386–407.

Wilson, Samuel. "An Account of the Province of Carolina, in America." In *Narratives of Early Carolina*, edited by Alexander S. Salley, 164–76. New York: Charles Scribner's Sons, 1911.

Wood, Peter H. *Black Majority: Negroes in Colonial South Carolina from 1670 through the Stono Rebellion.* New York: Alfred A. Knopf, 1974.

Woodman, H. D. "Sequel to Slavery: The New History Views the Postbellum South." *J South Hist* 43 (1977): 523–54.

Woodward, C. Vann. *The Burden of Southern History.* Baton Rouge: Louisiana State University Press, 1960.

Woodward, R. L., Jr. "Spanish Commercial Policy in Louisiana, 1763–1803." *Louisiana Hist* 44 (2003): 133–64.

Wyatt-Brown, Bertram. *The Shaping of Southern Culture.* Chapel Hill: University of North Carolina Press, 2001.

Yandell, L. P. "Remarks on Struma Africana, or the Disease Usually Called Negro Poison, or Negro Consumption." *Transylv J Med* 4 (1831): 83–103.

INDEX

ague, 11, 27
Albemarle, 12, 120
alcohol, 14, 27, 29, 95, 157
alder-bark, 101
almshouses, 130, 171
American Medical Association (AMA), 173, 186
amputations, 68, 151, 153, 155
anesthesia, 68, 117, 130, 180, 181, 184
antimonial (antimony), 35, 86
antisepsis, 180, 184
Antony, Milton, 116–20, 201
apothecaries, 24, 50, 69, 95, 145, 156
Arbuthnot, John, 5
Ashley River, 12, 13, 42, 77
asylums, 46, 105, 114, 121, 127, 172; Lunatic Asylum (New Orleans), 128
Atlanta Medical and Surgical Journal, 167, 168, 185
Augusta, Georgia: Civil War, 149, 151, 156, 167; medical education, 116–18, 168, 197; Revolutionary War, 53; sicknesses, 119

Barton, Benjamin Smith, 100
Bartram, John, 101, 102
Bassett, John, 107, 108
Battey, Robert, 183, 184, 189
Berkeley, John, 12
Best, George, 4
Biloxi, Mississippi, 15
blistering, 7, 8, 29, 32, 35, 93, 138, 177, 179
bloodletting ("therapeutic" bleeding), 7, 8, 30, 32, 35, 39, 40, 47, 68, 86, 93, 110, 177, 178

Boerhaave, Herman, 35, 47, 113
botanicals (botany), 94, 100–102, 123, 124, 156, 178
Brownfield, Robert, 58
burns, 101

Cabanis, Pierre Jean Georges, 99
calomel, 86, 102, 128
camphor, 84, 128
cancer, 182
Cape Fear, 12, 77
carbolic acid, 184
Carpenter, Jesse T., 3
Carteret, George, 12
Cartwright, Samuel, 19, 20, 84, 85, 87, 88, 178–80
castor oil, 86
cataplasms, 86
Catawba, 94, 100
cathartics, 22, 50, 86, 101
Chalmers, Lionel, 48, 49
charlatans, 21, 49, 93, 108, 112, 117, 131
Charleston, South Carolina: Charles Towne, 13, 36, 42; Civil War, 135–37, 144; epidemics, 30, 36, 37; medical community, 23, 45–47, 112–14, 128, 129; origins, 13; slavery and Black people, 77, 80, 82, 160, 171; Reconstruction, 166, 169; Revolutionary War, 53–57, 59, 60–62, 65, 66–68, 70
Charlottesville, Virginia, 23, 120–25, 143, 145, 168, 197
Cherokee, 36, 94, 99, 101
Chickasaw, 16, 17, 94

Chisolm, John Julian, 153–55
Chitimacha, 79
Choctaw, 81
cholera, 5, 38, 39, 53, 81, 83, 84, 88, 93, 119, 128, 141, 161, 182, 195
cinchona (*Cinchona officinalis*), 28, 29, 66, 67; as native *quina-quina*, 28
Clayton, John, 95, 96, 98
climate: Black people (Africans), 75, 83, 85, 88; Civil War, 150, 157; diseases, 18–21, 23, 45, 49, 78, 96, 111, 113, 115, 118; distinctiveness, 3–6, 13, 14, 42, 48, 104; Mississippi, 96; Native Americans, 80; New Orleans, 126, 127, 132, 191, 194, 195; Revolutionary War, 51–55, 59, 61, 62, 65, 66, 68; Virginia, 121, 123
Clinton, Henry, 53, 54, 56, 58–61, 64, 65
Clostridium tetani, 84
Colden, Cadwallader, 29
College of Philadelphia, 108
Combahee (River), 12
Confederate Medical and Surgical Journal, 138, 153, 156
contagion, 30, 34–37, 69, 119, 138, 152, 197
Cooper, Anthony Ashley, 12, 181
Cornwallis, Charles, 59–67, 70
Cox, William, 14
Craven, William, 12, 13
Creeks, 94
Cullen, William, 22, 32, 32, 35, 43, 47, 113
Current, Richard, 4

Dauphine Island, 79
Davis, Jefferson, 136, 137, 140, 157
Davis, John Daniel Sinkler, 187–90
Davis, William Elias Brownlee, 187–90
de Montigny, Jean-François-Benjamin Dumont, 97, 98
De Tocqueville, Alexis, 75, 82
Derham, James, 91
diarrhea, 32, 33, 38, 39, 49, 59, 65, 83, 84, 100, 148, 149, 152
Dickson, Samuel, 112, 113, 115
"dirt eating," 84, 85
distemper, 26, 29, 30, 47, 62, 94

distinctiveness (southern), 4, 6, 19, 48, 104, 159, 162, 175, 178, 187, 193, 194, 199; medical, 10, 21, 49, 111, 118, 155, 182
Drake, Daniel, 18, 19
Du Bois, William Edward Burghardt (W. E. B.), 163
Dunglison, Robley, 122–24
dysentery, 5, 14, 16, 22, 24, 39, 59, 61, 66, 83, 100, 126, 150, 195; bilious fever, 38; as bloody flux, 38, 80; camp dysentery (Civil War), 138, 144, 148, 149; cholera, 5, 53, 128; epidemic, 22, 150, 160; Revolutionary War, 59, 65; shipboard, 15; "summer (southern) fluxes," 24, 49; typhoid fever, 33

Emmet, John Patten, 123, 124
epidemics, 4, 7, 15, 23, 28, 34, 46, 48, 49, 52, 61, 105, 128, 138, 151, 152, 154, 185; cholera, 83, 84, 88; malaria, 22; smallpox, 22, 47, 61; yellow fever, 18, 22, 29, 30, 47, 146
Eve, Joseph, 106, 117
Eve, Paul Fitzsimmons, 181, 189

Fayssoux, Peter, 46, 47, 57, 58, 61, 112
Fenner, Erasmus Darwin, 9, 20, 83, 89, 104, 105, 133, 134, 170
fistulas, 97, 181, 183
Flexner, Abraham, 196, 197
flux (bloody), 14, 24, 38, 39, 53, 60, 62, 65, 80, 95, 96
folk healers, 111
Forry, Samuel, 5
Fort Maurepas, 15
Fort Rosalie, 16, 18
Freedmen's Bureau, 161, 164, 165, 168, 172, 173

gangrene, 39, 151–54, 179
Gates, Horatio, 37, 59, 60, 64, 70
Georgia Blister and Critic, 19, 135, 179
Great Dismal Swamp, 12
Greene, Nathaniel, 64, 67, 70
Gross, Samuel David, 130, 154, 180, 185

Hampden-Sydney College (Virginia), 124–26
hemorrhoids, 100

"heroic therapy," 177
Hillhouse, Augustus, 71
Hilton, William, 12
Hôpital des Pauvres de la Charité (Charity Hospital, New Orleans), 16, 127, 129, 130, 132, 146, 170
Hôpital du Roi, 16
Hopital San Carlos (New Orleans), 127
hospital gangrene, 151–53
hospitals: Augusta General, 116, 117, 151; Chimborazo (Richmond), 141–43; Continental, 56, 58, 70; Fair Ground (Atlanta), 146, 183; Freedmen's (Washington), 173; Gate City (Atlanta), 183; Johns Hopkins, 196, 197; Marine (Charleston), 113–15; Marine (Norfolk), 121, 122; Pennsylvania, 110; Philadelphia Almshouse, 110; Richmond, 126, 168; Roper (Charleston), 144, 169; slave, 16, 87
Howard, Oliver, 172–74
Hubbard, George Whipple, 174, 175
Hunt, Thomas, 128–32
Hyde, Edward, 12
hygiene, 30, 31, 89, 138, 152, 154, 174
hysteria, 183, 184

illnesses, 15, 18, 41, 42, 81, 83, 93, 110, 128, 199; camp fever, 137, 138, 160; cholera, 39, 128; the enslaved, 83, 86, 90, 174; malaria, 28; Native Americans, 95, 98, 100; periodic fevers, 194; Revolutionary War, 45, 49, 57, 60–63, 65, 66, 72, 87; smallpox, 35; southern climate, 7, 49, 104, 106, 113, 149, 178, 195; typhoid fever, 32, 84, 152; typhus, 31; yellow fever, 195
indentured servants (laborers), 7, 12, 74, 75, 76, 116, 159
influenza, 44, 84
insanity (the insane), 46, 114, 144, 183
intermittent fevers, 28, 61, 67, 158

Jackson, Robert, 59, 61, 64
Jamestown, 11, 73
jaundice, 25, 28, 29, 30, 100, 138
Jefferson, Thomas, 120–24

Jesuits' bark ("Bark"), 28, 66, 67, 150; cinchona, 28, 29, 66, 67
Jim Crow, 192, 198
Jones, John, 68, 69, 180
Jones, Joseph, 149–53, 160
jongleurs, 96–98
Josselyn, John, 101

Kalm, Pehr (Peter), 101, 102
Keen, William Williams, 151
Kentucky, 83, 94, 111, 142

laudanum, 29, 35, 39, 40, 63, 71, 86, 95, 157
lazaretto, 37
Le Conte, Joseph, 148, 149
Le Moyne, Jean-Baptiste (Sieur de Bienville), 15, 16, 17,
Le Moyne, Pierre (Sieur d'Iberville), 15, 16
Le Page du Pratz, Antoine-Simon, 15, 96, 98
lice, 32, 152
Lincoln, Benjamin, 55, 56, 58
Lining, John, 48
Lister, Joseph, 184
London Company, 11
Louisiana Territory, 16, 79, 96
Luzenberg, Charles, 129–32

magnesia, 86
malaria, 15, 22, 26, 27, 29, 32, 33, 54, 62, 65–67, 77, 81, 93, 138, 148, 150, 151, 158, 171, 195;
mal aria (Italian), 4, 26, 27
malnutrition, 80, 84, 152, 154, 159
materia medica, 24, 124
Mather, Cotton, 33, 34–36, 62
McCaw, James, 140–42
McDowell, Ephraim, 181
McDowell, William, 66, 67
McGuire, Hunter Holmes, 185, 189
measles, 34, 100, 123, 138, 150
medical colleges: Atlanta Medical College, 166, 167, 183; Howard University, 173, 197; Medical College of Georgia, 106, 119, 149, 150, 167, 168, 182, 187, 197; Medical College of Louisiana, 132, 133, 170; Medical College of New Orleans, 132;

Medical College of the State of South Carolina, 113, 115, 117, 123, 153, 155, 169, 197; Medical College of Virginia, 126, 168; Meharry Medical College, 175, 197, 198; University of Nashville, 174
Meharry, Samuel, 175
mercurials, 35, 102, 156, 178
miasmas, 5, 21, 29, 30, 49, 66, 68, 100, 149, 178, 193, 194
midwives (midwifery), 91, 111, 174
Minié ball, 153, 154
Mississippi Delta, 196
Mississippi River, 15, 17, 79, 81, 94, 126, 156
Mississippi Territory, 17, 18
Mississippi Valley, 19, 82, 170
Mobile, Alabama, 15, 79, 110, 111, 156, 170, 172
Monck, George, 12
Mooney, James, 100, 101
Moore, Samuel Preston, 137, 141, 142, 145, 152–57, 162
Moore Hospital (Richmond), 145
Mordecai, Solomon, 109–11, 137, 201
mosquitoes, 15, 18, 28–30, 73, 81, 194, 195, 199; *Aedes aegypti*, 29, 30, 195; *Anopheles* sp., 28
Moultrie, James, 113, 114
Moultrie, William, 53, 55, 56, 57, 59, 61

Nashville, Tennessee, 147, 174, 182, 183, 186, 189
Natchez (Native American tribe), 14, 16, 17, 94, 96, 97
Natchez, Mississippi, 15, 16, 18, 80, 81, 97, 161
Native Americans, 7, 12, 16, 22, 34, 74, 77, 79, 80, 86, 92–96, 98, 173
New Orleans, Louisiana, 195; Civil War, 137, 146, 148, 161; medical community, 91, 96, 127, 129, 130, 133; origins, 15–17; Reconstruction, 170; sicknesses, 126–28, 131, 132, 135; slavery, 79, 80
New Orleans Medical and Surgical Journal, 133, 170, 171
New Orleans School of Medicine, 134, 170, 171
Nightingale, Florence, 141
nursing, 85, 141, 142, 145, 148, 183; nursing homes, 114

Oglethorpe, James, 13, 14
Oliphant, David, 56, 59, 70, 112

oophorectomies, 183–84
opium, 29, 84, 95, 128, 157
Osler, William, 107, 195, 197, 198
Oxford, England, 50
Oxford, Mississippi, 23
Oyster Point, 13, 42

pain, 95–98, 148, 188; abdominal, 33, 38, 39, 152
Pember, Phoebe Yates, 142, 143
periodic fevers, 26, 27, 67, 150, 195
pestilence, 22, 30, 31, 37, 45, 47, 59, 127, 140, 159, 170
pharmaceuticals, 7, 102, 103, 124, 155, 156, 178, 179
Philadelphia, Pennsylvania, 21, 22, 53, 57, 69, 82, 108, 109, 111, 117, 179, 183, 195
physic, 8, 41, 49, 69, 112, 121, 134, 177, 179, 180; *Primitive Physic*, 49, 50
Pindell, Richard, 64
plague, 26, 30, 33, 34, 47, 49, 72, 84, 94, 106, 167
plantations, 6, 14, 29, 42, 46, 54, 75, 79, 80–86, 102, 161, 199
pneumonia, 84, 85, 144, 160
Pollack, Simon, 81
Porcher, Francis Peyre, 155–57
poultices, 30, 35, 64, 85, 96, 97, 101
Powhatan, 99
preceptorships, 111, 117
Pringle, John, 28, 38–40
protozoa, 26, 28, 83, 194–96
purges (purging), 7, 11, 35, 39, 93, 177, 178
pustules, 33–36, 100
putrefaction, 3, 18, 23, 26, 31, 34, 39, 53, 127
putrid fever, 31, 32, 59

quackery (quacks), 9, 21, 22, 47, 102, 106, 108, 116, 117
quarantine, 16, 36, 37, 47, 55, 87, 195
quinine, 28, 150, 155, 158

racism, 19, 172, 185
Ramsay, David, 3, 31, 36, 41–46, 55–57, 89, 111–15, 117, 118
Ramsay, James, 112, 113, 115
Ramsay, W. G., 89
Read, William, 69–71

Reed, Walter, 195
Richmond, Virginia, 109; Civil War, 139, 140, 142, 143, 145, 146, 154, 155, 156, 158, 162, 168; medical education, 121, 122, 124, 125, 126, 129
Rush, Benjamin, 22, 23, 30, 31, 39–45, 47, 55, 69, 98, 99

Salmonella typhi, 33, 39, 152
sanitation, 10; Civil War, 138, 148, 149, 152, 154, 160–62; Reconstruction, 172, 174, 182, 195, 196; Revolutionary War, 37, 39; southern sicknesses, 127, 129
São João Bautista (ship), 74
sarsaparilla, 101
Savannah, Georgia, 14, 30, 37, 49, 53–56, 66–69, 111, 115, 148, 149, 157, 172
Savannah River, 14, 37, 56
scrofula, 85
scurvy, 15, 80, 83, 94
sectionalism, 4, 9, 10, 106, 117, 134, 194
sepsis, 34, 39, 151
Sherman, William Tecumseh, 148, 158, 166, 167, 174
Sims, J. Marion, 181–84, 189
smallpox, 5, 16, 22, 24, 33–37, 46, 47, 55, 57, 59–61, 65, 66, 70, 81, 83, 93, 100, 123, 152, 161; inoculation, 35, 36, 37, 47, 59, 66, 70
Smith, James McCune, 90
Southern Medical and Surgical Journal, 118, 150, 168
Southern Medical Reports, 9
Southern Surgical and Gynecological Association, 188–90
sterility, 181
Stone, Warren, 128–31, 133, 146, 147
sweating, 7, 29, 32, 47, 70, 93, 177
Sydenham, Thomas, 31, 35, 38, 39, 47, 113

Tarleton, Banastre, 58, 59, 60, 62, 64, 67
Tennessee College, 175
tetanus ("lock jaw"), 84, 151
Thomson, Samuel, 102
Tidyman, Philip, 80, 81, 86
trismus nascentium, 84
tuberculosis, 42, 85, 86, 88, 171, 196, 197; known as consumption, 5, 42, 85, 86

typhoid fever, 33, 81, 83, 93, 144, 152, 160, 167, 195
typhus ("jail fever"), 5, 31–33, 59, 70, 84, 119, 152

University of Nashville, 174, 182
University of Pennsylvania, 108, 109, 117, 119, 122, 129, 146, 149, 181
University of South Carolina (Medical School), 169–70
University of Virginia, 23, 120, 123, 125, 143

vaccine (yellow fever), 195
Vanderbilt University, 174, 175, 183, 186–88, 196, 197
vapors (vapours), 4, 12, 13, 26, 30, 45, 48, 51, 96, 141, 150, 200
venereal disease, 16, 57, 83; gonorrhea, 16, 94; syphilis, 16, 24, 34, 171
Vicksburg, Mississippi, 18, 81, 147, 148
Virginia Commonwealth University, 126

Wando River, 13
Washington, George, 37, 52, 53, 64, 66, 68–70
Wayside Homes, 144, 146
Wesley, John, 49, 50
Williamsburg, Virginia, 22, 37, 121
Willis, Thomas, 32, 33
women, 16, 26, 45, 143, 173; castration, 184; Civil War, 142–45, 147, 159; folk medicine, 84, 86; medical education, 173; oophorectomy, 181, 183–84; Revolutionary War, 56, 60, 61
worms (intestinal), 57, 83
wounds and injuries, 46; Civil War, 139, 142, 143, 147, 151–55, 169, 182; Native healing, 95, 97–99, 101; Revolutionary War, 56, 58, 59, 63, 64, 68–72

yellow fever, 15, 18, 22, 29, 30, 38, 47, 59, 77, 82, 93, 119, 126, 133, 138, 146, 161, 195

ABOUT THE AUTHOR

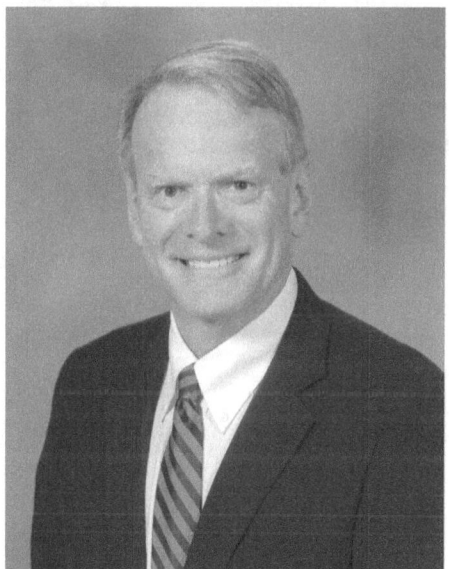

Photo by University of Mississippi Medical Center

THOMAS HELLING, MD, is a tenured professor of surgery at the University of Mississippi Medical Center in Jackson, Mississippi. He is clinically active and heads the Division of General Surgery. Dr. Helling is a graduate of the University of Kansas (undergraduate 1969, School of Medicine 1973). He has extensive experience in trauma care and served in the Army Medical Corps from 1991 to 2000, receiving an honorable discharge at the rank of lieutenant colonel. He completed various army schools, including the Combat Casualty Care Course, Advanced Officer School, and Command and General Staff College. Professionally, Dr. Helling is board certified in surgery and surgical critical care. He is a Fellow of the American College of Surgeons and a member of a number of prestigious societies, including the Southern Surgical Association, the American Surgical Association, and the American Association for the Surgery of Trauma. Dr. Helling also is a member of the American Association for the History of Medicine and is under consideration for membership in the esteemed American Osler Society. His intimate association with the unique challenges of southern medicine sparked an interest in the historical perspective of health care in the South, particularly the antebellum era. He is a reviewer for several scientific journals, including *Military Medicine*. Dr. Helling has authored or coauthored well over 110 scientific articles, including 5 in the field of history of medicine, and is the author of *Desperate Surgery in the Pacific War: Doctors, Damage Control, and America's Wounded, 1941–1945* (McFarland, 2017), for which he was awarded the Harry D. Langley Book Prize by the Society for the History of Navy Medicine in 2019, *The Agony of Heroes: Medical Care for America's Besieged Legions from Bataan to Khe Sanh* (Westholme, 2019), and *The Great War and the Birth of Modern Medicine* (Pegasus, 2022) and coauthor of *Historical Foundations of Liver Surgery* (Springer Nature, 2020). His publications are promoted at thomashelling.com. Dr. Helling currently resides in Madison, Mississippi.

www.ingramcontent.com/pod-product-compliance
Lightning Source LLC
Chambersburg PA
CBHW031803220426
43662CB00007B/505